GYNECOLOGIC ONCOLOGY

GYNECOLOGIC ONCOLOGY

FELIX RUTLEDGE, M.D.
Department of Gynecology
The University of Texas System Cancer Center
M. D. Anderson Hospital and Tumor Institute
Texas Medical Center
Houston, Texas

RICHARD C. BORONOW, M.D.
Director, Gynecologic Tumor Service
University of Mississippi Medical Center
Jackson, Mississippi

J. TAYLOR WHARTON, M.D.
Department of Gynecology
The University of Texas System Cancer Center
M. D. Anderson Hospital and Tumor Institute
Texas Medical Center
Houston, Texas

A WILEY BIOMEDICAL PUBLICATION

JOHN WILEY & SONS, New York · London · Sydney · Toronto

Library of Congress Cataloging in Publication Data:
Rutledge, Felix.
  Gynecologic oncology.

  (A Wiley biomedical publication)
  Includes bibliographies.
  1. Generative organs, Female—Cancer.

I. Wharton, James Taylor, 1938–   joint
author. II. Boronow, Richard C., joint author.
III. Title. [DNLM: 1. Gynecologic neoplasms—
Therapy. WP145 R981g]

RC280.G5R87   616.9′94′65   75-30951
ISBN 0-471-74720-3

Printed in the United States of America

10 9 8 7 6 5 4 3

TO

R. LEE CLARK, M.D., a physician whose deep compassion for human suffering has been the impetus for seeking the best means to alleviate the pain of cancer and allied diseases.

R. Lee Clark's abiding belief in the eventual medical and scientific control of cancer and, thereby, of numerous other human diseases, has sustained his lifelong and eminently successful efforts to build an institution dedicated to cancer research and education as well as patient care. The philosophy of The University of Texas M. D. Anderson Hospital and Tumor Institute in Houston, Texas, centers on a team of biomedical specialists from every discipline working in concert to develop innovative and increasingly better means for the control of cancer. This team of dedicated people, under the imaginative leadership of Dr. Clark, has attracted the admiration of other cancer specialists around the world. As a result, Dr. Clark has responded to numerous requests from national and international sources to participate in planning worldwide cooperative programs for better control of cancer and prevention of many types of cancer.

PREFACE

Any physician who receives women as patients has an opportunity to detect gynecologic cancer. Although the patient may be referred for treament when cancer is discovered, many physicians become involved in management in varying degrees. Thus a basic knowledge of gynecologic cancer must be part of all physician education. Although he may not be planning to participate in the treatment of gynecologic cancer, any physician may be obliged to counsel his patients and refer them for proper treatment. Gynecologic cancer crosses the boundaries of specialization in medical practice and may involve physicians in fields completely unrelated to gynecology. The generalist and the internist are alert to the possibilities of gynecologic cancer because they customarily approach the patient's complaint with a broad diagnostic view. Often the internist is the first to be consulted by a patient with ovarian cancer because the patient's complaints resemble those of intestinal tract disease. Sometimes the urologist or proctologist may be the first specialist consulted because the symptoms produced by a pelvic mass of ovarian carcinoma resemble a bladder problem; similar effects may distend the perirectal veins and cause hemorrhoids. The roentgenologist may be the first to see the shadow of an ovarian neoplasm. A gastrointestinal series is often requested for patients with carcinoma of the ovary before the diagnosis is known. Metastatic lesions of gynecologic cancer may involve lung, bone, lymph nodes, and liver. Like other types of cancer, metastasis may produce the initial symptoms of gynecologic cancer. Thus all physicians should be prepared to deal with cancer at any site, and because gynecologic cancer is one of the more common neoplasms, an overall view of the management of gynecologic cancer is basic information for clinicians.

In this book we plan to present such information in a straightforward manner, by using simple publication techniques that can be kept current. This book is not intended to be a textbook in gynecologic oncology, rather it is a collection of lectures that the three authors have presented as a postgraduate course on this subject.

We often share similar opinions, having worked together for several years, and consult one another frequently about clinical problems. Although we agree on many topics of treatment, each of us has individual preferences about some features of gynecologic cancer. We have deliberately presented our personal views as recommendations. If at times this seems didactic and opinionated, our aim is to provide positive and definite advice rather than a broad, indecisive, and more complete review of topics. We have left little opportunity for the reader to choose from a broad presentation of differing opinions.

We work in institutions in which special facilities are available for managing cancer patients. Since these facilities and the special situations we encounter influence our practice, our advice for management may not be applicable to physicians in other geographic areas. In presenting the material dealing with surgical techniques, we are likely to show considerable personal prejudice and clinical bias. The methods of radiation therapy are strongly representative of

Dr. Gilbert Fletcher's teachings at the M. D. Anderson Hospital. Our experiences in chemotherapy are personal ones. Since this is the newest of treatment modalities and the least settled, it is constantly changing.

Although we function primarily as pelvic surgeons, we are gynecologic oncologists, which implies a working knowledge of radiotherapy, and active participants in the use of chemotherapy for gynecologic cancer. The student planning a career in this field is therefore urged to prepare to treat these patients with all three modalities.

FELIX RUTLEDGE, M. D.
RICHARD C. BORONOW, M. D.
J. TAYLOR WHARTON, M. D.

Houston, Texas
August 1975

CONTENTS

GYNECOLOGIC ONCOLOGY

CARCINOMA OF THE CERVIX

CHAPTER 1 CURRENT CONCEPTS: CERVICAL INTRAEPITHELIAL NEOPLASIA (Carcinoma In Situ and Dysplasia)

RICHARD C. BORONOW, M.D.

CURRENT CONTROVERSIES

1. Should all patients with atypical cytology have cervical conization?
2. What is the significance of dysplasia?
3. Should vaginal "cuff" be excised when treating carcinoma in situ?

In the United States today fewer women die annually from carcinoma of the cervix than in any period in modern American medical history. Areas of clinical progress include (1) increased utilization of cervical cytology, (2) better assessment and evaluation of the patient with an abnormal Pap smear, (3) better primary therapy. In addition, certain areas of research progress include (1) the possible relationship of herpesvirus type 2 (HSV-2) to cervical neoplasia,[1] (2) a better understanding of the spectrum of cervical intraepithelial neoplasia, (3) clinical trials that lead to better primary therapy for invasive cervix cancer. While the mortality rate from this disease is constantly decreasing on the national level, we also see a reversal in the ratio of cases of carcinoma in situ and invasive cancer. Yet invasive cervical cancer remains a significant cause of morbidity and mortality. With currently available techniques and

methodology, however, death from invasive cancer of the cervix becomes theoretically preventable. This disease can be detected and cured in its preclinical and preinvasive phases.

To include dysplasia with carcinoma in situ of the cervix, from pathologic, diagnostic, clinical and therapeutic considerations, represents the embodiment of a number of relatively new concepts formulated in the last decade or so and only currently being validated by certain sophisticated techniques. Some of these concepts could not have been justifiably advanced ten years ago. Significantly, the major thrust in the conquest of cervical cancer is not with the gynecologic oncologist in a cancer center setting but rather with the obstetrician-gynecologist, the family practitioner, and the generalist who see many patients on a day-to-day basis. These same physicians are challenged to find means to extend their abilities beyond the relatively few patients now being routinely screened to the other two-thirds of the American population who, for both social and economic reasons, do not reap the benefit of cervical cytology. Indeed, the major thrust must be made here, for epidemiologic data suggest that this silent majority, more than the minority in our offices, represents the truly at risk population for cervix cancer. The spectrum of cytologic and histologic changes from normal cervical epithelium, dysplasia, carcinoma in situ, and invasive cancer are illustrated in Figures 1–8.

EPIDEMIOLOGY

A large body of data has accumulated regarding patient populations with high and low rates of cervical cancer. Although these data do not imply precise causative factors, they do alert the practitioner to certain patient populations that justify greater or lesser cytologic surveillance. Reported low-risk populations include nuns and women in other religious orders, Jewish women, and country women. Reported high-incidence groups in this country include Negroes as well as Puerto Rican, Mexican, and other immigrant populations. Included are also women of low socioeconomic status, early age at first marriage, and early age at first coitus; women of high parity, divorced, and separated women, prostitutes, those with a background of emotional unhappiness and depression; and, more recently, women with Herpes virus type 2 infection of the genital system.

The relationship of HSV-2 to cervical neoplasia has attracted considerable interest in recent years. The association of herpesvirus and animal oncogenesis with tumor systems in frogs, chickens, and monkeys provided some of the basic data. Currently HSV-2 appears to be the causative agent in infectious mononucleosis, and, from a variety of immunologic studies, related at least as a cofactor to Burkitt's lymphoma and perhaps nasopharyngeal carcinoma. Herpes simplex virus type 1 (oral, buccal mucosa, lip), and herpes simplex virus type 2

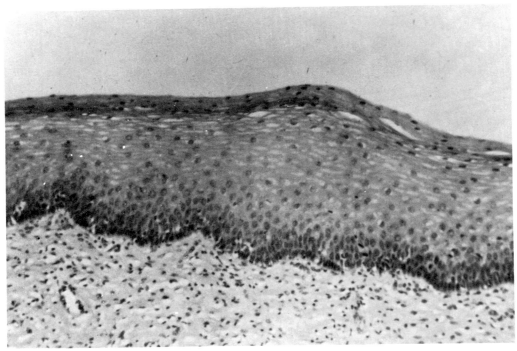

Figure 1   Biopsy of normal stratified squamous epithelium.

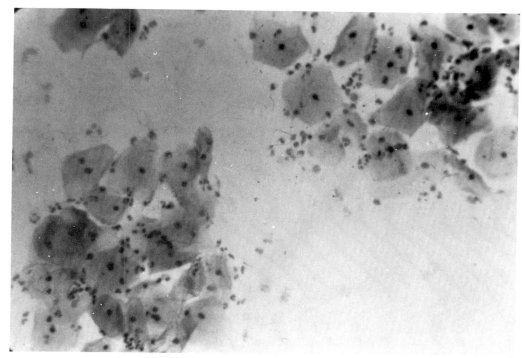

Figure 2 Pap smear of normal cervix with normal nuclear and cytoplasmic features.

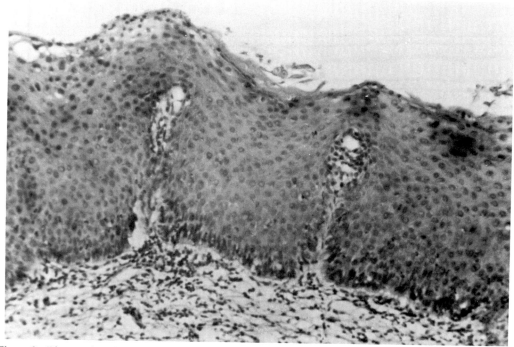

Figure 3 Biopsy of moderately severe keratinizing dysplasia.

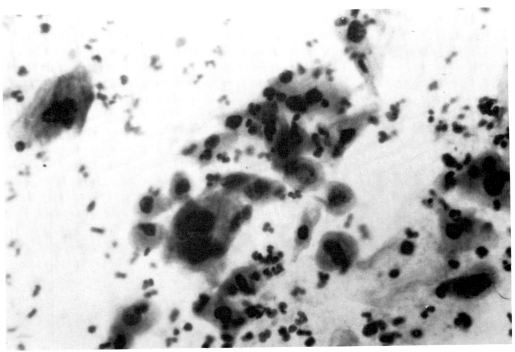

Figure 4 Pap smear with nuclear changes characteristic of moderate keratinizing dysplasia.

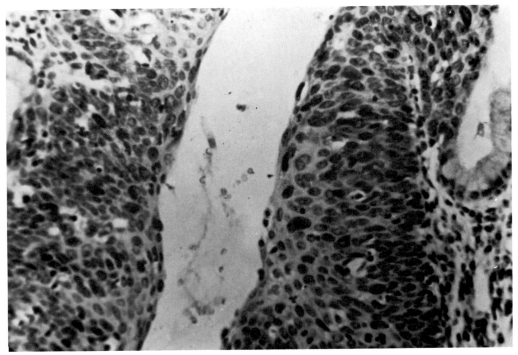

Figure 5 Biopsy of carcinoma in situ with full thickness atypia.

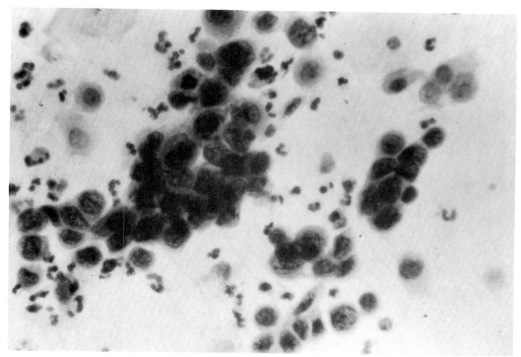

Figure 6 Pap smear of carcinoma in situ. Note characteristic syncytial arrangement, with "third type" cells (nuclear atypia, but retention of thin cytoplasmic rim). Note "clean" background.

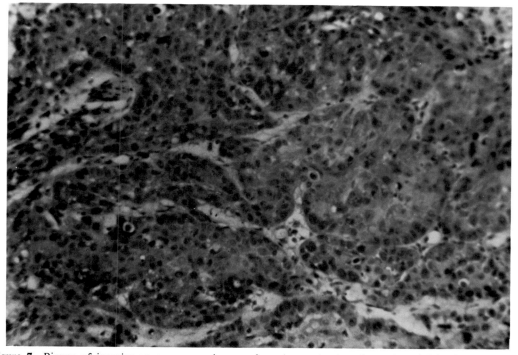

Figure 7 Biopsy of invasive squamous carcinoma of cervix, predominantly nonkeratinizing large cell type.

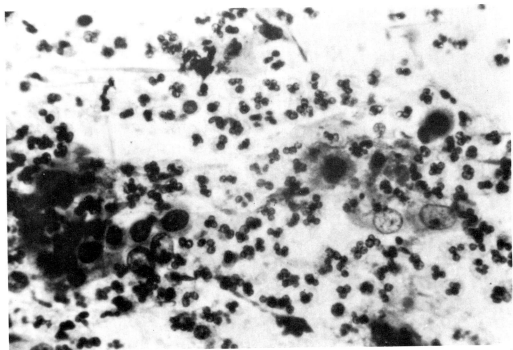

Figure 8 Pap smear of invasive cervix cancer. Note marked hyperchromatism, naked nuclei with occasional macronucleoli and "dirty" background of so-called "cancer diathesis" red cells, polymorphonuclear leukocytes, and necrotic debris, which suggest ulcerative infiltrative characteristics of the lesion.

(genital) are recognized to be different both from each other and from other herpes viruses (e.g., cytomegalovirus, varicella roster). The type 1 and type 2 strains differ from each other virologically and clinically (antigenically and biologically). There is a distinct age difference for populations with type 1 and type 2 antibodies. Antibodies to type 1 appear to be ubiquitous in all age populations, whereas antibodies to type 2 do not appear in the female populations studied until heterosexual activity begins. Not surprisingly, HSV-2 is associated with neonatal herpes infections.

In a study by Naib and associates in 1969,[2] of over 200 cases of active genital herpes, 24% had histologic cervical atypia; 12 of the 58 patients had carcinoma in situ, and 4 had invasive cervical cancer. In a comparable group of age and socioeconomic controls without herpes infection, the degree of cervical epithelial atypia was 1.6%

Sophisticated antibody determinations for HSV-2 are positive in from 80 to 100% of patients with invasive cancer. This is in contrast to healthy, economically and age-matched controls with a 20% incidence of HSV-2 antibodies. However, it was observed that 50% of the patients with carcinoma in situ have antibodies to type 2 herpes and about 25% of the population with dysplasia have similar antibodies. This raises the question, "Why do these rates vary if the same factors are thought to be causative?" No answer is apparent. It has been speculated that these preinvasive lesions progress to invasive cancer only among cases with type 2 antibodies. To date, however, this does not appear to be a sufficient explanation.

Cultures of herpesvirus in invasive cervical cancer and carcinoma in situ have proved unrewarding. However, in animal DNA virus tumors there is a long delay between infection and onset of the malignancy, and at that point the identifiable virus has disappeared. Recently, however, "fingerprints" of the viral infection have been found in tissue cultures of cervical malignancy (viral genome in the DNA) by one group of investigators,[3] but this has not yet been confirmed.

Prospective studies are needed for patients with HSV-2 antibodies and with matched controls (if it is possible to assume an adequate biologic control by this method). Patients should, of course, be followed prospectively to see if they develop cervical atypia. Another approach to prospective analysis is to follow patients with cytologic evidence of herpes infection (multinucleated giant cells with distinct nuclear molding and acidophilic intranuclear inclusions, often surrounded by a halo, by large single hypertrophic basal or endocervical cells with bland nuclei and scanty cytoplasm) to determine the incidence of those who develop atypia. (The reader is directed to the current and comprehensive review cited in Reference 1.)

Recently the role of immunologic suppression in oncogenesis has received considerable attention.[4] Clearly an increased incidence of malignancy, particularly of the reticuloendothelial system, has been identified among patients in long-term follow-up for kidney transplantation. In such a population, 1 case of invasive cancer, 3 cases of carcinoma in situ, and 3 cases of dysplasia have been mentioned in the literature.

The role of oral contraceptives in cervical oncogenesis has been clouded by studies subject to many questions regarding methodology, design, and the like. An obvious bias is the recognition that many studies have been reported from low-income family planning clinic populations, thus introducing several at-risk factors at the outset. Currently there are no data to indict the oral contraceptives as a carcinogen.

With regard to the general body of data on the epidemiology of cervical cancer, it must be stated that although the cause is unknown, certain populations appear at risk, the disease can be produced in animals, and venereal factors seem prevalent.

PATHOLOGY AND CYTOLOGY

Carcinoma In Situ

This is designated Stage 0 in the International Federation of Gynecologists and Obstetricians (FIGO) staging system. It has also been referred to as incipient cancer, preinvasive cancer, Bowen's disease of the cervix, intraepithelial cancer, precancerous metaplasia, and noninvasive cancer. There is no characteristic gross appearance, although there may be some redness due to vascular changes in the epithelium. An iodine stain may identify target areas for biopsy.

The International Committee on Histologic Terminology for Lesions of the Cervix defines carcinoma in situ as follows: "Only those cases should be classified as carcinoma in situ which, in the absence of invasion, show surface epithelium, in which, throughout its whole thickness, no differentiation takes place. The process may involve the cervical glands without hereby creating a new group. It is recognized that the cells of the uppermost layer may show some flattening [Figure 5]. The very rare case of an otherwise characteristic carcinoma in situ which shows a greater degree of differentiation belongs to the exception for which no classification provides."[5] Interpretation of the semantics of the last two sentences provides the basis for significant controversy among pathologists.

The hallmark of neoplasia is the nucleus. Cytologic manifestations of carcinoma in situ have been analyzed in detail. One excellent reference is Patten's monograph.[5] The cells are usually arranged in a syncytium, and there is a coarse or sometimes fine granular chromatin pattern. There may be disruption of the nuclear membrane, reflecting mitotic activity. Many feel that the finding of prominent oval nucleoli in an otherwise in situ cell spread suggests microinvasion. There may be nuclear indentation and grooving, and an eosinophilic cytoplasm. Consistently the atypical cells have a high nuclear-cytoplasmic ratio; usually a thin rim of cytoplasm is retained (the characteristic "third type" cell, Figure 6).

Dysplasia

Cervical dysplasia also has been called by a variety of names such as atypical hyperplasia, dyskaryosis, basal cell hyperplasia, atypical basal cell hyperplasia, anaplasia. This lesion shows no gross characteristic appearance, but may be suggested by nonstaining or relative nonstaining after application of an iodine preparation.

The International Committee follows its definition of carcinoma in situ with this definition of dysplasia: "All other disturbances of differentiation in the squamous epithelial lining, the glands or the covering of the surface, are to be classified as dysplasia. They may be characterized as a high or low degree, terms which are preferable to suspicious and nonsuspicious as the proposed terms describe the histologic appearance and do not express an opinion." It can be seen that the dysplastic reaction is characterized by disordered maturation at various levels of the epithelium, frequently abnormal differentiation of the uppermost cell layers, and abnormally large nuclei in association with varying degrees of cytoplasmic maturation (Figure 3).

Cytologically the cells may appear in a syncytium, and there is a less pronounced alteration of the nuclear-cytoplasmic ratio than in carcinoma in situ. The chromatin pattern tends to be more finely granular (Figure 4). Patten comments that "while correlation is not absolute, the sole feature of these cellular samples which seems to

provide consistent data for predicting the severity and ultimate course of a dysplastic reaction is an evaluation of the number of abnormal cells." This quantitative assessment assumes completely uniform sampling in all instances; therefore, many pathologists feel that a better criterion is the severity of the individual cellular atypia. Patten also observes that "any dysplastic reaction, regardless of initial severity, is potentially a lesion which *may* antedate a more serious process." There can be little disagreement with this statement.

DIAGNOSIS

Cytology

Although some believe it may be premature to suggest that cytology is responsible for the decrease in death rate in cervical cancer, it is nevertheless important to assess the data of Boyes.[6] In a 20-year study of the screening program in British Columbia, Canada, he indicates that 350,000 cases a year are currently being screened. When the program began in 1949, fewer than 1,000 patients were screened. In evaluating the impact of cytology on the incidence of invasive cancer, the author postulates that if in situ carcinoma is removed from the population it can be projected over subsequent years to reduce the incidence of invasive cancer. Indeed, the incidence of invasive cancer has sharply decreased in British Columbia and the death rate is also declining.

In the past decades the recommended age at which cervical cytologic studies are initiated has continually declined. Although it has been suggested that any woman 20 years of age or over should be screened (under 20 if married or ever married, or if pregnant or ever pregnant), once heterosexual activity begins the patient appears to be at risk and cytologic studies should be performed routinely. If we concede that cytologic screening is the best method for detecting dysplasia and carcinoma in situ, it becomes important to evaluate the best method to use to obtain a cytologic sample. Richart and his co-workers have provided a statistical basis for the selection of a method. He reports a false-negative rate for a single slide sample for histologic in situ carcinoma and dysplasia as follows: vaginal pool 50%, cervical scrape 15%, endocervical sample 8%, os apiration and scrape 3%.[7] From the medicolegal standpoint, a precedent has been set that the cytologic spread must include endocervical cells. Thus, while it seems clear that an endocervical sample is essential, there is no absolute consensus among responsible pathologists.[8]

Biopsy Techniques

When an atypical cytologic report is obtained, regardless of the cytologic diagnosis from the pathology laboratory, it is the duty of the physician to establish the precise histologic diagnosis before instituting any form of treatment. Figure 9 shows a standard type of flow sheet for evaluation of the patient with an abnormal cervical cytology. Inherent in this method is the outpatient component in much of this workup. Clearly, if there is a gross lesion it should be biopsied; assuming no gross lesion, an iodine stain is useful for identifying target areas for biopsy. One should remember that normal endocervical epithelium does not take the iodine stain, but varying degrees of cervical atypia will either stain poorly or not at all. This helps to assure that with the multiple biopsy technique, areas likely to harbor cervical atypia will be sampled or removed. We use the Wittner cervical biopsy punch (Figure 10 and 10a).

An experienced colposcopist can further define the target areas for sampling. The role

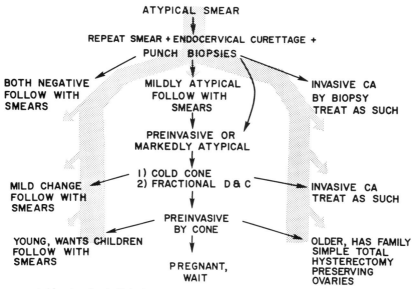

Figure 9 An acceptable, standard clinical approach for evaluation of abnormal cervical cytology. In most cases the center arm will be followed to reach the final diagnosis by conization, then move appropriately to the left or right arm, as the findings and clinical picture suggest. When initial outpatient biopsies reveal invasive cancer, one mover directly to the left arm, and the cone is avoided. Cone may also be avoided when the lesser atypia of the Pap smear are corroborated by histologic findings in comprehensive outpatient biopsy studies.

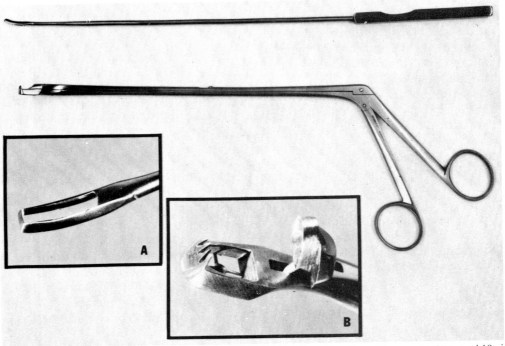

Figure 10 Outpatient cervical biopsy instruments used by the author. The Kevorkian curette (top, and 10*a* inset) has a 2mm, sharp cutting edge. The Wittner cervical biopsy punch instrument (bottom, and 10*b* inset) has an angled jaw and lower jaw teeth to secure a biopsy of 4.5 × 8 mm.

of colposcopy in evaluating patients with abnormal cervical cytology and no gross lesion has undergone a resurgence of interest in the last decade. There are a number of factors responsible: (1) the yield of serious pathology, as severe dysplasia, carcinoma in situ, or very superficial invasion comprises about 10% of these cases, (2) the total cost for conization is about $600, whereas the outpatient colposcopy and biopsy cost is about one-tenth of this figure, (3) there are distinct differences in morbidity between the two approaches, (4) the subject has benefited by an improvement in the scientific scholarship of its contemporary proponents, such as Coppleson, Stafl, and Townsend.

For the colposcopic technique to replace the more standard approaches, however, requires considerable experience and exper-

tise. First of all, the colposcopic examination must be satisfactory; that is, the transformation zone or squamocolumnar junction must be seen entirely, and thorough endocervical curettage must contain no fragments of atypical epithelium. Secondly, the colposcopist must be able to identify the most atypical area for biopsy with a high degree of accuracy: 99% in Stafl's Wisconsin satellite clinic.[9] In less than 1% of cases were the final cone-hysterectomy pathologic findings significantly more advanced (two grades or more difference among their grades: mild dysplasia, moderate dysplasia, severe dysplasia, carcinoma in situ, microcarcinoma and frank invasive carcinoma) than the findings in the colposcopically directed biopsies.[9] This 99% accuracy in identifying the most atypical area assures its safety. Until other clinicians can develop such accuracy, the safety of their patients is best served by following more traditional and standard biopsy procedures.

An essential step in the outpatient work-up is thorough endocervical curettage. We follow the recommendation of Townsend and associates[10] and use the Kevorkian curette, which is very sharp and small enough to be accommodated without dilatation. The ultimate diagnostic procedure—after repeat cytology and appropriate office biopsies—is cervical conization, to exclude the presence of invasive cancer of the cervix. The importance of avoiding conservative hysterectomy when invasive cervical cancer is unrecognized is emphasized by the tendency toward local pelvic recurrence when the paracervical channels of the pelvic lymphatic spread pattern are transected. This type of local resection, which we refer to as a "cut-through hysterectomy" is analogous to the use of segmental resection as definite treatment for colon cancer, or local excision ("lumpectomy") of a breast lump when breast cancer is present. All these situations are characterized by tragic local recurrence.

CLINICAL SIGNIFICANCE

Carcinoma In Situ

When intraepithelial carcinoma of the cervix was recognized as a precursor of invasive cancer, the following important clinical questions were raised: How often does carcinoma in situ progress to invasive cancer? How much time is required for this progression?

Incidence data suggest a peak of carcinoma in situ in the range of 35 to 40 years of age and for invasive cancer of 45 to 50 years, the implication being that a 10-year interval is a reasonable figure for the progression. Some authors suggest it may be as little as eight or even six years. An immediate consideration is that when carci-

noma is situ is diagnosed, one may not be certain how long it has existed. Other issues involve the certainty and method of diagnosis. Related to the last two points are considerations regarding the possibility of progression of untreated carcinoma in situ to invasive cancer. With data available today, there is no longer any ethical medical justification for the prospective follow-up of untreated carcinoma in situ patients. In the past data have accumulated in the literature suggesting that from 10 to 15% to 60% or more will develop into invasive cancer. Two relevant questions must be asked regarding such data: How long are patients followed? How was the diagnosis established?

If the diagnosis is established by cone biopsy and the cone appears to include the whole lesion, the patient may be cured by the diagnostic procedure alone. Similarly, multiple cevical biopsies may have removed the lesion completely. Even if they are not removed completely, the important study of Richart[11] indicates that biopsy will influence the natural history of the cervical changes.* Another consideration relating to the fact that apparently not every carcinoma in situ will become an invasive cancer is the question of the actual malignancy of the

---

* In the next section there is further discussion of Richart's unifying concept of dysplasia and carcinoma in situ as representing a continuum, which he designates as cervical intraepithelium neoplasia (CIN). He has observed that: "One or more punch biopsies may eradicate an area of CIN completely and may be therapeutic as well as diagnostic; the biopsy wound lying in the center of an area of CIN will be reepithelialized by CIN; the biopsy wound with an area of CIN which includes a junction of normal squamous epithelium will tend to be re-epithelialized by normal squamous epithelium and any remaining areas of CIN will tend to assume a smooth convex border, or, if only a small area remains, will tend to regress completely over a relatively long period of time; areas of CIN isolated in normal squamous epithelium without continuity with the squamo-columnar junction may regress spontaneously."

process itself. The controversial views of Green[12] imply that few if any in situ cancers actually become invasive. His reports are provocative, but are at present accepted by only a few authorities. The herpesvirus proponents suggest that although virtually all invasive cancers have antibodies to HSV-2 and fewer than half of in situ carcinomas have these antibodies, perhaps those that do represent those in situ carcinomas destined to become invasive cancer. This implies a dissimilarity in behavior among histologically similar lesions. There are more questions than firm answers on the subject.

Dysplasia

An understanding of the biologic significance of dysplasia is considerably more difficult than that for in situ carcinoma. It has been noted that many clinical studies have confirmed that carcinoma in situ generally peaks

at an earlier age than invasive cancer; the peak incidence of dysplasia also occurs at a younger age than that for carcinoma in situ. These clinical observations, coupled with the apparent morphologic progression of cellular atypia seen in cell spreads shed through mild, moderate, and severe dysplasia and carcinoma in situ, all suggest a continuum of these processes.

Nevertheless, contributions to the literature have been variable, and it has been suggested that approximately 20 to 50% of cervical dysplasias will regress to normal, whereas from 1 to 20% of dysplasias and as many as 65% of severe dysplasias will progress to carcinoma in situ. The bulk of the data in the literature is based on biopsy material (Table 1). These data are subject to technical artifacts and to misinterpretations of reparative metaplasias and other benign cervical conditions. As was noted earlier, these studies fail to recognize that biopsies of the cervix alter the natural his-

Table 1   Fate of Biopsy Diagnosed Dysplasia[25]

Author	Total Cases	Progression to Carcinoma In Situ (%)	Regression to Normal (%)
Galvin, Jones, Telinde (1955)[13]	191		
Grade I	93	2	54
Grade II	63	11	44
Grade III	35	65	17
Greene (1955)[14]	142	10	37
Peckham, Greene (1957)[15]	489	10.7	40
Rawson, Knoblich (1957)[16]	56	17 (3 cases, invasion)	75
McKay et al. (1959)[17]	129	3.8 (1 case, invasion)	20
Johnson et al. (1960)[18]	89	1.1	40
McLaren, Attwood (1961)[19]	39	10	32
Dougherty, Torres, Cotton (1961)[20] ("epithelial instability")	293	3	51
Lambert, Woodruff (1963)[21] ("spinal cell atypias")	108	12	
Jordan, Bader, Day (1964)[22] ("major atypical lesions")	95	8.4	

tory of the intraepithelial process. Thus, only a few studies (Table 2) have directed attention to the undisturbed natural history of these epithelial changes. These have been cytologic, colposcopic, and colpomicroscopic evaluations without biopsy.

The most comprehensive study of this type, and also the most provocative, is that of Richart and Barron.[25] They graded dysplasias by cytologic means into a variety of subdivisions utilizing their nonbiopsy technique, and were able to project progression rates with time. This was done only after the methodology of relying on the nonbiopsy technique had been validated by critical assessment of the consistency of their cytologic interpretations and the accuracy of these interpretations compared with final histologic material. The progression rates that developed represented a composite of the total material and recognized that in any given case one was not permitted to predict the ultimate fate of each lesion. Their data (Figure 11) did, however, document the tendency of dysplasia to progress, and suggested that dysplasias of all degrees and carcinoma in situ represent a continuum that might better be referred to as cervical intraepithelial neoplasia, and that the lesion be graded cytologically and histologically from 1 to 3 on the basis of the severity of atypia.

TREATMENT

Carcinoma In Situ

Carcinoma in situ may be successfully eradicated by hysterectomy, cervical conization, local excision, cryosurgery, hot cautery, radiation therapy, and even chemotherapy. Although the lesion may be removed or destroyed, the particular causative and host factors may still be operative and all patients must be followed cytologically since they are at risk for developing additional epithelial atypias (Tables 3 and 4).

HYSTERECTOMY

By the abdominal or the vaginal route, hysterectomy has been the standard American method of management and is probably the most definitive. The recurrence and reoccurrence rates are lower (Tables 3 and 4). In the past authors have recommended excision of a 1 or 2 cm of vaginal cuff as prophylaxis against the occasional vaginal cuff recurrence. Although vaginal recurrence has been reported, it is so infrequent that there are no satisfactory data to justify resection of a portion of the cuff. (But the technical effort required to obtain 1 cm of tissue will assure complete removal of the cervix!) There are no data to justify more

Table 2   Fate of Cytologically Diagnosed Dysplasia[25]

Author	Total Cases	Progression to Carcinoma In Situ (%)	Regression to Normal (%)
Lerch et al. (1963)[23]	80	2.5 (in 3-year follow-up	0
Fox (1967)[24]	278	60 (167 CIS or severe dysplasia; 2 micro-invasion, 1 early invasion)	31

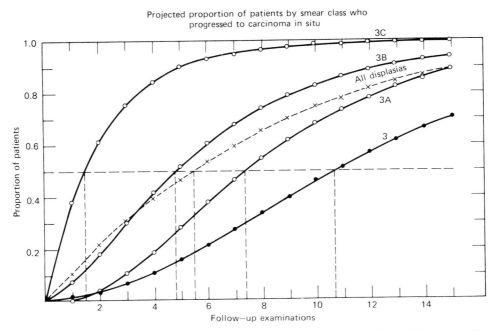

Figure 11 Graphic representation of the progression rates to carcinoma in situ of patients with entering diagnoses of 3 (very mild dysplasia), 3*A* (mild dysplasia,) 3*B* (moderate dysplasia), and 3*C* (severe dysplasia), and for all dysplasias. Dotted lines represent medians where each follow-up examination is 8 months. The projected median transit time to carcinoma in situ is about 86 months for a patient with very mild dysplasia, 58 months for mild dysplasia, 38 months for moderate dysplasia, 12 months for severe dysplasia, and 44 months for all dysplasias taken together. Note that these curves approach a limit, implying that a substantial proportion of patients will remain in the stage in which they were detected and not progress to a higher stage over a definite period of time. The progression rate cannot be used at any one time to predict the rate at a subsequent time. From Richart, and Barron, A follow-up study of patients with cervical dysplasia. *Am. J. Obstet. Gynecol.* **105**: 386 (1969). Reproduced by permission.

extensive surgery, and it has been argued that if a lesser procedure is sufficient it might be more appropriate.

CERVICAL CONIZATION

Although this is a diagnostic study, if the proximal and distal margins of the cone are free of intraepithelial neoplasia, the procedure is probably definitive. In a reliable population group that avails itself of cytologic follow-up (Table 3) and desires further child-bearing capability, cervical conization is a valid approach to management.

Table 3 Rates of Subsequent Disease for In Situ Squamous Carcinoma Related to Initial Therapy and Patient-Years of Follow-up[26]

Method of Treatment	Patient-Years	Persistent Disease	New Disease
Cone biopsy	2,448	7.4/1000	5.3/1000
Hysterectomy	13,436	0.9/1000	0.9/1000

LOCAL EXCISION

By punch biopsy or incisional biopsy, with colposcopic guidance, local excision has been recommended by some. This requires

Table 4   Type and Site of 67 Cases of Subsequent Disease Found in the Follow-up of 3688 Cases of In Situ Squamous Carcinoma of the Cervix[26]

Method of Treatment	Total Cases Treated	Cases of Subsequent Disease	Carcinoma In Situ		Carcinoma In Situ with Microscopic Foci of Invasion		Occult Invasive Carcinoma		Clinically Invasive Carcinoma		
			Cervix	Vagina	Cervix	Vagina	Cervix	Vagina	Cervix	Vagina	Other
Wedge biopsy	11	9	6[a]	0	1	0	2	0	0	0	0
Cone biopsy	808	31	28[a]	0	0	0	1	0	1	1	0
Hysterectomy	2849	24	0	19[b]	0	0	0	2	0	1	2[c]
Radiotherapy	20	3	1	1	0	0	0	0	1	0	0
Totals	3688	67	35	20	1	0	3	2	2	2	2

[a] One case involving cervix and vagina.

[b] Two cases involving labia also.

[c] One case had metastasis on pelvic side wall, and one case had a new focus of invasive perianal disease.

precise localization of the lesion and strict follow-up. Table 4 documents the weakness of this approach even in skilled hands; we believe it is inadequate.

CRYOSURGERY

Utilized on a large scale in only a limited number of clinics, available followup data suggest only that cryosurgery may be as useful and as efficient relatively as cervical conization. This method depends, however, on a sophisticated ability to accurately exclude the presence of invasive cancer colposcopically prior to treatment, and is not available in the vast majority of institutions or physicians's offices. Until further data are available cryosurgery should be limited to centers that study the technique critically.

RADIATION THERAPY

Occasionally, in the patient unsuitable for operation, radiation therapy (usually with radium application) has been employed successfully.

CHEMOTHERAPY

A limited experience with topical chemotherapy is being accumulated in several treatment centers, and short-term preliminary results suggest a favorable outcome. Long-term followup data are not yet available, and this technique should also be confined to treatment centers maintaining precise follow-up.

EXPECTED RESULTS

A wealth of significant clinical information is available in the report of Boyes and associates[26] who review 4389 cases of preclinical cervical squamous carcinoma (this includes mainly carcinoma in situ and some preclinical invasive cancer). Some of this information is recorded in Tables 3 and 4.

Of 808 cases of carcinoma in situ treated by cone biopsy only, 31 cases of persistent or subsequent disease were found. Their report notes that 18 cases represented persistent disease, and 16 of the 18 developed within the first five years (of 643 patients followed for five years); the other 2 cases of persistent disease developed in the next five-year interval (of 142 patients followed for 10 years). New disease was found in 13 patients, 10 in the first five years and 3 in the second five-year interval.

Of 2849 cases treated by hysterectomy, 24 cases developed persistent or subsequent disease; 12 had persistent disease (8 in the first five-year interval and 3 in the second five years). These data suggest (1) that the risk for new disease remains at a relatively level rate throughout any interval of follow-up, and (2) that many new recurrences reported in small numbers in other reports may represent actual persistence of initially unrecognized intraepithelial neoplasia.

Of a small series of patients treated initially by wedge biopsy alone, the majority developed subsequent disease.

Dysplasia

While there is increasing acceptance that severe dysplasia (and particularly those cases in which the pathologist is troubled over the distinction between severe dysplasia or carcinoma in situ) are successfully treated by hysterectomy (provided the patient has completed her family), it is clear that the majority of dysplasias can be managed satisfactorily by lesser procedures.

In general clinical practice, one follows an atypical Pap smear report with a repeat smear, appropriate staining, and biopsy techniques that include endocervical curettage. There are then two alternatives. If the cytologic and histologic material show mild dysplasia, these procedures may suffice until healing is complete and follow-up cytology can be utilized. If the cytologic atypia is more severe, and if biopsies also reflect more severe dysplasia, most clinicians will proceed with conization. Similarly, if either the histologic or cytologic material suggests a greater degree of atypia, conization should be done; this diagnostic procedure may be therapeutic as well. Again, when careful follow-up is assured, this treatment may be definitive if cytologic studies continue to be normal. The addition of cryosurgery or hot cautery may also be considered at this time if the cytologic and histologic interpretation is of a less severe degree of dysplasia. Generally, unless sophisticated expertise is available to exclude invasive cancer without conization, the practioner should not utilize primary cryosurgery, cautery, or other modalities at this time.

REFERENCES

1. Symposium: Herpesvirus and cervical cancer. *Cancer Res.* **33:** 1345 (1973).

2. Naib, A. M., A. J. Nahmias, W. E. Josey, and J. H. Kramer: Genital herpetic infection associated with cervical dysplasia and carcinoma. *Cancer* **23:** 940 (1969).

3. Frenken, N., B. Roizman, E. Cassai, and A. Nahmias: A DNA fragment of herpes simplex 2 and its transcription in human cervical cancer tissue. *Proc. Natl. Acad. Sci. U.S.A.* **69:** 3784 (1972).

4. Kay, S., W. J. Frable, D. M. Hume: Cervical dysplasia and cancer developing in women on immunosuppression therapy for renal homotransplantation. *Cancer* **26:** 1048 (1970).

5. Patten, S. F., Jr.: *Diagnostic Cytology of the Uterine Cervix,* The Williams and Wilkins Company, Baltimore, 1969.

6. Boyes, D. A.: The British Columbia screening program. *Obstet. Gynecol. Surv.* **24:** 1005 (1969).

7. Richart, R. M.: Techniques for the detection and diagnosis of cervical neoplasia. In *Gynecologic Oncology.* H. R. Barber, and E. A. Graber Eds., Excerpta Medica Foundation, Amsterdam, and the Williams and Wilkins Company, Baltimore, 1970.

8. Gilbert, F. E., M. D. Hicklin, S. L. Inhorn et al.: Conclusion of study group on stand-

ards of adequacy of cytologic examination of the female genital tract. *Gynecol. Oncol.* **1:** 271 (1973).

9. Stafl, A., and R. F. Mattingly: Colposcopic diagnosis of cervical neoplasia. *Obstet. Gynecol.* **41:** 168 (1973).

10. Townsend, D. E., D. R. Ostergard, and D. R. Mishell: Abnormal papanicolaou smears. *Am. J. Obstet. Gynecol.* **108:** 429 (1970).

11. Richart, R. M.: Influence of diagnostic and therapeutic procedures on the distribution of cervical intraepithelial neoplasia. *Cancer* **19:** 1635 (1966).

12. Green, G. H.: Invasive potentiality of cervical carcinoma in-situ. *Int. J. Gynaecol. Obstet.* **7:** 157 (1969).

13. Galvin, G. A., H. W. Jones, and R. W. TeLinde: The significance of basal-cell hyperactivity in cervical biopsies. *Am. J. Obstet. Gynecol.* **70:** 808 (1955).

14. Greene, R. R.: Discussion of Galvin, G. A., H. W. Jones, and R. W. TeLinde. *Am. J. Obstet. Gynecol.* **70:** 808 (1955).

15. Peckham, B., and R. R. Greene: Followup on cervical epithelial abnormalities. *Am. J. Obstet. Gynecol.* **73:** 120 (1957).

16. Rawson, A. J., and R. Knoblich: A clinicopathologic study of 56 cases showing atypical epithelial changes of the cervix uteri. *Am. J. Obstet. Gynecol.* **73:** 120 (1957).

17. McKay, D. G., B. Terjanian, D. Poschyacinda, P. A. Younge, and A. T. Hertig: Clinical and pathologic significance of anaplasia (atypical hyperplasia) of the cervix uteri. *Obstet. Gynecol.* **13:** 2 (1959).

18. Johnson, L. D., A. T. Hertig, C. H. Hinman, and C. L. Easterday: Preinvasive cervical lesions in obstetrical patients: methods of diagnosis, course and clinical management. *Obstet. Gynecol.* **16:** 133 (1960).

19. McLaren, H. C., and M. D. Attwood: The movement of cells in pregnancy. Proc. First International Congress of Exfoliative Cytology, 1961, pp. 133–135.

20. Dougherty, C. M., J. Torres, and N. Cotton: The fate of atypical hyperplasia of the uterine cervical epithelium. Proc. First International Congress of Exfoliative Cytology, 1961, pp. 103–109.

21. Lambert, B., and J. D. Woodruff: Spinal cell atypia of the cervix: a clinicopathological study. *Cancer* **16:** 1141 (1963).

22. Jordan, M. J., G. M. Bader, and E. Day: Carcinoma in-situ of the cervix and related lesions. *Am. J. Obstet. Gynecol.* **89:** 160 (1964).

23. Lerch, V., T. Okagaki, J. H. Austin, A. Y. Kevorkian, and P. A. Younge: Cytologic findings in progression of anaplasia (dysplasia) to carcinoma in-situ: a progress report. *Acta Cytol.* **7:** 183 (1963).

24. Fox, C. H.: Biologic behavior of dysplasia and carcinoma in-situ. *Am. J. Obstet. Gynecol.* **99:** 960 (1967).

25. Richart, R. M., and B. A. Barron: A followup study of patients with cervical dysplasia. *Am. J. Obstet. Gynecol.* **105:** 386 (1969).

26. Boyes, D. A., A. J. Worth, and H. K. Fidler: The results of treatment of 4389 cases of preclinical cervical squamous carcinoma. *J. Obstet Gynecol. Br. Commonw.* **77:** 769 (1970).

CHAPTER 2 PRETREATMENT EVALUATION AND THERAPY SELECTION FOR PATIENTS WITH INVASIVE CARCINOMA OF THE CERVIX

J. TAYLOR WHARTON, M.D.

The number of deaths caused each year by carcinoma of the cervix is decreasing as a result of improved medical knowledge and skills by physicians responsible for the care of these women. Early detection has contributed to this success. A more meaningful factor is the better understanding of the principles of irradiation therapy and radical surgery. A thorough pretreatment evaluation of patients with invasive carcinoma is essential in order to properly select and apply these treatment modalities.

The purpose of pretreatment evaluation is to determine the volume and extent of the cervical neoplasm. It is equally important to detect accompanying medical and psychological disorders that might hinder the completion of the planned therapy. Poor evaluation of either the cervix cancer or medical reserve can result in therapy failure and unnecessary suffering for the patient.

PATHOLOGY

Lesions that arise at the squamocolumnar junction or from the epithelium of the external surface of the portio vaginalis are of the squamous (epidermoid) variety and account for 95% of cervical cancers. Usually squamous carcinoma is moderately undifferentiated histologically, contains many pleomorphic cells of varying size, and numerous mitoses can be seen. Epithelial pearl formation is rare in this form. A well-differentiated carcinoma can also develop and is characterized by large abnormal cells with keratinization, forming epithelial pearls. An undifferentiated form consisting of uniform, small basophilic cells and having a high mitotic count has been described and is considered to be anaplastic and associated with a poor prognosis.[10]

Adenocarcinomas account for 5% of cervical malignancies and are thought to originate in the endocervical glands. The usual carcinoma contains mucin-producing cells of variable differentiation. A "clear cell" or mesonephric pattern is observed. Gallager and his associates and others have described an adenoid cystic carcinoma of the cervix that consists of basal cells in a cylindromatous glandular pattern.[5]

Although there are many histologic patterns, it is our impression that these cervix carcinomas grow and spread in a similar manner and respond equally to irradiation or surgical therapy. As a rule, therefore, we do not vary treatment techniques because of cell type or histologic differentiation, nor do we try to predict radiosensitivity or radioresistance on the basis of cytological characteristics.

SPREAD PATTERN

Carcinoma of the cervix spreads primarily by direct extension to adjacent structures and by lymphatic metastases. Table 2.1 categorizes this aspect of the disease.

Table 1　Spread Pattern Carcinoma of the Cervix, The M. D. Anderson Hospital[a]

Continuous

1. Beneath or onto the vaginal mucosa, possibly extending a considerable distance beyond palpable or visible disease.
2. Into the myometrium of the lower uterine segment producing a "barrel-shaped" configuration (Fig. 2).
3. Directly into the paracervical tissue with extension to pelvic wall, bladder, or rectum.

Discontinuous

1. Into the major lymphatic trunks
   a. frequent initial involvement of interiliac group (obturator nodes) and other pelvic nodes;
   b. progressive spread to common iliac and aortic nodes in patients with more extensive primary cancer;
   c. infrequent involvement of aortic nodes without involvement of pelvic nodes.
2. Vascular metastases.

[a]Reprinted, with permission, from reference II.

The lymphatics draining the cervix have been described in detail by Plentyl and Friedman and consist of three main trunks: lateral, posterior, and anterior.[8] The middle branches of the lateral collecting trunks are among the largest that drain the cervix. These branches pass posterior to the hypogastric artery and terminate in the interiliac nodes on the obturator nerve. These nodes, referred to as obturator nodes by most gynecologists, represent early sites of metastatic carcinoma. We have been impressed with the frequency in which this node group contains metastatic cancer in patients with bulky primaries who have a preirradiation exploratory celiotomy and removal of these nodes for histologic examination.

Branches of the lateral trunk lymphatics also drain into the gluteal, sacral, and aortic nodes. The posterior trunk drains into the common iliac and aortic nodes, whereas the anterior trunk drains into the iliac nodes.

An additional practical point has evolved from exploratory celiotomy preceding irradiation. Cancer of the cervix spreads in an orderly manner, and it is unusual to find common iliac and aortic metastases in patients with Stages IB and IIA carcinomas (Table 2). Those patients with more advanced cancers have common iliac and aortic metastases, but usually the pelvic nodes are extensively involved.

Table 2　Spread Pattern of Carcinoma of the Cervix Status of Lymph Nodes at Surgery, The M. D. Anderson Hospital

Stage	Negative	Pelvic	External Iliac	Common Iliac	Paraaortic	Total
IB	14	5	2	0	0	21
IIA	9	0	1	0	0	10
IIB	13	7	10	3	7	40
IIIA	12	3	7	1	10	33
IIIB	2	0	1	1	4	8
IV	1	0	0	0	0	1
Total	51	15	21	5	21	113

The practitioner can gain valuable information from studying lymphangiograms and relating the various node groups to pelvic structures and lumbar vertebrae. Figure 1 shows the distribution of the external iliac, common iliac, and periaortic nodes. Note that the proximal common iliac nodes extend to the level of the fourth lumbar vertebra.

PATIENT EVALUATION

Cytological evaluation of smears taken from the vagina and cervix will frequently in-

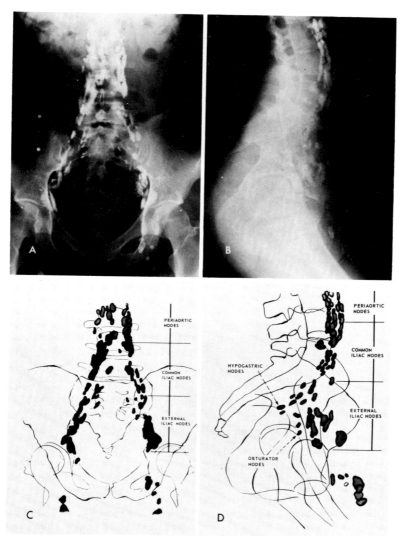

Figure 1 Anteroposterior (A) and cross-table lateral (B) orthogonal radiographs of a patient with a normal lymphangiogram of the lower extremity. Parts (C) and (D) illustrate the regional lymphatics of the pelvis and lower lumbar area, and the terminology used in this chapter. With the exception of the obturator nodes located inside the acetabula, and some of the hypogastric and uterosacral nodes, the nodes are not on the pelvic walls. From Durrance, F. Y., and Fletcher, G. H.: Computer calculation of dose contribution to regional lymphatics from gynecological radium insertions. *Radiology* **91**: 141 (1968). Reproduced by permission.

dicate that a neoplasm is present in the genital tract. The smear is only a diagnostic test and is not a substitute for a careful examination. A suspicious cervical lesion is always biopsied, even if the cytological evaluation of the exfoliated cells is negative for malignancy. If there is no visible lesion, random biopsies of the cervix are performed. The anterior and posterior lips are always sampled since carcinomas tend to start in these areas. Lugol's solution (Schiller's test) is helpful in locating abnormal areas for biopsy because abnormal epithelium is usually devoid of glycogen and is not stained by the iodine.

The endocervix is curetted because a lesion arising high in the endocervix can be missed by the usual cervical biopsy. This latter procedure is particularly useful in the older patient, since the squamocolumnar junction may be quite high.

The colposcope is a valuable instrument for examining the entire lower genital tract and accurately locates abnormal areas for biopsy. The need for hospitalization and cold knife conization will be less frequent for the patient of a skilled colposcopist. The colposcope is particularly useful in examining the cervix of a pregnant patient. Interested physicians may consult the excellent texts on colposcopy by Coppleson and co-workers[1] or Per Kolstad and Stafl.[7]

Conization may be necessary to rule out invasive cancer if random biopsies or, preferably, colposcopically directed biopsies fail to explain the origin of the cytologically abnormal cells. When a tissue diagnosis of invasive carcinoma is established, a comprehensive evaluation of the patient follows. The complete medical history is taken, and diseases such as hypertension, anemia, pyelonephritis, diabetes, and pulmonary disorders are recorded. A history of previous pelvic infections or abdominal operations is important because both conditions adversely affect pelvic irradiation therapy. Any process that produces pelvic fibrosis and adhesions may cause the bowel to become fixed in the pelvis and receive more intense radiation than the patient can tolerate.

Particular attention should be given to direct palpation of lymph nodes in the inguinal node groups and left supraclavicular area during the physical examination. Direct palpation allows detection of metastatic disease that would otherwise be missed. When supraclavicular nodes are palpable, they usually contain metastatic disease.

The extent of the cervical neoplasm is determined by pelvic examination. These findings are correlated with the other physical and x-ray examinations, and the cancer is then staged according to the criteria of the International Federation of Gynecologists and Obstetricians (FIGO) (Table 3).

An equally important factor that influences therapy planning and survival is the volume of tumor involving the cervix. Pretherapy assessment by palpation and probing of the cervix is essential if maximum efficiency of irradiation therapy is to be obtained. The gynecologist must accurately detect the large, bulky lesions, since these are always treated first with external irradiation, in order to induce the regression in tumor volume essential for successful intracavitary irradiation. In such situations, the use of intracavitary radium first squanders this necessary part of the therapy.

The tumor volume factor can be further demonstrated by an advanced carcinoma of endocervical origin. Certain growth patterns (barrel-shaped lesions) may concentrically enlarge the cervix to a diameter equal to or greater than the uterine fundus (Figure 2). The examiner, on passing a uterine probe, frequently observes that the endocervical canal is irregular and enlarged due to necrosis caused by the tumor outgrowing its blood supply. The cells near the necrotic center are hypoxic and require more intense radiotherapy for destruction. Further evaluation by fractional curettage frequently

Table 3 Definitions of the Different Clinical Stages in Carcinoma of the Cervix Uteri to Be Used from January 1, 1971

Preinvasive Carcinoma

Stage 0	Carcinoma in situ, intraepithelial carcinoma.
	Cases of Stage 0 should not be included in any therapeutic statistics.

Invasive Carcinoma

Stage I	Carcinoma strictly confined to the cervix (extension to the corpus should be disregarded).
Stage IA	The cancer cannot be diagnosed by clinical examination; it includes (1) early stromal invasion, and (2) occult cancer.
Stage IB	All other cases of Stage I disease.
Stage II	The carcinoma extends beyond the cervic but has not extended to the pelvic wall. The carcinoma involves the vagina, but not the lower third.
Stage IIA	No obvious parametrial involvement.
Stage IIB	Obvious parametrial involvement.
Stage III	The carcinoma has extended to the pelvic wall. On rectal examination there is no cancer-free space between the tumor and the pelvic wall. The tumor involves the lower third of the vagina.
Stage IIIA	No extension to the pelvic wall.
Stage IIIB	Extension to the pelvic wall.
Stage IV	The carcinoma has extended beyond the true pelvis or has involved the mucosa of the bladder or rectum.
	A bullous edema as such does not permit allotment of a case to Stage IV.

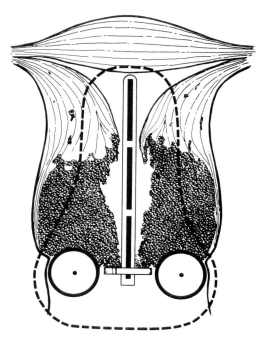

Figure 2 Invasion of the myometrium of the isthmus ("barrel-shaped" lesion). Tumor cells are too far from the radium sources for adequate dose distribution. Even after 4,000 rads, shrinkage may not bring disease in the periphery close enough to the radium sources. Modified from Fletcher, G. H.: *Textbook of Radiotheraphy*, Lea & Febiger, Philadelphia, 1966, p. 479. Reproduced by permission.

reveals that the carcinoma extends into the lower uterine segment. Recognition of such growth patterns during pretherapy evaluation identifies the patient who has a greater chance for developing a central recurrence following standard radiation therapy. The potential for a central failure can be eliminated by combining an extrafascial hysterectomy following slightly less intense intracavitary irradiation.[6,9]

Minimal laboratory and roentgenographic studies consist of a complete blood count, urinalysis, automated analytic blood chemistry determination (SMA 12/60) or its equivalent, electrocardiogram (EKG), cystoscopic examination, chest x-ray, and intravenous pyelogram (IVP). The IVP is useful in staging cervical cancer because obstruction of a ureter indicates Stage III carcinoma.

If the patient is allergic to contrast material it will be necessary to obtain a renal scan or to perform retrograde pyelograms, to insure that the kidneys are not in the pelvis or otherwise abnormal. Knowledge of the status and anatomic features of the urinary tract is essential whether radical surgery or radiation therapy is the selected therapy.

Lymphangiography is a particularly useful diagnostic procedure. The external iliac, common iliac, and aortic nodes are consistently visualized on the lymphagiogram. A defect in a node (usually crescent-shaped) not traversed by lymphatics is a highly reliable criterion that metastatic disease is present. The presacral and internal iliac nodes are not consistently visualized, and experience obtained by performing preirradiation celiotomy shows that extensive disease may involve the interiliac (obturator) nodes and escape detection by lymphangiography.

Lymphangiography is used mainly to determine the presence and extent of lymph node metastasis. Detection of proximal common iliac and aortic node metastases is important because these nodes are not routinely irradiated when a standard 15×15 cm pelvic field (superior border at level of the fifth lumbar vertebra) is irradiated (Figure 1).

Additional diagnostic procedures such as proctoscopic examination, barium enema, liver scan, and metastatic bone x-ray survey are not routinely recommended.

PRETHERAPY EXPLORATORY CELIOTOMY

The causes of irradiation therapy failures in patients with carcinoma of the cervix are summarized in Table 4. In our experience central failures do not represent the major problem (Table 5). The 1.5%, 5%, and 7.5% central recurrence rates for Stages

Table 4   Causes of Irradiation Therapy Failures in Carcinoma of the Cervix, The M. D. Anderson Hospital

1. Geographic failure—metastatic cancer outside the standard 15×15 cm pelvic irradiation therapy fields.
2. Regional failure—inability to destroy metastatic cancer in regional lymph nodes that received full intensity radiation therapy.
3. Central failure—failure to control cancer in the cervix.

Table 5   Status of Disease in Patients Dead up to 5 Years: 1705 Patients with Megavoltage External Irradiation, September 1954–December 1963 (Analysis March 1966)[a][b]

Stage	Number of Patients	Patients with Central Active Disease Alone or at Other Sites
I	407	
IIA	327	1.5% (12)
IIB	291	5.0% (15)
IIIA	324	7.5% (24)
IIIB	275	17.0% (49)
IV	81	39.0% (32)
Total	1705[c]	132

[a] Reprinted, with permission, from reference 4.
[b] Includes patients treated incompletely or for palliation.
[c] Three cardiac patients in Stages IIB, IIIA, and IIIB died during treatment.

I, II, and IIIA, respectively reflect the excellent qualities of intracavitary radiation.

The two areas of failure about which we have primary concern are (1) outside the pelvis (geographic failure) and (2) the pelvic lymph nodes (regional failure). These two areas were shown to be significant in an analysis of failure sites in 148 patients who had exploratory celiotomy and pelvic lymphadenectomy following full intensity irradiation therapy (Table 6). Further study suggested that those patients with residual

Table 6 Failure Sites Carcinoma of the Cervix: Incidence of Positive Nodes 3 Months after Completion of Radical Irradiation in 148 Unselected Stage III Patients[a]

Positive Nodes	Number of Patients
1. Geographic failure (outside treated area)	10
2. Regional failure (within treated area)	7
3. Both within and outside treated area	11
Total	28 (20%)

[a] Reprinted, with permission, from reference 2.

Table 7 Squamous Carcinoma Dose—Tumor Volume Relationships: 90% Control[a]

Tumor Volume (cm)	Dose (rads)
Subclinical disease	5000
<2	6000
2–4	6800
4–6	7300
>6	7890

[a] Reprinted, with permission, from reference 3.

cancer in the pelvic nodes following irradiation had extensive involvement prior to initiation of treatment. Thus, the volume of cancer in lymph nodes evolves as a critical factor in determining curability.

An exploratory celiotomy performed prior to initiating irradiation therapy would provide histologic proof of the extent of metastatic cancer in lymph nodes and other abdominal organs. Those patients with disease in lymph nodes outside of the standard pelvic irradiation fields (usually 15 × 15 cm) would be candidates for experimental extended-field irradiation therapy. An additional benefit would be gained by removing enlarged lymph nodes containing cancer: following excision, the remaining cancer would consist only of microscopic cell aggregates in the lymph node site. The cell aggregates, termed "subclinical disease," are well oxygenated and easily killed by doses of irradiation well within normal tissue tolerance. The subclinical disease concept has been proven in the treatment of head and neck and breast malignancies and may be applicable to pelvic malignancies. Table 7 shows the dose of irradiation required to obtain a 90% control rate for various volumes of cancer and may be used as a guide in therapy planning.

A detailed explanation of the subclinical disease concept has been published by Fletcher.[4] Clearly lymph nodes containing masses of cancer >2 cm in diameter, whether in the neck, axilla, or pelvis require more than 5000 rads in five weeks to obtain a high control rate. Doses in excess of 5000 rads given to the lower abdomen and pelvis are associated wth a higher incidence of bowel complications. In summary, an additional use of exploratory celiotomy before irradiation, surgically reducing tumor volume in these nodes, is an experiment to determine if cancer control in the pelvis can be improved while maintaining standard doses of irradiation.

THE M. D. ANDERSON EXPERIENCE

In our institution, 113 patients in good physical condition, with carcinomas of the cervix 5 cm or more in diameter, had exploratory celiotomy prior to initiation of irradiation therapy (Table 8). A midline incision was used and extended cephalad as much as necessary for proper exposure of the abdominal aorta and inferior vena cava. The accessible anterior and lateral node groups on these vessels were removed en bloc. Selected common iliac, external iliac, and hypogastric nodes were also removed and placed on a plastic template to facilitate accurate anatomical localization (Figure 3). An attempt was made to remove clinically

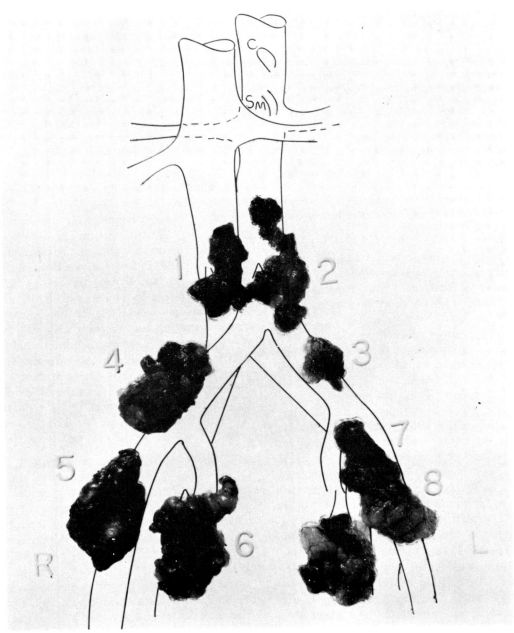

Figure 3 Nodes in place on the plastic template. This patient with Stage IIB cervic cancer had 45 nodes removed and had metastatic disease in the obturator, external iliac, and common iilac nodes bilaterally. From Fletcher G. H., *Textbook of Radiotherapy*, 2nd edit. Lea & Febiger, Philadelphia, 1973, p. 712. Reproduced by permission.

Table 8 Distribution of Patients by Stage, July 1971–December 1973

Stage[c]	Patients
IB	21
IIA	10
IIB	40
IIIA[a]	33
IIIB[b]	8
IV	1
Total	113

[a] Tumor extends to one pelvic wall.
[b] Tumor extends to both pelvic walls.
[c] M. D. Anderson staging system.

suspicious nodes. The number of pelvic nodes removed varied greatly, and in some patients dissection was extensive.

The size of the treatment field was selected with regard to the findings at laparotomy. A standard 15 × 15 cm field was used for those patients with negative nodes or metastatic nodes in the obturator or hypogastric group. Patients who had positive nodes in the external iliac area were treated with an extended field which covered the common iliac chain (Figure 4). This field extends to the bottom of the L-4 vertebra and provides a margin of one normal node chain above the group proven positive at laparotomy. A T-12 field extending to the diaphragm was used when positive common iliac or paraaortic nodes were encountered (Figure 5). Patients receiving extended field therapy were treated with the 25-MeV linear accelerator for a total dose of 5500 rads (850 rads/week). Intracavitary radium was used as part of the treatment, depending on the volume and anatomy of the lesion. Patients unsuitable for intracavitary radium received additional external therapy with reduced field size.

Results

At laparotomy intraabdominal spread of disease was found in 11 patients: 7 patients had perforation of the tumor through the cervix into the cul-de-sac; 1 patient had an ovarian metastasis, 1 a sigmoid implant, 1 had an omental nodule, and 1 had metastases to the terminal ileum.

At lymphadenectomy, 51 patients had negative nodes and 62 patients had metastatic carcinoma in one or more lymph nodes (Table 2). Metastasis occurred in a progressive stepwise order, involving proximal node groups before spreading to the more distal chains. All patients with Stages IB and IIA cervical carcinoma with positive nodes had these nodes well within the standard pelvic treatment field.

Patients with more advanced lesions had a higher incidence of positive nodes and distant metastases. Two-thirds of the patients with Stage IIB lesions or greater had positive nodes, and in 10 the nodes were in the common iliac and/or paraaortic groups. In all, 26 (23%) of the 113 patients had disease above the standard pelvic irradiation field that would have been left untreated.

Intraoperative and serious, immediate postoperative complications were rare. The major problems of combination pretherapy exploratory celiotomy and extended-field irradiation therapy have been late complications related to bowel and urinary tract injury: 4 patients developed gastric ulcers in the T-12 radiation field, 2 patients developed small bowel obstruction due to adhesions alone, and 15 had small bowel problems due to combination adhesions and irradiation injury. Of these 15 patients who required reoperation, 5 had intestinal perforation and only 1 survived. Small bowel bypass or resection with or without colostomy was carried out on the other 10 patients, and 8 are alive at the present time. Of the 3 patients who developed bilateral

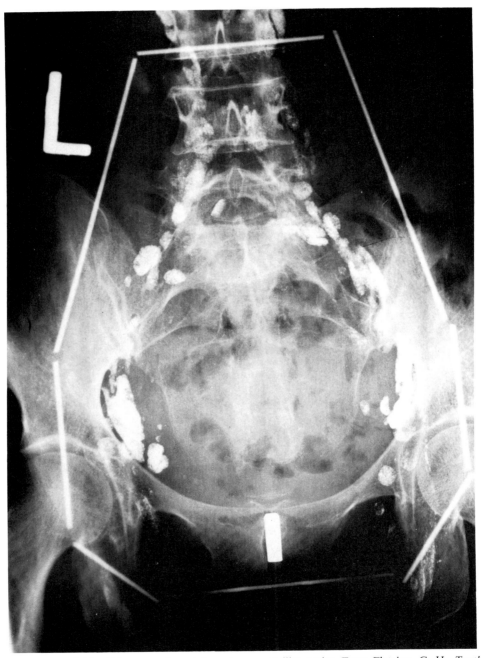

Figure 4 The L-4 field which covers the pelvic and common iliac nodes. From Fletcher, G. H., *Textbook of Radiotherapy*, 2nd edit. Lea & Febiger, Philadelphia, 1973, p. 654. Reproduced by permission.

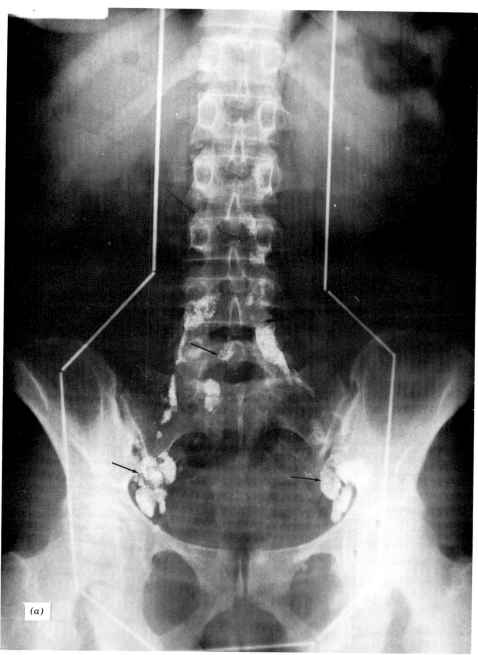

(a)

Figure 5 The T_{12} field covers the paraaortic nodes to the level of the diaphragm. Figures 5*B* (anterior view) and 5*C* (posterior view) show the radiation therapy portals drawn on the patients' abdomen. The dotted line crosses the 4th lumbar vertebra. The T_{12} extension usually measures 8 cm in width and 15 cm in height. From Fletcher, G. H., *Textbook of Radiotherapy*, 2nd edit. Lea & Febiger, Philadelphia, 1973, p. 655.

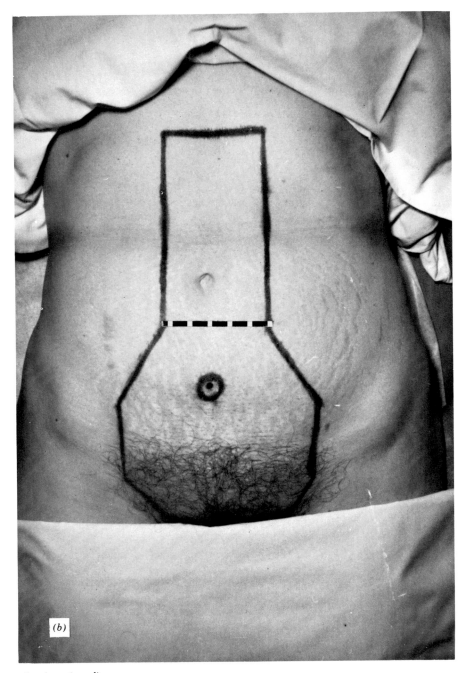

(b)

Figure 5 (*continued*)

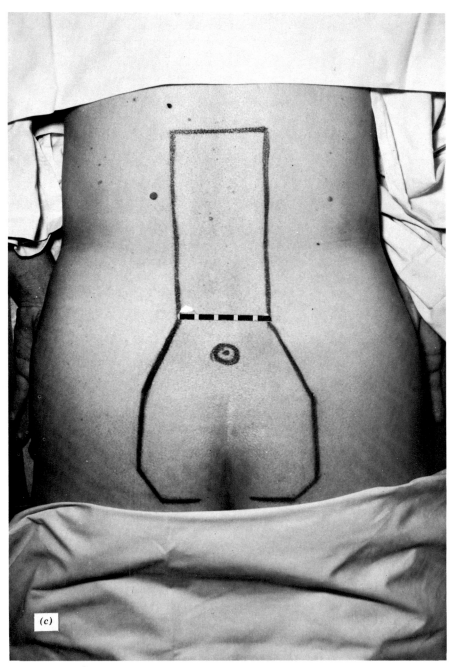

Figure 5 (*continued*)

Table 9 Results of Treatment

Stage	Alive NED[a]	Alive (Cancer)	Dead (Cancer)	Dead (Complications)	Not Evaluated[b]	Total
IB	13	1	3	4	0	21
IIA	6	1	2	1	0	10
IIB	15	4	11	7	3	40
IIIA	16	3	4	3	7	33
IIIB	2	0	2	0	4	8
IV	1	0	0	0	0	1
Total	53	9	22	15	14	113

[a] No evidence of disease.
[b] Less than 6 months follow-up.

ureteral obstruction due to intense retroperitoneal fibrosis, 2 had ileal conduits, and 1 underwent a ureteroileoneocystostomy.

The current status of these patients is shown in Table 9. 53 patients are active, with no evidence of disease for a period of 6 to 30 months; 22 have died of cancer, 9 are alive with recurrent disease, and 15 have died of complications related to their therapy.

In conclusion, preirradiation exploratory celiotomy as a special surgical procedure used to evaluate the extent of cancer spread is not without serious complications. Our first experience has clearly shown that surgical dissection in the pelvis must be kept to an absolute minimum, and that the surgeon should remove individual suspicious nodes selectively. The paraaortic dissection should also be conservative, since radical dissection anywhere creates disruption of lymphatic flow and widespread adhesions.

Since January 1, 1974, the dose for extended field irradiation has been reduced to 4500 rads (850 rads/week). Surgical dissection has decreased to the minimal amount necessary to remove suspicious lymph nodes. The complication rate has also decreased dramatically as a result of the plan described, and the work continues. These

studies are considered an experiment in operative gynecology and extended-field irradiation therapy and are not routine in the pretreatment evaluation for patients with invasive carcinoma of the cervix.

REFERENCES

1. Coppleson, Malcolm, Ellis Pixley, and Bevan Reid, *Colposcopy, A Scientific and Practical Approach to the Cervix in Health and Disease,* Charles C Thomas, Springfield Illinois, 1971.

2. Fletcher, G. H., and F. N. Rutledge. *Amer. J. Roentgen.* **114,** 116 (1972).

3. Fletcher, Gilbert, Clinical dose response curves of human malignant epithelial tumors. *Br. J. Radiol.* **46,** 1–12 (1973).

4. Fletcher, G. H., *Textbook of Radiotherapy,* Lea & Febiger, Philadelphia, 1973, p. 713.

5. Gallagher, H., Stephen, C. B., Simpson, and Alberto C. Ayala, Adenoid cystic carcinoma of the uterine cervix. Report of four cases, *Cancer* **27,** 1398–1402, 1406 (1971).

6. Nelson, Alvan J., Gilbert H. Fletcher, and J. Taylor Wharton, Indications for adjunctive conservative extrafascial hysterectomy in selected cases of carcinoma of the uterine cervix, *Am. J. Roent. Ra Therapy Nucl. Med.,* **123,** 1, 91–99, 1975.

7. Kolstad, Per, and Adolf Stafl, *Atlas of Colposcopy,* University Park Press, Baltimore, 1972.

8. Plentyl, A. A., and E. A. Friedman, *Lymphatic System of the Female Genitalia,* W. B. Saunders & Company, 1971, p. 5.

9. Rutledge, F. N., and J. T. Wharton, Surgical procedures Associated with radiation therapy for cervical cancer. In *Textbook of Radiotherapy,* Fletcher, G. H., Ed., Lea & Febiger, Philadelphia, 1973, p. 711.

10. Wentz, W. B., and J. W. Reagan, Survival in cervical cancer with respect to cell type, *Cancer,* **12,** 384 (1959).

11. Wharton, J. Taylor, Julian P. Smith, Luis Delclos, and Gilbert H. Fletcher. In *Gynecology and Obstetrics,* Vol. II, Davis, Harper & Row, Hagerstown, Maryland, 1972, Chap. 73, p. 2.

CHAPTER 3 MANAGEMENT: STAGES I AND II CARCINOMA OF THE CERVIX

FELIX RUTLEDGE, M.D.

The importance of early detection in the outcome of gynecologic cancer has often been emphasized, but less attention has been given to the adequacy of initial treatment. In cancer therapy, the first treatment is important to prognosis. This is particularly true in cancer of the cervix, a common type of cancer in an area accessible to examination. With the knowledge and treatment methods currently available, cure is possible in most cases. The physician who has a patient with gynecologic cancer is responsible for ensuring the best possible treatment for his patient the first time she is treated, since the way in which he discharges this responsibility can literally make the difference between life and death.

Treatment for cervical cancer that is adequate by modern standards is by no means a simple, routine affair. It is complicated by the need for individualization, which usually demands the services of physicians representing several specialties and also requires the availability of a wide range of tools and skills. Such desirable arrangements do not simply occur; they must be planned for. To ensure that a patient is given the treatment which is best suited for her, services must be organized to provide: (1) a multidisciplinary approach to management (close cooperation between the gynecologist and the radiotherapist is necessary), (2) tools and skills adequate for any contin-

gency, including those needed for advanced, persistent, and recurrent cancer, and (3) organization to ensure continuous follow-up, so that the first sign of recurrent or persistent cancer can be detected and remedial measures taken. Unless these requirements are fulfilled, good individualized treatment will not be possible, and satisfactory results will not be obtained.

MULTIDISCIPLINARY APPROACH TO MANAGEMENT

Before treatment, the patient's general health and her cancer must be studied thoroughly. The cancer type, extent, and direction of spread of the disease must be determined. The amount of damage to the genitourinary and gastrointestinal tract and to the lungs must be assessed. Obviously, although the aid of the pathologist and the diagnostic radiologist is essential, this type of consultation does not fulfill the real meaning of the multidisciplinary approach to management. It is in therapy planning that the combined knowledge and skills of several disciplines are more productive.

About 20 years ago, we organized the Gynecology and Radiotherapy Services in our institution to provide joint care for gynecologic patients. The M. D. Anderson Hospital is a state-supported, specialized cancer institution, and all of our patients are referrals. Therefore, although our particular plan might not be suitable for other institutions, it has worked so well for us that only minor changes have been made in the original organizational plan. Good communication, we found, was essential, and the usual means—notes, diagrams, letters in the charts—were not adequate. The best solution was a series of conferences, planned and held on a regular schedule. Figure 1 shows the organization used in joint service care for cervical cancer.

The preliminary diagnostic workup is done by the gynecologist because members

of this service are more experienced in performing cystoscopies and proctoscopies, and are more familiar with the unusual manifestations of cancer. At the disposition clinic, the next step toward treatment, members of both gynecology and radiotherapy services reexamine the patient and study her medical history and her present state of health. At this time, the cancer is staged, the decision for additional studies is made, the biopsy is repeated if necessary, and a plan of treatment is formulated. Alternate therapeutic plans may also be arranged. These are decisions to be made jointly by the gynecologist and the radiotherapist.

At the weekly dosimetry clinic attended by the gynecologist, the radiotherapist, and other staff members, the progress of each patient who received radium (members of both services perform radium insertion) is reviewed; localization radiographs of each application are studied; the dosage to the bladder and rectum and regional node groups is noted from computerized isodose graphs; and plans are made to correct any deficiencies.

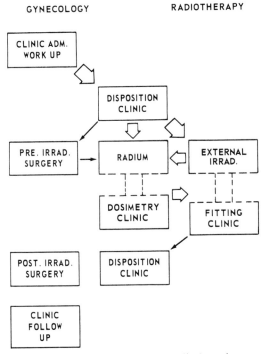

Figure 1 The gynecologist and radiotherapist team each contribute to the care of patients with cervical cancer. Gynecology functions individually, as noted in the left column, radiotherapy in the right column. They work together in selecting treatment and deciding new problems (Disposition Clinic). The application of radium is equally divided. There is a review of the control data of radium application (Dosimetry Clinic). Old problems are rereviewed in the Disposition Clinic.

ADEQUATE TOOLS AND SKILLS

Individualized treatment and meticulous attention to detail are very important in cervical cancer because anatomic variations among patients require adjustment in the position and type of applicator for radium. Several effective radium applicators and systems have been devised, each with its advocates. These designs differ basically in the arrangement and intensity of the sources of radium, the proportion of radium in total milligrams in the uterus to that in the vagina, the hourly dose rate from the radium system, and the number of radium insertions that constitute the treatment plan. All systems share some essential elements. A stock of radium sources of varying intensity and a complement of versatile applicator sizes are basic requirements for good intracavitary therapy (Figure 2). Since a properly fitted radium system is vital to success, a large selection of tandem applicators in different lengths and curves and vaginal ovoids in a range of diameters must be available. Any compromise may mean that treatment will be inadequate or the hazards of complication will increase.

A wide range of surgical knowledge and skills must also be available. Occasionally, with cervical cancer, urinary or fecal diversion must be accomplished before irradiation is begun. Sometimes a combination of irradiation and surgery, in which neither modality is used at full strength, is necessary. Occasionally, some type of pelvic exenteration may be indicated for a patient with massive, centralized cancer. As is true

with irradiation, the therapeutic plan may have to be altered in the operating room, and the surgeon should have the knowledge and skill to make the necessary adjustment. A need for a more extended resection than planned may be discovered during laparotomy.

FOLLOW-UP

The follow-up period for the patient with gynecologic cancer has received less attention than the diagnostic and treatment phases. Even today, some physicians do not recognize the importance of periodic examinations after treatment. They seem to believe that if the patient is cured, she needs no further attention, and that if the disease

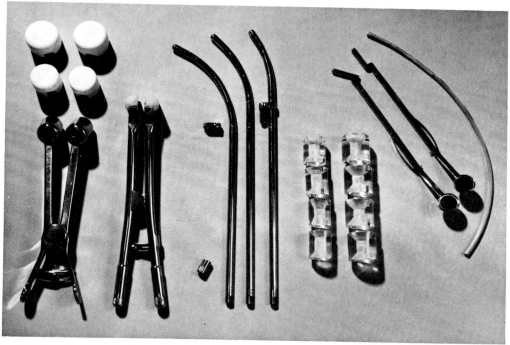

Figure 2 Variation among different patients in the size of the upper vagina and the length and position of the uterine cavity requires colpostats of several diameters, and a selection of uterine tandems with facilities for varying the length and degree of curvature. Expanders may be applied to the colpostats. A guard may be set along the tandem to control the insertion depth. Cylindrical expanders may be threaded along the tandem to distend the vagina when colpostats cannot be used. Provision for after-loading has important advantages.

is not controlled by the initial treatment, nothing else can be done. This pessimistic outlook is incompatible with the possibilites inherent in present day treatment and should be replaced by one of tenacity and optimism. Much can be done to control persistent or recurrent cancer. Furthermore, if the patient is incurable, palliation is as much a part of the physician's responsibility as is treatment for the original lesion. No physician should undertake the treatment of a gynecologic cancer patient unless he is willing to be her medical counselor throughout the course of her disease.

ANATOMIC VARIETIES: THEIR CLINICAL SIGNIFICANCE

The growth pattern of the cancer and the sites of regional involvement influence a choice of primary treatment by either surgery or irradiation. These anatomic features not only indicate the best single treatment but, when a combination of operation and irradiation is to be used, the growth forms may also dictate the sequence of therapy. Preoperative radium before radical hysterectomy is such an example. Although the clinical appearance of the lesion around the cervix may not always indicate the severity of the prognosis it does supply important information about the difficulty in determining treatment; thus descriptive terms are clinically useful.

The shape, firmness, and size of the gross lesions in Stages I and II cervical cancer patients varies because these features depend upon the growth rate of the neoplasm, the adequacy of the blood supply, the site of origin, the age (duration) of the cancer, and perhaps some poorly understood ability of the cancer to invade or of the host to resist spread.

The common descriptions of cervical cancer are exophytic and endophytic, plaque or ulcerative. Recognizing that mixed forms are more common and that additional growth will in time change the shape, these descriptions are still worth recording in each patient's record on examination. Observation of change in the features of the cancer should also be noted, that is, conversions from exophytic to ulcerative, or from ulcerative to more proliferative (Figure 3).

Exophytic Type

This growth type of cervical cancer extends outward into the vagina and has clinical significance for the following reasons:

1. It is a friable polypoid lesion that bleeds with slight trauma and may produce a spontaneous serosanguineous exudate as a vaginal discharge. Coitus induces bleeding. These signs of cancer alert the patient and may be responsible for earlier detection of exophytic cancer.

2. Examination and manipulation may produce frightening, but rarely threatening, hemorrhage.

3. When the exophytic mass is quite large, it occupies the upper part of the vagina and may obstruct satisfactory bimanual examination. The tumor mass may hamper the examiner's effort to define the amount, location, and limits of the spread. It may conceal the cervical os and thwart measurement of the cervical canal.

4. The large exophytic mass is a condition which is unsuited for immediate application of radium, for the tumor may hold the irradiation source away from the tumor base attachment.

5. This growth form is especially vulnerable to transvaginal irradiation, and the response may be prompt with rapid regression of tumor mass and control of hemorrhage.

Endophytic (Infiltrative) Type

1. Some cancers, after establishing a primary lesion, push into the surrounding

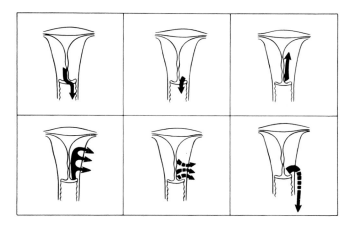

Figure 3 (1) Cancer develops along the surface of the endocervical portion of cervix and vagina simultaneously. This neogenesis covers a large area but may not be metastatic. (2) Outward growth "cauliflower type" fungating type. (3) Spread toward corpus (unusual). Bottom, left to right: (1) Endocervical compact origin, replaces the stroma expanding the lower uterine segment to produce barrel-shaped lesions. (2) Discontinuous metastasis through the stroma with small islands of cancer. (3) Metastasis to the lower vagina with normal segment of vagina intervening.

tissues with tentacles of neoplasia that crowd the host tissue and expand the cervix and lower uterine segment, making it much larger and firmer than normal. The ulcerative lesion may appear small when viewed from the vagina, but this view can be deceptive.

2. The stony, hard, distorted cervix may be misinterpreted as a cervical fibroid, endometriosis, or some other benign change that could also produce unusually firm consistency.

3. Since only a small amount of neoplastic tissue is visible, the pelvic surgeon may be misled into performing a conventional hysterectomy, a too conservative procedure for this lesion. The operation will be inadequate for the primary tumor and also for the regional nodes, for when there is a larger portion of the primary tumor it infiltrates throughout the stroma of the cervix and there is often lymph node metastasis.

4. Special dosimetry is necessary for this growth pattern. The larger amount of tumor infiltration present requires a higher dosage of irradiation. Even when the additional

bulkiness is considered in planning irradiation dosimetry, these patients are more likely to develop local recurrences because the tumor is not completely destroyed. A tumor with this growth pattern could require a dose that exceeds the tolerance of the normal tissue. To lessen the risk of irradiation injury in trying to reach this dosage, these patients may be better treated by a combination of irradiation and more conservative hysterectomy. The major part of the cell population is destroyed by irradiation; the remainder is excised. When the endophytic lesion is large, the physician should be aware that a special treatment plan may be needed.

The Ulcerative (Crater) Lesion

These lesions can change in appearance if observed long enough, for they may form an exophytic lesion that loses its protruding part. As the base portion of the tumor grows and usurps the blood supply, the exophytic part sloughs. Eventually, the central part of the base also sloughs, leaving a crater. Thus, what was originally an exophytic lesion may become an ulcerative crater.

To some physicians, this form suggests a compact, more contained, perhaps more indolent lesion. Clinical behavior does not however, support such an assumption.

The crater, especially when it is within the endocervical canal, causes a problem in intracavitary radium dosimetry. As with the exophytic type, the radium action is weakened because its energy is dissipated by the added distance to the neoplastic cells. The inability to apply the radium intimate to the base of the lesion lessens its power; thus one must prepare the endocervical crater by giving x-ray therapy before the radium application. Preradium x-ray therapy shrinks the tumor, making it possible to bring the intrauterine tandems closer to the neoplasm.

The Endocervical Type

Because squamous cell carcinomas develop inside the external os and remain hidden there, the cancers are usually large when found, they differ from the endophytic type which spreads to the endocervix by characteristic infiltrating growth.

Endocervical lesions penetrate deeply into the vascular levels of the cervix and the lower uterine segment of the uterus, and metastases to the lymph nodes on the pelvic wall and periaortic region are common. Severe hemorrhage may plague the course of irradiation because arteries of larger diameter are reached in the depths of the cervical stroma.

Endocervical lesions may become bulky; the population of cancer cells seeking nourishment strains the vasculature supplying the lesion, causing some cells to survive in a hypoxic state. These cancer cells are more resistant to irradiation, making it difficult to obtain total destruction of the cancer by irradiation alone.

The Surface Lesion (Plaque)

If the neoplastic conversion of squamous epithelium develops over a broad area of the cervical portio and contiguous vaginal mucosa, there may be invasion of the underlying tissue, although not as deeply as in other forms of cervical cancer primary lesions.

The plaque type of lesion may be favorable for the invasion into deeper vascular channels that may not have been reached. Although the total population of neoplastic cells may be large, they extend over a broad base and are less thick. These conditions are more favorable for a short-range course of radium treatment. The lesion may be very radiosensitive, since the blood supply is good and the oxygenation favorable for cancerocidal action of the ionizing energy.

One might suspect that these patients would have more late recurrences, since they develop new carcinomas in a new location of the vaginal mucosa; the wide area of cancer genesis makes the uninvolved vaginal mucosa especially susceptible for the development of other neoplastic lesions. Such patients should be marked for high risk and and observed carefully for 10 years or more after irradiation for a new cancer site within the vagina. If the amount of vaginal involvement is fairly widespread, it should influence the physician against using radical hysterectomy as the primary treatment because shortening of the vagina will be severe.

The clinical terms discussed here are used frequently to document anatomic conditions. They are stressed in individualized treatment plans, and although we appreciate the limitations of accuracy in forecasting success, words are conserved by their use. The terms supply a picture of the primary site and are often used as a framework for schematic presentations of treatment policies; thus there is justification for perpetuating what may be criticized as nonspecific terminology.

Features of Management

In discussing the management of cancer of the cervix, I have separated Stage I and

Stage II carcinomas from the more advanced lesions because in these stages there is an opportunity to choose between irradiation and surgery as primary treatment. Stages I and II carcinoma of the cervix may be treated successfully by: (1) radical hysterectomy, (2) radium and x-ray therapy, and (3) irradiation followed by operation. To decide the most appropriate method of therapy for the individual patient, the size of the primary lesion and the ease of performing the operation must be compared with the efficiency and suitability of applying radium. The preference for either radical hysterectomy or irradiation for a given patient will be influenced by the age and health of the patient, and any physical obstacles for the operation (e.g. obesity) that would be a much greater problem for treatment by radical hysterectomy than by irradiation therapy.

The availability of only one of these methods of treatment of patients should not be the deciding factor, for each patient should have access to either radical hysterectomy or irradiation therapy. If the chosen treatment is not available, the physician should refer the patient to the appropriate center for therapy. Unfortunately, the emphasis on radiotherapy or operation for cancer of the cervix still varies geographically. The reasons may be individual physician preference, but often local, practical, and economic factors are decisive. Many patients are still treated on the basis of available facilities, without sufficient regard for their true needs. Although these conditions are being rectified, we must still acquaint the family physician with the factors of the disease which determine correct management, so that he can refer the patient to a treatment center that will suit her needs.

RADICAL HYSTERECTOMY

The extended hysterectomy is an effective treatment for carcinoma of the cervix,

Stages I and II.[1,7,8,11] Its success has been defined and its limitations exposed by comparison with an able competitor for this role, irradiation therapy. That radical hysterectomy has survived as a complete treatment for this disease affirms some advantages over irradiation therapy, which are evident only when the operation is used properly.

Advantages

The advantages of the radical hysterectomy are (1) excision of the cervix and uterus prevents recurrence of disease in these organs, (2) the radioresistance factor is avoided, (3) the ovaries are not removed and continue to supply hormones, thus benefiting younger patients, (4) late irradiation complications of the bladder and rectum are avoided, (5) the treatment is less prolonged, (6) infected adnexa may be removed, and the hazards of irradiation of a chronic pelvic inflammatory disease avoided, (7) irradiation of normal organs is avoided, (8) surgical treatment is a more positive action, and the information obtained by laparotomy provides a more certain prognosis.

Indications

For the early stage carcinoma of the cervix, the cure rate will be as good with radical hysterectomy as with irradiation therapy. Radical hysterectomy is preferred for the young patient, since the ovarian function can be conserved and the pliability of the vaginal canal maintained. For selected patients in whom complications are rare, radical hysterectomy yields good results; however, the cancer must be small. With few exceptions, moderately advanced cervical cancer is better treated by irradiation. Other exceptional situations in which radical hysterectomy is preferred include (1) individuals with prior pelvic inflammatory disease, (2) patients in whom cancer obstructs the proper application of the radium system, (3) pregnant patients, where Cesarean section and radical hysterectomy offer an opportunity for delivery and removal of the cancer in a single operation, and (4) special histologic types of tumors which have a reputation for radioresistance. This last category is still open to controversy, and involves such problems as management of adenocarcinoma of the cervix.

Whether treatment for adenocarcinoma of the cervix should differ from that of squamous cell carcinoma is still unresolved. Our experience indicates that there is some dissimilarity in the site of origin and development, pattern of growth, frequency of local recurrence, and rate of dissemination of primary adenocarcinoma. We doubt, however, that there is any difference in radiosensitivity of the tumor cells per se. Therefore, primary surgical treatment for adenocarcinoma of the cervix is not routinely advocated.

Errors

The most frequent mistake in primary surgical treatment for carcinoma of the cervix is misapplication of the hysterectomy. The able surgeon may attempt to excise too advanced lesions, and by doing so may diminish the margin around the specimen. The resection is insufficient and fails to cure because recurrences appear. The uncertain surgeon resects too narrowly around even the earlier and smaller lesions, and also fails because the cancer recurs at the margin. In either situation, nothing is accomplished and much is lost because the patient's disease has now disseminated, and the opportunity for intracavitary radium is irretrievably lost. Unless the surgeon can encompass the cancer and provide a margin of normal tissue which is clinically negative at the periphery, the outcome will be poor. (Figure 4)

The cervical cancer which is suitable for treatment by radical hysterectomy must either be confined to the cervix or have only a minimal spread to the vagina in the immediate vicinity of the cervix. Lesions which extend a distance into the parametrium involve the ureter and the base of the bladder with cancer which cannot be resected by this operation. The physician who chooses the operation for cancer of the cervix in stages more advanced than Stages I and II must have a special reason. Proper selection of the stage of the cancer greatly determines the percentage of cure by radical hysterectomy; therefore, thorough preoperative study of the disease must not be neglected.

Disadvantages

1. Only selected patients with carcinoma of the cervix are suitable for extended surgical treatment.

2. This form of treatment is more hazardous, with a greater risk of death from an acute surgical complication.

3. The vagina is shortened.

4. Urinary and rectal fistulae are more frequent after extended surgical treatment than after irradiation therapy.

5. Bladder dysfunction is common. Chronic urinary retention or bothersome incontinence are often consequences of the true radical hysterectomy.

6. Frequently, postoperative x-ray therapy is necessary because metastases are discovered at operation.

Preoperative Study

After establishing the patient as a suitable operative risk, a basic search for metastases is made. An intravenous pyelogram (IVP) is essential for all but very early lesions. In patients with ureteral obstruction not otherwise explained by benign causes, the physician must assume that this is due to cancer which is unsuitable for resection by radical hysterectomy. The value of the lymphangiogram remains controversial. At our institu-

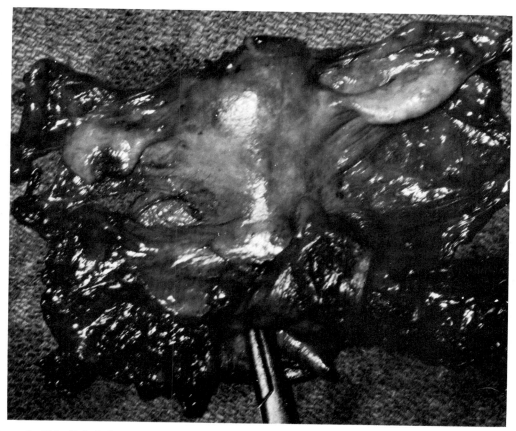

Figure 4 This clinical photograph of a specimen removed by radical hysterectomy shows the margins of tumor-free tissue excised around the cervix. Radical hysterectomy accomplishes this important requirement for all cancer operations: a margin of normal looking tissue in all directions around the primary lesion. This is only possible, when patients with small cervical cancers are selected for radical hysterectomy. Parson's doctrine stresses treatment of the primary lesion for unless this is done well the metastatic disease has no importance. This dictum is not in conflict, however, with the policy of individualized treatment of the cancer which does permit variations in the radicality of resection. Microinvasive carcinoma of the cervix have a minimal risk of metastasis and may be managed by less radical hysterectomy with obvious advantages. This excised specimen contained 3 cm of vagina. More could be excised, for after the ureters and bladder base have been freed from the cervix the length of vagina excised becomes optional.

tion, we have confidence in the study when signs of metastases are seen that clearly indicate the node is positive. Yet we realize that there are important nodes which are not opacified and, therefore, not assessed. The metastases must be a minimum size to be visible. We are aware that benign alterations may be misinterpreted, and positive nodes may not show. Thus only a portion of those patients examined are still the definitive answer. In preoperative evaluation, the lymphangiogram is a part of the basic evaluation of the patient with late Stages I and II carcinoma of the cervix. Chest x-rays and lymphangiograms provide a view of those bones most prone to metastasis, therefore, a bone survey for metastasis is not a routine procedure.

LAPAROTOMY

Preliminaries to Reaction

The surgeon cannot omit checking the sites within the abdomen for metastasis before proceeding with the hysterectomy, although the preoperative evaluation indicates that the lesion is small and confined near the cervix. Failure to inspect the abdominal viscera, to palpate the paraaortic nodes, and to lavage the peritoneal cavity for cytologic study of free cells may result in inadequate treatment and leave the prognosis more uncertain. The surgeon should avoid premature dissections of the blood supply to the uterus, which commits the treatment to hysterectomy before the avascular spaces along the pelvic wall are explored and a search is made for extension of tumor that could make the radical hysterectomy unwise. Preliminary dissection in the region of the cervix where the base of the bladder and the rectum are attached should be checked to make sure that the lesion does not require an exenteration. The surgeon must remain alert to the discovery of cancer spread which could make removal of the uterus unfortunate. If cancer will remain around the bladder or rectum after radical hysterectomy, irradiation therapy should be reconsidered. Hysterectomy should then be omitted, since the uterus is essential as a receptacle for radium applications.

Technical Suggestions

Since lymphadenectomy is usually a part of the radical hysterectomy, the surgeon should perform this part of the procedure first. There are advantages in starting the operation with lymphadenectomy because information about the nodes and sites of metastases will be revealed early in the operation. Should an unfavorable cancer become evident by discovery of disseminated nodal metastasis, external therapy will be needed, and therefore the plan of treatment may be altered to favor irradiation of both the primary and the metastatic sites. A treatment plan can be changed even at laparotomy. The discovery of a large group of matted nodes should arouse suspicion that even the primary lesion may be larger than originally estimated. The surgeon should suspect that tissues surrounding the cervix are harboring subclinical metastases. This concern can be sufficient to consider termination of the operation, and irradiation therapy employing both intracavitary and external techniques can then be instituted without subjecting the patient to the side effects of both operation and irradiation. Unless there is an expectation of a definitive cure by operation, the risk of complications from radical hysterectomy and from subsequent irradiation is not justified.

COMPLICATIONS OF RADICAL HYSTERECTOMY AND LYMPHADENECTOMY

Lymphocyst

The gynecologic oncologist should be prepared for certain complications of radical hysterectomy that are caused by extensive dissection. Because there are many severed lymph vessels in the technique of pelvic lymphadenectomy, fluid-filled cysts usually develop postoperatively (Figure 5). These lymphocysts may form large masses and produce pain and blockage of the ureter by compression or angulation. The resulting threat to impaired renal function forces the surgeon to drain the lymphocysts, whereas the asymptomatic lymphocysts should be treated conservatively to await spontaneous resolution.

The surgeon must be aware of the threat of the lymphocysts and should ligate all identifiable lymphatic trunks leading to the dissection site. Suction evacuation of the

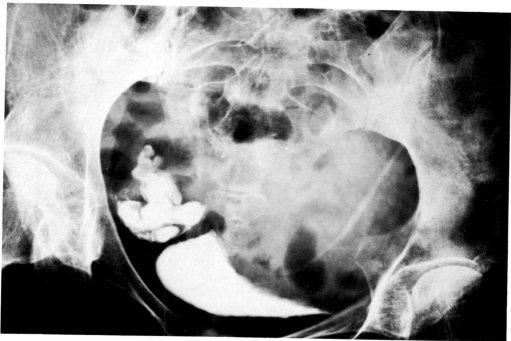

Figure 5 The average lymphocyst may be readily detected by bimanual examination. Some are too high to feel along the pelvic wall or above and may be evident only by their distortion of the colon, ureter, or by compression of large pelvic wall veins. Roentgenography will aid diagnosis. Intravenous pyelogram is probably the most useful and practical examination. The clinical importance of lymphocyst is determined by its size and position. Symptoms caused by lymphocyst (e. g., urinary frequency and constipation) are common because lymphocyst causes compression of the bladder and rectosigmoid. Edema of the external genitalia and lower extremities is common due to compression of the pelvic wall veins. Obstructive uropathy is the most serious complication and renal injury will follow unless obstruction is relieved. The condition of the ureter must be checked promptly when lymphocyst is discovered, since ureteral obstruction is a contraindication to conservative management of lymphocyst.

pelvic wall space for the first few days postoperatively has proved the most successful preventive measure. Tubes are placed at the termination of the operation into the retroperitoneal space and aspirated with a strong negative pressure as long as the drainage collects.

Fistulae

Within the boundaries resected by radical hysterectomy, some vessels to the ureter must be sacrificed. This diminished blood supply, combined with postoperative infection in the pelvis, with preoperative irradiation causes one of the more distressing complications of radical hysterectomy, the ureteral or the vesical fistula.[2] Preoperative irradiation impairs vascularity by occluding the smaller, more terminal arterioles, thus increasing the risk of fistulae from the ureter or the bladder through the vagina. In recent years, surgeons have become more aware of the blood supply to the ureter and its limited tolerance for dissection. Since the experience of Meigs,[8] they have sought to reduce the incidence of postoperative urinary fistulae and have been remarkably successful.

Stallworthy[15] has proved his theories for avoiding ureteral fistulae by successful clinical application, using a surgical technique by which the blood supply to the ureter is protected by preservation of mesial mesentery to the lower end of the ureter. Green and co-workers[5] advised splinting and supporting of the ureter to conserve its vasculature by attaching it to the superior vesicle artery. Symmonds and Pratt have suggested that more effective drainage of the dissection site will reduce the incidence of pelvic infection.[16] Novak has transplanted the lower ureter into the peritoneal cavity to protect it from surrounding infection and perhaps to restore an improved blood supply.[9] These techniques employed by individual surgeons have generally lessened the threat of ureteral vaginal fistulae.

Urinary Retention

Micturition disturbances with urinary retention or incontinence are well known but little understood consequences of radical hysterectomy. Since the corrective operations are seldom done and no effective prevention is known, the topic receives little attention. However, patients suffer much disability because of the atonic dysfunctional bladder. They are susceptible to recurrent cystitis; and unless attention is paid to the prevention and treatment of cystitis and pyelitis, patients who have undergone a successful operation for cervical cancer will die early of renal failure. If the kidney escapes damage, the patient may still be very disturbed for a long time by a poorly functioning bladder. The incidence of this dysfunction is directly related to the radicality of the operation and occurs often when the dissection is of the Meig's type in extent. More recently, a cystometric study of the bladder following radical hysterectomy has explained some of the mechanisms of the dysfunction.[12] An atonic bladder with diminished sensation leads to urinary retention. Incomplete micturition ultimately creates a large amount of residual urine with overdistention of the bladder, and this is responsible for the symptoms of frequency or urgency and compounds the problem because bladder contractility is impaired further. Cystometric studies help guide the physician in postoperative care, and indicate when bladder tone has returned sufficiently to remove the catheter. Improved postoperative management of the atonic bladder offers promise for less chronic disability.

PREOPERATIVE IRRADIATION

Preoperative irradiation of the primary lesion before radical hysterectomy is established as effective treatment for selected patients and has been employed successfully in some medical centers for many years. Preoperative irradiation offers the following advantages (1) By first irradiating the cervix, a necrosing lesion can be cleansed, lessening the risk of postoperative infection, (2) The bulky cancerous lesion may regress by preoperative irradiation, creating more favorable conditions for the surgeon, (3) Perhaps even a tolerant, conservative dose of irradiation administered before operation reduces the ability of the neoplastic cells to produce a new growth if the dissection site is contaminated by tumor fragments. Indirectly, preoperative irradiation may make benign tissues less favorable for cells to implant, another way to impair the survival ability of the cancer cells so that implantation does not occur. The threat of implantation during operation is real and is often a source of recurrence.

The distinction between preoperative irradiation followed by radical hysterectomy and combination therapy will be made clear in a subsequent chapter. The purpose of preoperative irradiation is to prepare the cancer for definitive treatment by excision. Although the dose alone is not enough for cure, a larger dose of irradiation within cancerocidal range followed by operation is combination therapy. Low-dose preoperative irradiation may add little to the incidence of complication in radical hysterectomy, whereas the more cancerocidal dose used for combination therapy seriously restrains the radicality of subsequent operation. A serious error can be made by the surgeon who chooses to perform a radical hysterectomy after high-dose irradiation. This applies to dosage delivered by radium and/or x-ray therapy. The postoperative complications are intolerable: frequent sloughing of tissues within the dissection site start quickly; infection gains an advantage; breakdown of the ureters, bladder, or rectum pours urine and feces into the degenerating sloughing region and compounds the problem of care, and the patient is miserable.

RADICALITY OF HYSTERECTOMY

A variety of operations may be termed radical hysterectomy, or Wertheim's operation. Variation in the radicality of the hysterectomy for different cancers of the cervix is useful because the treatment by operation should be an individualized plan based on the size of the cancer and whether this is primary treatment or treatment for recurrence (Figure 6). It is also necessary to consider whether allowance should be made in the radicality for the effects of preoperative irradiation that may be given. Radicality suggests the distance the surgeon extends the resection away from the cervix, and involves such factors as the nearness to the pelvic wall in which the parametrium is divided, the length of the upper vagina removed, the amount of mobilization of the ureter from its bed, and the sacrifice of ureteral vasculature. Early lesions may be cured with a less radical resection that would be inadequate for more advanced and complex problems.

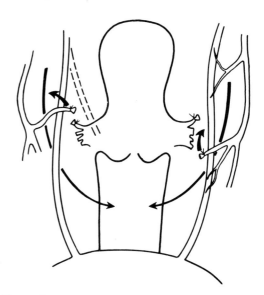

Figure 6 The line for excision for radical hysterectomy (Type III) may extend along the sides of the pelvic wall and to the midvagina (long curved arrows). The shorter arrows indicate the direction for retracting the mobilized ureters to accomplish this resection. There is less vagina excised and less mobilization of the ureters when resection is more conservative (Type II).

SURGICAL MANAGEMENT: SUMMARY

There are many difficulties that confront the surgeon who assumes the responsibility for curing a patient of cervical cancer by radical hysterectomy, and the number of possible errors introduced may seem discouraging. Radical hysterectomy is, however, a very valuable treatment method in gynecologic oncology, and its safety has been improved by recent experiences. The operation may become even more useful as current detection methods encourage young patients with smaller cancers of the cervix to seek treatment.[14]

Technically, the operation appeals to the pelvic surgeon as an exciting challenge. A radical hysterectomy performed on an otherwise healthy young woman whose cancer is confined to the cervix and whose postoperative course is uneventful is a rewarding experience for both the physician and the patient. The patient is rid of her disease and recovers sooner than if treatment were by irradiation. The ovaries continue to function and the vaginal membrane is unaltered.

Surgical intervention is the most decisive means of eradicating cervical cancer, whereas radiotherapy has a wider range of effective application. If a malignant tumor can be removed entirely with a margin of normal tissue, then obviously it cannot recur. In radiotherapy, there is a chance that viable cancer will remain. Operation insures control of the primary growth for only those patients whose lesions are small enough to be encompassed along with an extra margin of normal tissue. Both the physician and the patient feel more secure if the site of the disease is excised and the pathological specimen indicates that the boundaries are free of cancer cells.

IRRADIATION THERAPY

In general, we consider radiotherapy to be the preferred treatment for Stages I and II cervical cancer, although we recognize that extended hysterectomy may be used successfully for the young patient for whom preservation of the ovaries is desirable. Carefully applied intracavitary radium remains the most useful tool in irradiation treatment for Stages I and II cervical carcinoma because it delivers the greatest dose of irradiation to the developing cancer and, at the same time, spares the more radiosensitive rectum and bladder because of its limited range of penetration. The primary lesion can be controlled with radium in all but the more advanced Stage II lesions if the uterus is of normal depth and the vagina provides room for the larger radium holders. Since destruction of metastasis is necessary to control the disease,

almost all patients receive both radium and external irradiation.

RADIUM

The range for effective treatment from intracavitary radium is limited to a volume of tissue around the cervix that will encompass a moderate-sized primary lesion (Figure 7). Thus (1) late Stage I, II, or III disease cannot be effectively treated with radium alone, and a greater portion of the treatment for the late stage cancers must be external therapy, (2) metastasis to the parametrium and pelvic wall nodes will not receive an adequate dose of irradiation from the radium system alone, (3) the radium must be placed into the cancer close to the base of the tumor, otherwise the distance will lower the dose to an inadequate level, (4) the center of the primary lesion commonly receives 20,000 to 30,000 rads when radium is employed, and this is sufficient to destroy both normal and neoplastic tissue.

Table 1 Survival Rates of Squamous Cell Carcinoma on Intact Uterus: 1,705 Patients, September 1954–December 1967[a, b]

Stage	Five-Year Survival Rate[c] (MeV %)	Ten-Year Survival Rate[c] (MeV %)
I	91.5	90.0
IIA	83.5	79.0
IIB	66.5	57.0
IIIA	45.0	39.5
IIIB	36.0	30.0
IV	14.0	14.0

[a] Reprinted, with permission, from reference 4.
[b] Includes patients treated incompletely or for palliation.
[c] Modified life table. Patients dying from intercurrent disease are excluded.

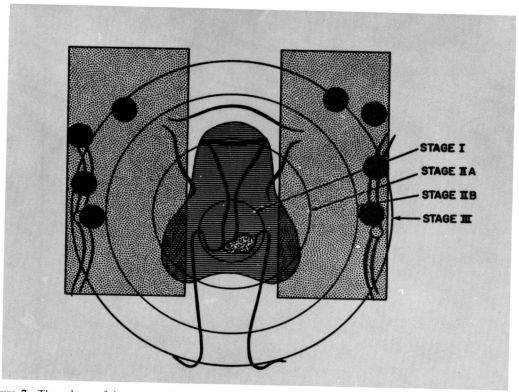

Figure 7 The volume of tissue around a cancer of the cervix that can be delivered a cancerocidal dose of irradiation when the anatomy is ideal is illustrated by the pear-shaped figure in the center. The fields for parametrial external therapy cover the pathway for metastases to pelvic wall lymph nodes (dark round spots).

This high dose is tolerated because the thick-walled uterus separates the radium from the surrounding normal tissue. Local destruction occurs in the cervix which heals with fibrosis. Being in the cervix, the dense fibrosis which develops with healing of the irradiation effects is tolerated, although the entry to the uterus is sealed. Since the endometrium is destroyed by radium, hematometra does not occur. This scarring must not extend into the bladder or rectum. This high dose will only be safe when the radium applicators are properly applied and maintained during the application time. Misapplication or displacement of the system may produce a slough of the vagina with ulceration and fistula in the bladder or rectum.

Although the central area receives the greatest intensity in dosage of irradiation, the level diminishes at the periphery of a moderate-sized cancer; still, a dose from 6000 to 7000 rads from a good radium system can be delivered to the periphery; and (5) radium is not immediately appropriate for all cancerous lesions of the cervix; but may be made suitable with preradium x-ray therapy.

Radium Dosimetry

Although the rapid diminution of irradiation intensity as it emanates from the radium may be advantageous for protecting the normal tissues around the carcinomatous

Table 2 Squamous Cell Carcinoma of the Cervix, Maxima for Combining Whole Pelvis Irradiation and Intracavitary Radium Therapy[a]

Stage	Whole Pelvis	Maximum Hours[b]	Maximum mg/hr[b,c]	Parametrial (rads)
1 < 1 cm		72—2 wk—72	10,000	
1 > 1 cm		72—2 wk—72	10,000	3000–4000
and	2000	48—2 wk—72[d]	9000	1000–2000
IIA	4000	48—2 wk—48	6500	
IIB[e]	4000	48—2 wk—48	6500	
IIIA	4000	48—2 wk—48	6500	1000–1500 on side in-volved
	5000	72[f] or	5000	Possibly 1000 on side involved
		48—2 wk—24–48[d]		
IIIB and	6000	72[f]	4000	
IV	7000			

[a] Reprinted, with permission, from reference 4.

[b] Used whichever maximum occurs first, either the time or the mg/hr.

[c] May be exceeded for unusual tumor size; then three insertions, each two weeks apart, are used.

[d] May use the longer time first, if the vault size does not permit two colpostats for the second application.

[e] Whole pelvis irradiation may be carried to 5000 rads if regression is slow.

[f] If indicated by the status of central disease, the time may be increased beyond 72 hr or above 5000 mg/hr, then split into 48—2 weeks—24 to 48 hr.

Note: A tandem with a protruding source and a 3 cm diameter vaginal cylinder should have a 20 mg source in the cylinder with 1½ sources protruding (e.g., 15, 10, and 20 mg, or 15, 10, 10, and 20 mg).

uterus and upper vagina, because of this limited range there can be no error in correctly locating the radium application. For patients with deformity of the vaginal axis and deviation of the uterus due to cancer, modification must be made for the standard inverted "T" arrangement of radium sources in the uterus and upper vagina. Sometimes the vaginal ovoids must be placed in staggered relationship to each other. The narrowed vagina with small fornices does not accommodate ovoids large enough to be advantageous over a straight line placement of the uterine and vaginal radium. Isodose distribution patterns should be employed for each patient to chart the range of effective dose to the primary lesion and to the regional pelvic wall nodes. Areas of excessive and inadequate treatment must be detected early and corrected either by changes in loading or postradium x-ray therapy given to supplement dosage to the deficient site.

Radium Applicators

The radium holders must provide a range of length and diameter to allow flexibility in associating the components, thus permitting them to be placed advantageously for the varied shapes and growth patterns of cancer. The system must allow loading after the patient has returned to her room. This after-loading eliminates exposure of the surgical team, technicians, and nurses, and haste during application to lessen irradiation exposure is unnecessary. Full care can be given to the placement and, after a satisfactory application is confirmed, the intensity of the radium sources can be decided while viewing the localization films.

THE PHYSICS OF APPLIED RADIUM

The physical principles necessary for maximum range of irradiation with intracavitary radium are:

1. Use of the longest tandem source possible within the uterus to expand the dosage contribution for the paracervical area.

2. Expansion of the vaginal radium sources as widely as possible to place radium near the regional pelvic lymph nodes.

3. Support of the radium applicators upward, high into the pelvic axis, by careful full packing of the vagina with gauze. Thus the ionizing energy is nearer to the pelvic wall nodes most commonly affected by metastasis and further away from the bladder and the rectum.

4. Certainty that the design of the radium applicator takes advantage of the inverse square law of irradiation physics by providing maximum distance between the radium sources and the vaginal mucosa. This reduces the risk of slough from excessive dose and produces a good functional result within the upper vagina without compromising the depth dose of irradiation to the paracervical and paravaginal tissues.

5. Provision of some shielding in the applicators to bladder and rectum.

6. Adjustment of the intensity and distribution of the sources of radium within the system to eliminate zones of excessive or inadequate dose.

7. Adjustment of the overall plan when the vagina is narrow, the uterine canal is short, or an exophytic growth is present on the cervix to deliver more external irradiation to the cervical region.

EXTERNAL THERAPY

The principles for use of external irradiation are:

1. When the stage is an earlier, small lesion, a good radium system is available and the dosage is adequate to the central part of the cancer, external irradiation is confined to the parametrium and lateral pelvic walls (8000 to 10,000 mg/hr of intracavitary radium, and 3500 to 4000 rads to the parametrium).

2. When adequate radium treatment is not possible, although the lesion is not large, some supplementary external irradiation is given to the primary site (first 2000 to 4000 rads x-ray therapy to the whole pelvic region followed by 8000 mg/hr of intracavitary radium, then by additional x-ray therapy to the lateral areas of the pelvic region for a dosage of 3000 to 4000 rads to the parametrium).

3. For late stage cancer of the cervix, external x-irradiation to the whole pelvic region is the majority treatment (4000 to 5000 rads of whole pelvis x-irradiation plus 4500 to 5500 mg/hr of radium are standard dosage levels). The amount of intracavitary radium has been reduced correspondingly as the dose of whole pelvis x-irradiation is increased.

It is the duty of the gynecologic oncologist to study the shape of the tumor and its growth pattern; if a portion of the tumor causes an obstacle to placing the radium system in proper proximity to the dominant portion of the lesion, some preparatory x-ray is necessary. Clinical experience indicates that there is often an obstacle to immediate application of radium for patients with late Stage I and II disease, and many of these patients should have preradium x-ray therapy.

PRERADIUM X-RAY THERAPY

External therapy in doses of 2000 to 4000 rads given first to the whole pelvis will destroy the forward portion of an exophytic cancer protruding into the vagina. Such lesions fill the upper vagina and obstruct application of radium because the tumor occupies the space needed for the radium applicator. The same dose of external x-irradiation can also be used for problems caused by endocervical excavations by cancer and for large bulky endocervical tumors because preradium x-ray therapy will regress the tumor within the cervical canal and open the obstruction to the insertion of a radium application while constricting the diameter of the cervical lesion. The reduction brings the periphery of the tumor within the improved range of the radium.

PRERADIUM TRANSVAGINAL X-RAY THERAPY

Another very useful technique for the preparation of exophytic lesions for radium application is transvaginal x-ray therapy. Fewer patients are suitable for transvaginal irradiation than for external therapy because the vagina needs to be large enough (4 cm or more in diameter) to accommodate the tube-type cone from the x-ray machine. Often, in the elderly patient, the vagina will not dilate sufficiently at the introitus. (Figure 8) The advantage of transvaginal irradiation therapy over external therapy is its tolerance. Most of the irradiation given by the transvaginal route is absorbed in the tumor. There is little side scatter to the bladder and rectum. The bowel behind the cervix is most vulnerable. Rapid and intense doses can be built up in the tumor by transvaginal x-ray therapy in less than a week of treatment. Daily treatment of 500 rads each allows a total of 1500 to 2000 rads within a week. This method is successful when the tumor is hemorrhaging. Transvaginal therapy stops bleeding while preparing the tumor for continued treatment. The lateral boundaries of the isodose dosage curves are sharp, so that very little treatment is delivered to the paracervical tissues or along the lateral vaginal walls of the vagina. The ionizing effects are forward, to

lessen irradiation of the intestines behind the cervix, low voltage x-ray machines are used.

WHOLE PELVIS X-RAY

Irradiation directed to the pelvis produces changes in all tissues, and the effects on the neoplastic and the normal tissues depend on a small difference in susceptibility of the cancer cells. The level from the surface where the maximum changes are induced, however, is governed by the type of machine. Currently, only megavoltage machines are used to irradiate the deeper pelvic structures. A minimum-intensity MeV x-ray machine, such as the Cobalt-60, delivers a dose of up to 4000 rads to the pelvis. Above this dosage, subcutaneous tissue fibrosis becomes severe. Other equipment, such as the betatron or the linear accelerator, is preferred when a dose to the pelvis in the range of 5000 to 6000 rads is needed.

PORTALS (FIELDS)

There is a variety of personal preference for portal sizes and shapes among radiotherapists for treatment of the pelvic area (Figure 9).

1. Usually the portal is designed to cover the assessment of cancer obtained by physical examination and the likelihood of the pathway for spread.

2. Unnecessary irradiation is avoided by reducing the x-ray field to just the essential tissues.

3. The portal of x-irradiation must consider the contribution of irradiation from the intracavitary radium to the total dosage for the bladder, bowel, and vagina. To avoid excessive dosage, these tissues may be shielded during part of the external therapy. Since the contribution from radium is central in the pelvis, a 4 cm block of lead is

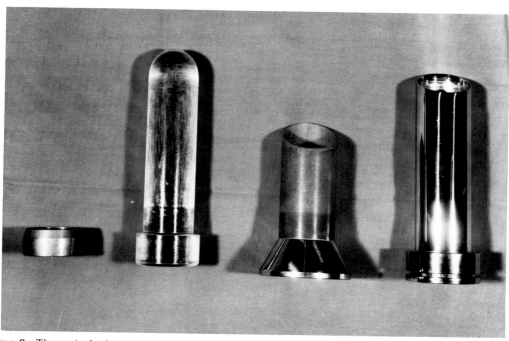

Figure 8 The vaginal adaptors for transvaginal x-ray therapy confine treatment to the upper vagina. Much of the dosage is absorbed in the cervix, which makes this method promptly effective to regress exophytic tumors and to stop hemmorhage. Transvaginal x-ray is especially useful for carcinoma of the cervical stump. Where opportunities for radium application are limited by the short canal, small cancers of the vagina are suited for transvaginal x-ray therapy.

interposed over the middle of the portal. Thus the external therapy field may cover the remaining pelvis, being excluded from the midline area.

4. The irradiation field need not be isometric, nor the dosage equal. The pelvic side where most of the known cancer is located may be emphasized. Such decisions are determined by pelvic examination, angiograms, or by a finding at preirradiation laparotomy. For example, 1000 rads more may be delivered to a side of the pelvis known to have metastasis in comparison to the opposite side which seems negative.

5. Eccentric contributions from the intracavitary radium created when the cancer distorts the position of the uterus may be balanced by additional x-ray therapy to the deficient side.

6. The lower boundary of the external therapy field is determined by the lowest level of palpable cancer. This may be represented by the cancer growth extending either into or along the vaginal wall or down the pelvic wall. This level is determined by pelvic examination, and is marked with radiopaque material to confirm adequate coverage by the treatment portal with localization x-rays.

7. The upper limit to which the external field extends usually reaches the pelvic brim or L-5. Evidence of metastasis above this level, determined by preradium laparotomy or lymphography, may warrant a higher level for external therapy. Routinely, the irradiation is designed to include all the external iliac nodes, the mid or lower common iliac nodes, the principal iliac nodes,

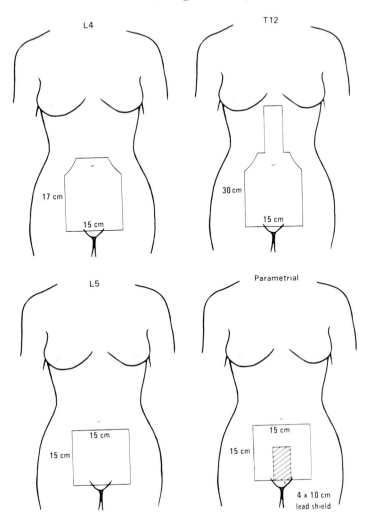

Figure 9   The conventional portals for external therapy to the pelvic region: the area covered by whole pelvis field (lower left), and a screen for the central region of the pelvis, for the patient who has had a high dose of irradiation from intracavitary radium. The upper diagrams show portals used when lymph node metastases are proven.

hypogastric nodes, and the internal iliac nodes. The upper common iliac and aortic nodes may be added by larger than standard fields when there is evidence that metastasis has reached this height.

In general, for Stages I and II cancer of the cervix, irradiation of the pelvic region with external therapy is planned either as a preliminary to radium or to augment the

contribution of intracavitary radium. If the lesion is especially large, a greater portion of the total irradiation will be by external therapy.

TREATMENT RATE

The time span during which a given dose is delivered is a factor that influences tolerance in the pelvic tissue. Protraction of therapy over a longer period of time has radiobiologic purposes.

Multiple fractions of a given dose extending over three, four, or five weeks is preferred to rapid, intensive external therapy. Protraction improves the oxygenation of a large, bulky tumor by bringing about regression of its general size and improvement in its vascularity. Dose fractionation also allows neoplastic cells to cycle into a more irradiation-sensitive phase. In addition, fractionation permits normal cells in the irradiated field to recover between treatments, thus lessening the side effects from complications.

WHOLE PELVIS PRERADIUM DOSAGE

Standard irradiation for Stage IIB lesions of the cervix is 4000 rads whole pelvis therapy. When high-dosage whole pelvis irradiation is given, reduction in the duration of radium treatment becomes necessary. Large, bulky primary lesions require a larger, more cancerocidal dose to the whole pelvis because the lateral spread into the parametrium is beyond the range of intracavitary radium. If positive pelvic wall nodes are present, an additional dose in the range of 5000 rads is necesary.

PARAMETRIAL PRERADIUM DOSAGE

Even when a good system of intrauterine radium is permitted by local anatomy, a smaller tumor mass, and a vaginal vault adequate to allow larger ovoids with separation, the radium dose to the parametrium and pelvic wall tissues is still not cancerocidal for all nodes usually involved. Thus in even the better radium systems, an additional 3000 rads of external therapy is given to the parametrium to augment the dosage from intracavitary radium.

REFERENCES

1. Averette, H. E., D. R. LaPlatney, and W. A. Little, *Am. J. Obstet. Gynecol.*, **105**, 79–89 (1969).
2. Calame, Richard J., and James H. Nelson, *Arch Surg.* **94**, 87, (1967).
3. Dodd, Gerald D., Felix Rutledge, and Sidney Wallace, *Am. J. Roentgenol., Radiat. Ther., & Nucl. Med.*, **108**, 312–323 (1970).
4. Fletcher, G. H., and F. N. Rutledge, *Modern Radiotherapy: Gynaecological Cancer*, Butterworths, London, 1971.
5. Green, T. H., J. V. Meigs, H. Ulfelder, and R. R. Curtin, *Am. J. Obstet. Gynecol.*, **20**, 293–312 (1962).
6. Hsu, Chien-Tien, and Yung Sheng Cheng, *Am. J. Obstet. Gynecol.*, **111**, 391–397 (1971).
7. Kazumasa, Masubuchi, Yoshio Tenjin, Hisamitsu Kubo, and Mitsuo Kimura, *Am. J. Obstet. Gynecol.*, **103**, 567–573 (1969).
8. Meigs, J. V., *Am. J. Obstet. Gynecol.*, **49**, 542 (1945).
9. Novak, F., *Am. J. Obstet. Gynecol.*, **72**, 506–510 (1956).
10. Novak, Franc, *Int. J. Gynecol. Obstet.*, **7**, 301–305 (1969).
11. Park, R. C., W. E. Patow, and R. E. Roger, *Obstet. Gynecol.*, **41**, 117–122 (1973).
12. Roman-Lopez, Juan J., and David L. Barclay, *Am. J. Obstet. Gynecol.*, **115**, 81–89 (1973).
13. Rutledge, F., *Prog. Gynecol.* **4**, 619–636 (1963).
14. Rutledge, F.: In *Controversy in Obstetrics and Gynecology*, Duncan E. Reid and T. C. Barton, Eds., Philadelphia, Pennsylvania, (1969).
15. Stallworthy, John, *Ann. R. Coll. Surg. Engl.*, **34**, 161–178 (1964).
16. Symmonds R. E., and J. H. Pratt, *Obstet. Gynecol.*, **17**, 57–64 (1961).

CHAPTER 4

MANAGEMENT: STAGES III AND IV
CARCINOMA OF THE CERVIX

FELIX RUTLEDGE, M.D.

The topic of treatment for carcinoma of the cervix has been separated into two parts, Stages I and II together and then Stages III and IV, because management involves different types of operations and different sources and methods of irradiation. A discussion of treatment by surgery for Stages I and II involves radical hysterectomy; treatment by irradiation deals with intracavitary radium predominately. For Stages III and IV, treatment by surgery concerns pelvic exenteration and by irradiation, external x-ray therapy (Figure 1).

TREATMENT FACTORS

The treatment of patients with advanced cancer of the cervix is complex and hazardous. External therapy is responsible for the majority of cures and is more applicable than radical operation. More patients are physically able to tolerate irradiation treatment. Also, external therapy can encompass metastases which cannot be excised. Yet there is a role for extended surgery when the conditions are complicated by pelvic diseases which interfere with irradiation effectiveness, such as pelvic infections, adnexal masses, ureteral obstruction, ulcerative colitis, acute diverticulitis, or prior irradiation to the pelvic area. Another indication for surgery is failure of the tumor to regress during irradiation. Such an assessment of

radioresistance cannot be made, however, without first giving high-dose irradiation to a large area of the pelvic viscera. This in turn is a contraindication to radical hysterectomy, and suggests exenteration as the operation of choice.

Special reasons are needed to justify the selection of surgery as the primary treatment for Stages III and IV carcinoma of the cervix, since the cure rate by irradiation is competitive and irradiation is better tolerated by the patient. There is a strong argument for pelvic exenteration for Stage IV carcinoma of the cervix with metastasis to the bladder or rectum without more distant spread (Figure 2). Yet these conditions are not an absolute indication for exenteration because irradiation, mainly external therapy, may cure such metastases while preserving bladder function. As the cancer becomes more advanced, the surgeon has fewer opportunities to excise the lesion totally without sacrifice of urinary, bowel, or sexual function. Still, the surgeon has an important role in caring for these patients even though he may be excluded from the primary treatment. Radiotherapy would not be successful without the contribution of the pelvic surgeon. To discover this role, the surgeon must first learn irradiation management of these advanced diseases.

We will emphasize external therapy, since intracavitary radium alone cannot encom-

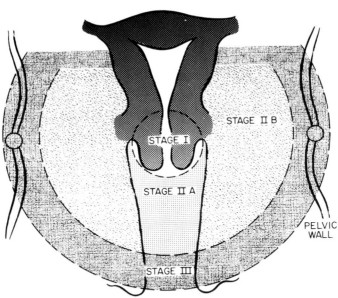

Figure 1   Some factors of FIGO system staging portrayed schematically to show the relationship of the cervix to neighboring structures which have been chosen as landmarks for their extent of spread and amount of metastasis. In addition to its primary purpose and function, staging aids in prognosis. It may also imply the complexity of the treatment. Sometimes a routine for management can be tied to staging. Many factors which influence treatment selection and plans can be related to staging. For example, cancer which is fixed by metastasis to the pelvic wall is not suitable for resection; that which spreads to the lower vagina is also less resectable because the bladder and rectum are proximally involved. The FIGO system has limitations and is incomplete for depicting all the clinical features of cancer. Within Stage I with cancer confined to the cervix there is a large size range, and substaging into IA and IB is advised. Localized cancer that does not extend and grows large may be difficult to sterilize with irradiation alone but might be resectable. Cancer confined to the cervix (a Stage I lesion) could be small and favorable, or the cervix and lower corpus replaced and enlarged by cancer with a graver prognosis. Deficiencies in Stage II cancers also represent a large parametrial and vaginal spread, a small extension from the cervix or throughout the parametrium just short of the pelvic wall. Unfortunately, there is no anatomical midpoint to subdivide the parametrium into inner and outer divisions. Thus it is not feasible to represent these findings as Stage IIA or IIB. Also, the cervix is not always in the middle. Often the uterus is pulled or pushed by disease nearer to one pelvic wall.

pass the total disease in advanced cervical cancer. Although both external therapy and intracavitary radium are used, that portion given by intracavitary radium is less than for Stages I and II of the disease. The dose of radium must be restrained to protect the normal tissues of the vagina, bladder, and rectum, because x-rays contribute their own injurious side effects. Therefore, in Stage III we are more concerned with external therapy and will adjust the radium dose to the preceding x-ray dose, which is the re-

verse of the management procedures for Stage I and II lesions.

When expressing the cancerocidal dose and also the injurious effects of x-ray treatment, three factors should be noted for accuracy. We must always know the tumor dose given to a specific volume of tissue and how rapidly it was administered. Without this information, the dosage has little meaning. The dose should also express the anatomic point selected for its calculation, or the depth to which the dosage refers. In

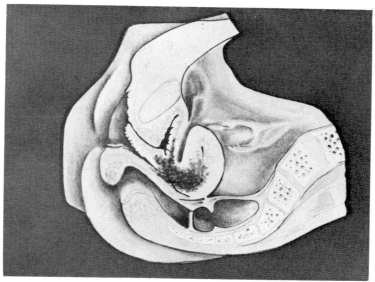

Figure 2 Cervical cancer is more prone to extend forward into the bladder than backward toward the rectum, and this condition often influences selection of anterior exenteration for treatment. This type, Stage IV carcinoma of the cervix, has a more favorable prognosis than most Stage IV cancers with distant metastasis that are not suitable for resection. The treatment problem is illustrated schematically to show the relatively compact distribution of Stage IV carcinoma of the cervix. If confined within the area included in whole pelvis x-ray therapy, with much of the cancer close enough to the uterus to be affected by intracavitary radium some Stage IV cervix cancers are curable without operation. Successful irradiation therapy shows reasonable prospects for success unless the disease is massive. Where there is a large cancer cell population although the tumor is still local, irradiation therapy may not completely sterilize the tumor and excision would ultimately be required. Anterior exenteration was designed for such a treatment problem. It has proved effective and is an acceptable and recommended treatment for patients with Stage IV disease due mainly to bladder invasion. Loss of bladder function is necessary handicap for the anterior exenteration operation. If the odds for a cure are good, the urinary conduit is a tolerable price to pay. Loss of much of the vagina is an additional sacrifice by the patient who undergoes anterior exenteration. This defect may be remedied if vaginal reconstruction is part of the planned management, that is, if provisions are made for maintaining a cavity for the vagina that can be developed from a skin graft after recovery from the exenteration procedure.

the new era of megavoltage therapy, measurements expressed as dose in air and skin dose are replaced by more specific tumor dose expressions; for gynecologists this means the amount of irradiation at depth in the pelvis. In Stages III and IV carcinoma of the cervix, we deal with the dose to the uterus, vagina, parametrium, and pelvic walls because all of these structures probably contain cancer. Generally, the cancerocidal dose will exceed 5000 rads given in approximately five weeks. A smaller percentage of patients with more radiosensitive

cancers can be treated with a lower dose, but we cannot identify these patients before therapy and they must, therefore, be treated as a group to an arbitrary but clinically established cancerocidal dose.

STANDARD EXTERNAL PORTALS

The area to be treated could be specifically calculated for each individual if only the palpable cancer were considered, but each patient with a large, palpable primary mass is also threatened by subclinical metastatic cancer. The cancer composed of the primary and its metastasis must be assumed to be larger than can be estimated by examination; therefore, we cannot safely direct the beam to the obvious cancer alone. (Figure 3) For example, although the spread pattern may seem to be on one side of the pelvis, the opposite more normal side to palpation must also receive a cancerocidal dose. Where the spread is asymmetrical, the parametrium with thick infiltration may warrant additional treatment to deliver a larger than standard dose.

External therapy to the pelvic region is directed to cover the primary, its obvious extensions, and the tissues in the pathway of metastasis. Thus, a basic or routine zone has been established for treatment for all patients with late stage cancer of the cervix. An augmented dose may be fitted to an individual on the basis of clinical examination.

Since one-third to one-half of patients will have lymphatic metastasis, the regional nodes must be treated routinely, although the risk of irradiation injury to the terminal ileum and sigmoid colon is increased. Lacking a reliable test to implicate metastasis in lymph nodes, a more precise direction for external therapy is prohibited. Although the individual cancer will somewhat modify the shape of the field used for standard treatment, it usually does so by expansion of the routine field rather than by diminishing it. This routine field of whole pelvis irradiation purposefully covers the uterus, much of the vagina, and the pelvic wall nodes. Unavoidably the bladder, rectosigmoid, and small intestine are also irradiated.

The radiotherapist may exercise some personal preference in the rate at which external therapy is given. Among criteria to be considered are: known radiobiological principles, local conditions, practical aspects of the work load, output of the x-ray ma-

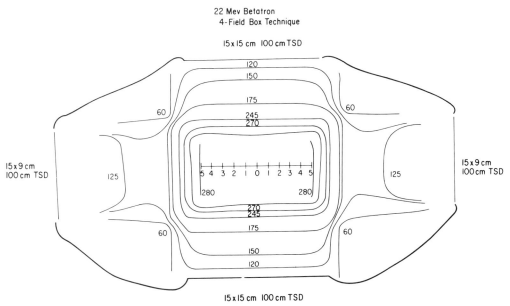

Figure 3   Whole pelvis irradiation. The portals for anterior and posterior irradiation measure 15 × 15 cm, the laterals 15 × 9 cm. The 15 × 15 cm size covers the pelvic wall nodes which become positive first. The lateral fields augment the dose, sparing of the subcutaneous tissues of the abdomen and the back. The various curves indicate the percentage dose at the respective level.

chine and, mainly, the patient's ability to tolerate x-ray therapy. Acute intolerance (nausea, vomiting, diarrhea, cystitis, malaise, and anemia) and the chronic consequent complications in the bowel, bladder, and vagina (e.g., hemorrhagic colitis, cystitis, vault necrosis, fistulae, and stenosis) are definitely influenced by the rapidity with which irradiation is administered. The side effects of external therapy are related to the rapidity of treatment in that a large total dose may be better tolerated if delivered over a longer period of time, although the cancerocidal effects may be correspondingly diminished. The common dose rate of x-ray therapy to a large field, such as whole pelvis irradiation (15 × 15 cm), is 800 to 1000 rads/week, so that x-ray therapy for Stage III or IV cervical cancer is given for five to six weeks.

An area of current clinical investigation in radiotherapy is variation in the dose fraction that makes up the course. These variations range from treatment schemes of a large dose given in a short period of time, usually to patients who have incurable disease or who cannot tolerate treatment because of physical disability (treatment is thus designed as palliation), to schemes that provide protracted, multiple treatment over a period of two to three months, sometimes interrupted entirely for intervals. Generally however, radiotherapists wish to maintain a continuous treatment scheme for there is some cumulative cancerocidal action in not allowing the neoplastic cells enough time to repair injury.

For the gynecologic oncologist, some basic knowledge of the technical details of external therapy is essential, since he will often need to assess the treatment from other centers that practice unfamiliar schemes of therapy. Often he must evaluate the adequacy of patient treatment to determine whether there is sufficient reserve tolerance for more irradiation, and to judge the possible effects of prior irradiation therapy on contemplated operations for recurrent cancer.

TRANSVAGINAL X-RAY THERAPY

Transvaginal x-ray therapy cannot be used as effectively for Stages III and IV lesions as for earlier stage cervical cancers for several reasons:

1. The Stage III and IV cancers are too large to be encompassed by the restricted area of exposure possible with the transvaginal beam.

2. Spread of cancer along the vaginal wall frequently obstructs the insertion of the treatment cone through which the x-ray beam is directed into the vagina.

3. Transvaginal therapy is used mainly as a preliminary treatment to regress an exophytic lesion in preparation for radium application, and radium application is not the first form of treatment for stage III and IV cancers.

4. Transvaginal therapy is less effective in Stages III and IV as a method for stopping hemorrhage from the vaginal portion of the cancer, since open blood vessels are deeply located and more laterally placed.

The definition of Stage III carcinoma of the cervix includes a wide range of problems for external therapy. Spread of cancer from the cervix into one or more parametria to the pelvic wall, with or without spread down the vagina to the lower third, defines a wide range of cancer for external therapy. Within the definition of Stage III carcinoma of the cervix, the distribution, direction, extension, and bulkiness of the tumor vary among patients. Some patients require a more extensive area of treatment and a more intensive dose, while others within the same Stage III can be controlled by a safer portal size and dose level. The plan for irradiation is dictated by the clinician's assessment of the treatment problem and should not be decided automatically by the categorical stage; for example, all patients with Stage III cancer should not be subjected to the same high risk of serious injury if this risk is unnecesary. While qualifying as Stage III carcinoma of the cervix, the cancer may still be confined to a lesser total size. Conservatism in dosage for safety is possible. For other patients in whom the problem is more desperate the gynecologic oncologist must be bold in managing the disease, for only by radical management with a high dose and wide range of external therapy can patients with very advanced lesions be cured. The need for individualization of management continues into the more advanced stages of cervical cancer.

Field Size

The field size for whole pelvis irradiation at M.D. Anderson Hospital is 15 × 15 cm. This is a conservative size determined partly because it was the maximum feasible for the 22-MeV betatron, which we have employed since 1954 as the main source of external therapy, and also because this field is sufficient to cover both parametrial and vaginal extension for Stage III and IV carcinoma of the cervix. The regional lymph nodes most commonly involved are also treated. When large portals are needed, a different type of x-ray machine is required. For extended field therapy, the linear accelerator is preferred over the Cobalt-60 machine because the dose level for the Cobalt-60 must be limited near the 4000 rad level to avoid subcutaneous fibrosis. However, both machines provide a larger field than the 15 × 15 cm restriction of the betatron.

Current interest in treating node groups above the pelvic brim to the paraaortic region has stimulated the use of new and larger portals for external therapy. This extension has assumed various shapes. Recently we adopted a planned program to include metastasis above the pelvic brim in

irradiation therapy (Figure 4). The benefits and safety in this large treatment field must still be tested by clinical use. In the past although we have sporadically directed x-ray treatment to known positive nodes in this region around the aorta with encouraging results, an organized approach to include these nodes regularly when indicated by lymphography or pretreatment laparotomy is still being explored. Some catastrophic injury to the small and large bowels has already been observed in our treatment by this method. Since other workers may have similar experiences, caution is advised when treating patients with extended field therapy. This is mentioned as a preliminary announcement to general information because several radiotherapist centers are developing new plans to extend the field of irradiation to the paraaortic nodes as they are found positive, and this will probably be a topic of current investigative interest for discussion over the next few years.

New interest in extended field therapy to a higher level has been stimulated by several factors:

1. New higher energy megavoltage x-ray machines are now available.

2. Posttreatment laparotomy and lymphadenectomy findings have shown that irradiation therapy is fairly successful, but there is incomplete eradication of the cancer because the treatment fields are not high enough to cover all the positive nodes. Positive nodes have been sterilized just below the level of the treatment field and in the area treated, indicating radiosensitive cancers.

3. Studies of the sites where recurrences first appear have shown that the pelvic area remains free, but abdominal recurrences suggest that failure was attributable to the upper common iliac and lower aortic nodes containing metastases and not irradiated.

4. More frequent use of pretreatment lymphography has identified positive nodes which are outside the standard treatment

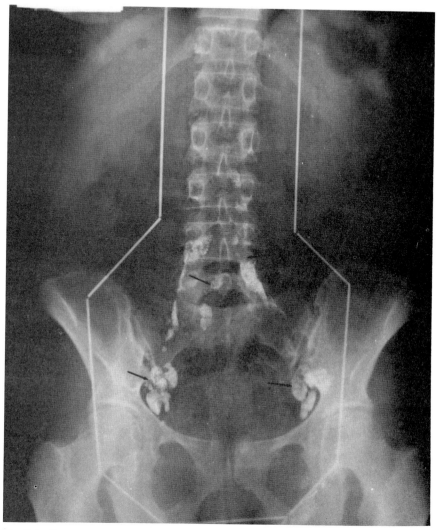

Figure 4   The light line represents the external therapy portal superimposed on a late-phase lymphangiogram. Roentgenographic shadows indicative of metastasis are shown in the positive nodes (arrows). Such evidence is currently confirmed by pretreatment laparotomy if extended field irradiation is contemplated. This operation may prove unnecessary where there is strong clinical and x-ray evidence of aortic node metastases.

area. Such patients, with a known increased risk for more distant spread, can be selected for extended field therapy (Figure 5). This may justify prescribing the more radical and possibly more hazardous external therapy.

Extended field irradiation is an effort to increase cure rates and is most appropriate for Stage III and IV cancers. Improvements are expected to be in small percentages.

Irradiation injury can nullify the salvage from cancer by adding deaths from complications.

INTRACAVITARY RADIUM

Inability to attain the desired application is a major reason that intracavitary radium

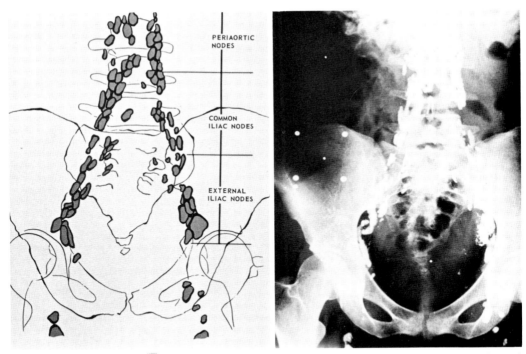

PERIAORTIC NODES

COMMON ILIAC NODES

EXTERNAL ILIAC NODES

Figure 5   Cancer of the cervix follows a pathway of spread up the chain of lymph nodes with predictable regularity. If a node group is known to be positive, the next group of greatest risk can be anticipated with sufficient accuracy to be useful in treatment. Using our knowledge of these spread patterns, external therapy can be directed to those nodes most vulnerable for metastases. Since most of the metastases are asymptomatic beyond reach by pelvic examination, and many are too small to be shown by lymphangiogram, external therapy is based upon probability. This practice can be supported by statistical frequency of pelvic node involvement. Less information is available about the aortic nodes. Since spread to aortic nodes is responsible for some treatment failures, we extend the fields to the level of L-4 vertebrae when the iliac nodes are positive or to T-12 when the lower aortic nodes are positive. Only selected patients receive this treatment because its advantages are not established and safety not yet confirmed. Pretreatment laparotomy proves the positive nodes histologically before this treatment plan is initiated.

has a lesser role in the treatment for advanced disease than for earlier stages. The tandem and ovoid applicators for intracavitary radium are used in more advanced Stage III and IV patients by a method similar to that employed for Stage I and II patients. The radium is less efficient, however, because the cancer encroaches on the needed space and alters the normal position of the uterus for a less efficient dosimetry.

The vaginal ovoids are hampered by less space in the upper vagina. Inability to expand the vagina makes ovoids less effective and the range of dosage is diminished to the midpelvic structures. Limitation to a set of small ovoids in the vagina is common, and for some patients a single ovoid is the most that can be fitted into the narrow space of the upper vagina. When these problems are present the inverted T-shaped arrangement of the uterine and vaginal sources is changed. When an extended tandem arrangement for linear distribution of radium from the uterus to the vagina is used, the sources are assembled in a single applicator. This protruding tandem contributes beneficially to the overall irradiation, but is less efficient and more threatening to the rectovaginal septum. Since the pelvic anatomy in Stages III and IV cervical cancer is less ideal for maximum intra-cavitary radium dosimetry, and because more external irradiation is needed to encompass the larger cancer, the maximum dose in mg/hr from intracavitary radium is less than that given in earlier stages of squamous cell carcinoma of the cervix.

Our radiotherapists are not enthusiastic about interstitial radium needles as a routine technique. This method is reserved for special problem cases not treated with the usual intracavitary radium applicators.

STANDARD TREATMENT SCHEMES AT M. D. ANDERSON HOSPITAL

At M. D. Anderson Hospital to fit the external therapy to the amount of cancer, we have for many years subdivided Stage III into Stage IIIA and Stage IIIB. These subdivisions serve to identify the treatment problem.

Stage IIIA (Favorable)

Definition: The primary lesion is not especially massive. The spread is to one pelvic wall or to the lower vagina. Treatment consists of whole pelvis irradiation of 15 × 15 cm portals, 4000 rads tumor dose in four weeks, plus radium 5500 to 6500 mg/hr total for both the uterus and vaginal sources. Parametrial irradiation through a 15 × 6 cm portal covering 1000 to 1500 rads is added if:

1. The cancer is predominately toward one side of the pelvis. The above additional treatment may be given to one parametrium.
2. The cervical canal and/or the vagina restrict the dosage contribution to the pelvic wall tissues from the radium system, and there is concern that the level for the parametrium is insufficient. An additional 1000

to 1500 rads may be given to one or both sides.

3. The radium system is satisfactory but diverted by anatomic changes away from the midpelvis and toward one side. This creates a deficiency in the opposite side; thus this opposite side dosage must be boosted more than the dose already delivered by whole pelvis treatment. The plan mentioned above for giving an additional 1000 to 1500 rads to the 15 × 6 cm field may be employed unilaterally.

Stage IIIA (Unfavorable)

Definition: This is a large primary lesion with thick parametrial infiltration, or the parametrial infiltration is fixed along the pelvic wall over a broad base, or this is combined with an obstructed ureter (a general indicator of bad prognosis).

Whole pelvis irradiation of 15 × 15 cm portals, 5000 rads in five weeks is the basic external therapy. An additional dose of 1000 to 1500 rads to boost the treatment to the parametrium through 15 × 6 cm portals may be elected. An intracavitary radium dose of 4000 to 6000 mg/hr is standard. (A larger optimal dose of radium is used when the primary lesion is bulky, especially when this bulky lesion regresses slowly during the course of external therapy treatment.)

Stage IIIB

Definition: The infiltration of parametrium is so massive that the primary lesion on the cervix and the parametrial infiltration now compose a single, large tumor mass, spread to both pelvic walls or spread to one pelvic wall plus the lower third of the vagina, or involvement of all areas with spread to both pelvic walls and to the lower third of the vagina.

The basic external treatment is whole pelvis x-ray therapy of 15 × 15 cm portals, 5000 rads in five weeks, plus whole pelvis therapy of 12 × 12 cm portals, 1000 rads for one additional week. Radium dose is 3000 to 4000 mg/hr (depending upon the bulkiness of the primary lesion, as mentioned earlier. External therapy for doses higher than 6000 rads is occasionally given after reducing the portal to 10 × 10 cm field for the final 1000 rads. The continuation of irradiation therapy at these high-dose levels is called for when there is a massive primary lesion and an unsuitable situation for a radium system.

SPECIAL TREATMENT SCHEMES

As mentioned previously, the value and safety of the extended portal for external therapy to the aortic nodes has not been established.[2] Radiotherapists have some experience with irradiation of the aortic nodes for metastasis from cancer of the cervix. A few patients have remained well, which indicates that a cancerocidal dose to the paraaortic nodes is feasible. Additional observations on patients' tolerance of this type of irradiation has been made by irradiating aortic nodes in other diseases. Only recently, however, has this type of irradiation become a project for improving our overall cure rate for cervical cancer.

METHOD

The width of the external field above the pelvis is narrowed to confine the irradiation to the immediate vicinity of the aorta, thus lessening the intestinal and liver injury, and avoiding the kidney. Early in this study at M. D. Anderson Hospital, x-ray therapy dosage was 5000 rads given at the rate of 800 rads/week using the linear accelerator to treat the upper abdominal fields. As anticipated, bowel disturbances were more severe during treatment.

COMPLICATIONS

Urinary Fistulae

Most patients who develop vesicovaginal fistulae following irradiation have advanced disease. Involvement of the anterior wall of the vagina by cancer weakens the vaginal wall and predisposes the patient to subsequent fistula development. Additional patients develop fistulae more directly caused by the radium system when the tolerance dose is exceeded. A "hot spot" of excessive dose is created by the compact relationship of the radium to a contracted vaginal vault. A more common cause and frequent threat of fistulae is the failure to consider the combined dosage of whole pelvis irradiation and radium. The combination of these contributors exceeds tissue tolerance.

We have had patients in whom fistulae were precipitated by trauma from vaginal wall biopsy after full dose irradiation therapy. Physicians should be cautious when biopsying the irradiated bladder or the vaginal wall. This is not said to discourage the gynecologic oncologist or urologist from searching for recurrent cancer in the abnormal bladder, but only to suggest that squamous cell carcinoma seldom recurs in the bladder without being evident in the vagina. Although single biopsy of the bladder mucosa may be warranted, rarely is there a need for repeating the procedure. A trauma to the tissues that are attempting to survive prior irradiation injury may precipitate a breakdown and a vesicovaginal fistula may result.

In recent years our experience with vaginal fistula incidence has declined. This is perhaps due to:

1. A preference for whole pelvis irradiation for advanced lesions, instead of the intense dose of intracavitary radium. The anatomy is generally less favorable for intracavitary radium because of changes caused by advanced cancer.

2. Less frequent use of the protruding tandem.

3. Improved retention of the vaginal applicator in the proper location during the entire application period.

Management of Fistulae

A vaginal fistula usually occurs within 6 to 24 months posttreatment. More often, there is preceding vaginal vault necrosis with ulcer, which usually indicates excessive irradiation. The diligent treatment of vaginal necrosis to reduce associated infection may avoid a fistula (3% hydrogen peroxide diluted in 3 parts water as a douche), and antiseptic vaginal cream or suppositories are beneficial. The presence of anaerobic infections in these tissues aggravates the tissue necrosis. The accumulation of necrotic exudate facilitates the growth of these bacteria, therefore vaginal douches two or three times a day with ¾% hydrogen peroxide not only destroys the anaerobic bacteria, but also removes conditions favorable for their survival. Using a half strength Dakin's solution may be preferable when the area of slough is quite large. This 0.25% sodium hypochlorite solution is readily available. Combined rectovaginal and vesicovaginal fistulae are common, since both the anterior and posterior vaginal wall are injured by the high dose of radium. Vaginal necrosis is aggravated by the presence of urine in the vagina if the vesical fistula develops first, and this increases necrosis that leads to the development of a second rectovaginal fistula. These conditions sometime force a decision for earlier repair.

Some patients develop fistulae 10 or more years after treatment. The process that causes these late appearing fistulae is not understood; perhaps systemic, vascular sclerosing diseases that further embarrass the blood supply to the bladder are responsible. Aging of the bladder wall tissue or

trauma may also be contributing factors. Recurrent cancer or new growth of cancer can be responsible for the fistula and must be excluded by biopsy of the fistula margin.

Management of Vaginal Fistulae

Repair of fistulae is usually unsuccessful if undertaken too soon after their appearance. When the necrosis has resolved, a small fistula high in the vagina may be repaired by partial colpocleisis (Latzko procedure). The larger fistulae surrounded by tissue markedly altered by irradiation changes are difficult to close primarily, even though acute necrosis has subsided. Greater success will be obtained by interposition of a gracilis muscle transplant or of a bulbocavernosus labial fat pad pedicle. By these techniques, a difficult closure may be accomplished with preservation of continence.

Proctosigmoiditis

Proctosigmoiditis with diarrhea, tenesmus, and rectal bleeding develops regularly near the end of whole pelvis irradiation.[6] (Figure 6) The intensity of the symptoms varies from transient changes caused by inflammation, edema, and mild ulceration of the mucosa with rectal bleeding to moderate diarrhea and lower abdominal pain due to spasm. These symptoms are successfully managed by paregoric, 4 cc/hr, until loose stools stop, or diphenoxylate hydrochloride with atropine sulfate (Lomotil), adequate fluid replacement, a low-residue bland diet, and topical application of medication for localized infection around the anus. Proctosigmoiditis may also occur in more severe forms, such as ulceration, stenosis, and obstruction. These serious changes are the result of higher doses delivered at a greater depth in the pelvic area, facilitated by the development of megavoltage techniques and irradiation. Disabling proctosigmoiditis may

Operations for Radiation Injuries of the Ileum

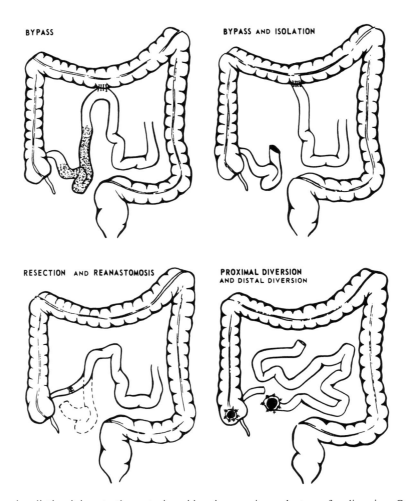

Figure 6   Some irradiation injury to the rectosigmoid region requires colostomy for diversion. Only rarely can segmental resection and anastomosis be done safely, because irradiation impairs healing severely. Although a sigmoid colostomy serves best, the bowel may not be suitable and transverse colostomy is then necessary. Injury to the ileum may be managed by different operations to relieve intestinal obstruction. Bowel resection and anastomosis are most physiologic. Bypass procedures may be simpler and surer. Ileostomy is least desirable, but may be advisable when bowel perforation is present.

last for many months and severely disrupt bowel function, often producing significant bleeding which leads to anemia and requires blood transfusion. The bowel is narrowed with ulceration, forcing marked changes in the stool. A low-residue diet is advised to reduce the trauma to the region of the bowel. Fecal impaction frequently results from bowel stenosis and, unless stool softeners are provided and good hydration is maintained, the symptoms are very distressing. Psyllium hydrophilic mucilloids (e.g., Metamucil) facilitate passage of the stool through a narrowed channel. Cholinergic drugs to counteract bowel spasm and disabling dysfunction in the area provide comfort. More severe proctosigmoiditis usually heals with some chronic alteration in bowel habits. Although repeated episodes of rectal bleeding may continue, colostomy can usually be avoided. The clinician should not be premature in performing colostomy for proctosigmoiditis, since the majority of the patients will respond to more conservative management. However, conservatism should cease when obstruction is evident or when clinical signs suggest that perforation is imminent; then a colostomy must be performed promptly to prevent life-threatening developments. Life-threatening perforation of the sigmoid results when obstruction is more complete. There are some situations in which segmental resection of the sigmoid bowel may be indicated at the time colostomy is performed. The more severe changes in the proctosigmoid region that appear between 6 and 24 months after irradiation can often be reconstructed by review of the irradiation treatment plan.

Mechanism of Sigmoiditis

This injury is related to the high dose delivered to the whole pelvis region by external irradiation. The incidence increases from 11 percent when the dose is 5000 rads to 16% with 6000 rads, and 31% at the 7000 rad level. Contributing to this is the intracavitary radium system, especially if the tandem is a long, linear arrangement of the radium sources, which extends down into the vagina (protruding tandem). The latter effect will be more damaging if the uterus and cervix are pulled backward by contracture of the pelvic tissues during treatment, bringing the radium sources nearer to the rectosigmoid. These observations confirm the usefulness of precise dosimetry in intracavitary radium therapy. Localization x-rays and computer dosimetry are examples of special dosage control that add safety and effectiveness to the irradiation treatment of Stages III and IV cancer of the cervix.

Small Intestinal Injury

The terminal small intestine, like the terminal large bowel, must receive a large dose of external therapy if the pelvic portal of treatment is to encompass the important pathways of spread from late stage cervical cancer. The frequency of injury to the small intestine coincides with the development and popularity of the greater field size for external treatment, using portals that extend higher into the abdomen. The prospects of still more serious injury to the small intestine as we contemplate expanding the pelvic portal to incorporate more of the lower aortic nodes are disturbing. At present, the occurrence of irradiation stenosis and obstruction of the terminal ileum after using standard whole pelvis portals for irradiation is infrequent, but it is a very serious complication. If therapy through a larger field becomes common practice, the problem of small bowel injury may prove to be intolerable.

Acute Symptoms

The mucosa of the small intestine has a rapid cyclic activity and is therefore especially susceptible to irradiation injury. However, since they heal very rapidly, the patient suffers relatively transient symptoms. The susceptibility of these cells shows up in the course of therapy as nausea, vomiting, abdominal pains, and diarrhea which may become persistent. If antiemetics fail and oral hydration is inadequate, irradiation should be discontinued until hydration is restored by intravenous fluid supplement. Resolution of this acute irradiation sickness is rapid after stopping the treatment. The majority of patients experience little long-term alteration of intestinal function. Other patients, for poorly understood causes, have more severe damage and develop small bowel obstruction.

Chronic Symptoms

Signs of small bowel obstruction are indicators of more permanent injury; however, conservative treatment may be warranted. Conservative management of small bowel obstruction with a long tube intubation is standard practice, but when it occurs repeatedly it should serve as a warning that the patient is particularly vulnerable to perforation. Necrosis of bowel segment that leads eventually to perforation is a serious aspect of this complication. The physician must decide when to abandon conservatism and attempt surgical relief by segmental resection or ileocolostomy bypass.

LYMPHADENECTOMY

From 1954 to 1962, more than 450 pelvic lymphadenectomies were performed at our institution as part of the management of cervical cancer. This represents several studies done during that time to obtain information about lymphatic spread. For all patients, the operation was performed only when it seemed probable that an additional benefit would be derived from excising the lymph nodes, and that any complication from operation would be minimal and would not hamper or nullify the desirable effects of prior irradiation therapy. These operations yielded much data about the metastatic pattern from carcinoma of the cervix, the action of high-dose x-ray therapy directed to the nodes, and the number and location of residual positive nodes. The patients tolerated the retroperitoneal dissection well and there were no unusual technical problems encountered by the surgeon because of prior irradiation. A clean anatomical dissection was accomplished, but treatment was marred by lymphocysts which complicated the patients' early postoperative

recovery. This formation of encysted lymph fluid caused by disruption of the lymphatic system creates a mass large enough to cause symptoms by pressure. Bladder and rectal capacity may be reduced and obstruction of the ureters occurs.

Before we were aware that complications would be troublesome, a formal program was designed to prescribe lymphadenectomy regularly for late stage disease because available information was inadequate. A systematic study was made to obtain quantitative information of positive nodes in late stage cervical cancer and to learn the response to irradiation. A transperitoneal lymphadenectomy was performed a few weeks after completion of irradiation in 100 consecutive Stage III patients who were medically suitable for operation.[4] We expected to find the same incidence of positive nodes for Stage III carcinoma of the cervix as that reported in the literature. We were pleased to find that the number of nodes recovered after irradiation was about one half that noted by authors who had collected data from node dissections associated with radical hysterectomy in nonirradiated conditions.

Signs of the cancerocidal action of irradiation were found in the microscopic evidence of sterilization in the nodes recovered; and this, combined with the reduction of expected incidence of positive nodes excised along the pathway of spread, proved that irradiation was effective. Careful dissection up to the bifurcation level of the aorta recovered 19% positive nodes for Stage III disease, much less than might be expected if the dissection had been performed without prior irradiation therapy. Thus, any doubts we may have had about the beneficial effects of high-dose irradiation therapy on positive nodes were resolved.

One question remained: Is lymphadenectomy following irradiation more curative? Since lymphadenectomy after irradiation in the 100 consecutive Stage III patients was performed without a clinical control for comparison, this group of patients could not be used to resolve the question. To justify the lymphadenectomy as routine treatment, sufficient proof was needed that the operation was adding to the overall cure rate, since lymphadenectomy exposes patients to additional risk. Therefore, a randomized study was performed to determine whether giving a group irradiation followed by pelvic lymphadenectomy produced an improved cure rate over a control group treated by irradiation alone. This study[5] included 142 patients in the lymphadenectomy group and 169 in the control group. Again, the incidence of positive nodes was low in all stages and particularly in Stage III, when compared to the published

data. The conditions at operation were also noteworthy. Positive nodes in patients were usually multiple, large, matted, and adherent to adjacent structures (Figure 7). Patients with less massive metastasis to the nodes were susceptible to external therapy, and were sterilized by the treatment. Although their operative specimens were negative for viable cancer cells, occasionally ghosts of cancer cells remained.

Evidence showed that metastatic nodal disease could not be resected with adequate margin to remove the neoplasm totally. Thus, lymphadenectomy did not produce additional cures. Approximately 1 patient in 5 who had lymphadenectomy had a complicated postoperative course.

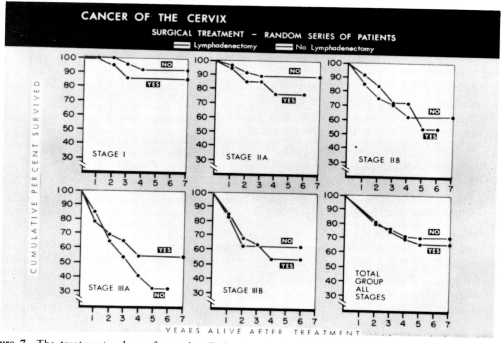

Figure 7 The treatment values of post irradiation lymphadenectomy were investigated by a clinical study which selected two groups of patients by random allocation. Both received the same irradiation plan, and one group had the pelvic nodes excised about six weeks afterward. The study also randomized the groups by stage, so that additional conclusions could be established for lymphadenectomy for early and later cancer of the cervix. The survival curves for each treatment plan are not statistically different when compared, although patients with Stage IIIA lesions showed a more favorable curve when lymphadenectomy was used. Lacking any clear benefit while adding much morbidity, lymphadenectomy as an addition to full irradiation was discontinued at our institution.

Originally, planning this study, we did not anticipate these postoperative problems, and they have since lessened our enthusiasm for such combined treatment. Based on our experience with lymphadenectomies, we have reached the following conclusions:

1. Pelvic node metastasis can be sterilized by external irradiation. This is not, however, accomplished in all patients.

2. Survival rates are not appreciably improved by postirradiation lymphadenectomy. In our first study of 100 consecutive patients with Stage III carcinoma of the cervix, no patient with positive nodes was cured by lymphadenectomy. In the second study (randomized Stages I through III), the survival times of the lymphedenectomy group and the irradiation only group of patients in all stages were almost identical.

3. Lymphadenectomy after high-dose irradiation causes serious complications. Lymphocysts developed in 20% of the patients, producing a variety of disabilities.

4. Failure of lymphadenectomy to improve survival rates can be attributed partly to the bulky metastatic disease in the lymph nodes surviving irradiation and the frequent involvement of the paraaortic nodes. Patients with few positive nodes and with small deposits of cancer within the nodes seemed to be sterilized by irradiation, leaving those patients with gross masses virtually impossible to resect with a margin of cancer-free tissue.

The positive result obtained from these studies was new information, for we learned much about the location of lymph node metastasis. This directed us to focus greater attention on the lymph nodes in the area of the abdominal aorta. Our systematic sampling of these lymph nodes during lymphadenectomy showed a surprisingly high incidence of positive nodes above the pelvic brim. Since aortic lymphadenectomy cannot be done with the ease and completeness possible in the pelvic region, irradiation, with extended-field external therapy, will be attempted in an effort to control metastasis.

The lymphadenectomy procedure should not be discarded altogether. Its usefulness must be tested by others, since lymphadenectomy in combination with resection of the primary lesion has been used favorably as part of the primary surgical treatment for cervical cancer. Since removal of the lymph nodes has been an essential part of surgical treatment, lymphadenectomy cannot be discredited when used properly .

Failure to cure metastasis in the lymph nodes still accounts for many of the failures in Stage III disease, since the failure rate and lymph node metastasis incidence approach each other. Modern irradiation methods provide an excellent prospect for curing positive nodes, especially smaller size deposits; and possibly by extending the irradiation to the lower aortic region, additional patients may be cured in the future.

HYPOGASTRIC ARTERY INFUSION

Infusion of the tumor area within the pelvis with chemotherapeutic agents by cannulating the arterial supply shows some promise.[7] Dramatic regression of advanced cervical cancer was produced by this technique in the initial work reported by Sullivan.[8] After further experience many tumors were shown unresponsive to this method of chemotherapy; those that did regress regrew promptly upon discontinuation of treatment. The classic agents used were methotrexate through the arterial catheter and citrovorum factor given systemically to neutralize the escaped drug, to prevent injury to the bone marrow, liver, and gastrointestinal tract. (Figure 8)

When regression induced by Methotrexate was shown to be of short duration, new agents were sought. Fluorouracil gained popularity because some synergistic action was observed by combining hypogastric infusion with external irradiation therapy. Other agents such as Actinomycin-D, Vin-

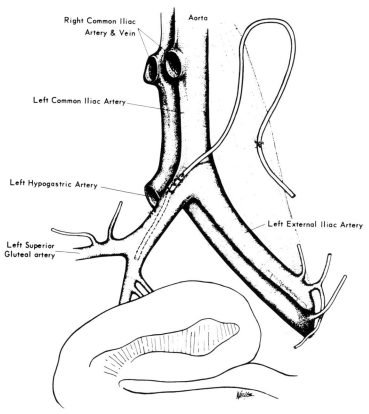

Figure 8 The left hypogastric artery is catheterized for infusion of chemotherapy. The catheter is secured near entry into the vessel and to the fascia of the psoas muscle. The catheter tip lies beyond the superior gluteal to lessen chemotherapy distribution to the buttocks.

cristine, and Cytoxan have been used in such plans, alone or in combination. The latter drugs are preferred for sarcoma in the pelvic region.

Our experience with infusion therapy spans a variety of problem patients. Some patients were usually unsuitable for the more standard irradiation treatment or radical surgery alone; others were treated by drug infusion for recurrent cancer after irradiation, and surgery when this therapy could not be repeated. Still others had special cell type cancers that were known to be unresponsive to irradiation, and surgery was not feasible.

Our first experience was in seeking palliation for recurrent tumor within the pelvis.

We used either hypogastric artery cannulation at the time of operation or percutaneous femoral catheterization directing the drug into the hypogastric system from a catheter lying with its tip in the internal iliac system. The percutaneous catheterization technique has proved effective, and may be employed for either inpatients or ambulatory patients since portable pumps have been devised. Entry of the femoral artery by cutaneous puncture permits passage of a catheter to the bifurcation of the aorta or along the iliac artery with entry into the internal iliac system. Catheters can be placed directly into the hypogastric artery at laparotomy, with some advantages over the percutaneous method. Distribution of the drug to the desired tissues can be controlled better because unwanted distribution can be limited by ligating some borders, and the catheter is made more secure if placed as an operative procedure. Although obvious disadvantage in major surgery, laparotomy is often necessary to establish the diagnosis and spread limits.

In 1965 a study was initiated at M.D. Anderson Hospital to determine whether continuous infusion of chemotherapeutic drugs into the hypogastric artery, and concurrent x-ray therapy, had additional therapeutic effects. The preliminary results suggested that patients treated with 5-fluorouracil with concomitant x-ray therapy for massive pelvic cancer benefited because there was a greater incidence of local clearance of the disease from the pelvis by irradiation. Patients treated with 5-fluorouracil had more sustained antitumor effect than patients treated similarly by Methotrexate with citrovorum factor; liver toxicity and bone marrow depression were also greater in the patients treated with Methotrexate.

Currently, we are using this method searching for better chemotherapeutic drugs to combine with irradiation therapy. Until newer drugs are produced for the systemic treatment of very advanced recurrent carcinoma of the cervix, the pelvic infusion technique will continue to be useful.

Technique of Hypogastric Artery Catheterization

Some technical aspects of placing catheters in the hypogastric arteries are worthy of note. The gluteal artery is isolated for ultimate ligation, and one must be careful not to injure major pelvic veins in this procedure. Minimal dissection of the hypogastric artery avoids spasm of this vessel. Spasm is undesirable because it increases the difficulty of inserting the catheter down the lumen of the artery. The catheter is introduced at a point 1.5 cm above the uterine artery and inserted past the ligated gluteal artery. A special catheter with a fused needle is used to enter the artery. The needle exits through the wall of the artery at a lower level and is cut from the catheter, whose tip is withdrawn into the lumen of the artery and extended downward into the lower pelvic area. To avoid clotting, the catheter is first filled with heparin solution and sealed until a continuous flow through the catheter can be established by connecting it to an infusion pump. Suture fixation for the catheter is essential. It is attached to the hypogastric artery, then to the psoas muscle and the abdominal wall, as the catheter continues its course retroperitoneally and out the lower abdominal incisions on each side respectively. The position of the catheter for the desired infusion of the involved zone may be confirmed by injecting fluorescein dye and testing the effect on the infused structures with ultraviolet light (Wood's light). The catheter position may also be confirmed by angiography, injecting radiopaque material into the catheter. The infusion rate will be adjusted to the quantity of fluid that the uterine and vesical arteries will accommodate within 24 hr and also to the amount of drug desired for the period.

STAGE IV CARCINOMA OF THE CERVIX

The majority of patients with Stage IV carcinoma of the cervix are incurable because they have distant metastasis. For these patients, therapy can only provide palliation. However, this discussion will be concerned only with the management expected to provide a cure. There is no concensus about the better method: pelvic exenteration or radical irradiation, applied alone or with adjunctive chemotherapy. A positive bladder biopsy for metastatic carcinoma of the cervix deserves special attention for treatment although it is often a cause for debate. The arguments against treatment with irradiation, like those in late Stage III cancers, are: (1) metastatic carcinoma in the bladder cannot be completely sterilized by irradiation, and (2) if irradiation is used, a vesicovaginal fistula will develop when the cancer in the bladder wall melts away after treatment. Since most cervical cancers that invade the bladder or rectum are also massive tumors, they often prove unresectable at laparotomy despite a favorable preoperative assessment.

Two recent publications are pertinent to this discussion. The report of Decker and Ketcham[1] from the National Institutes of Health deals with pelvic exenteration for Stages III and IV carcinoma of the cervix as primary treatment. They selected 65 out of 218 patients for pelvic exenteration and 24 for anterior pelvic exenteration. The actuarial five-year survival rate for the treated group was 48.5%, or an absolute survival of 25 out of 65 patients (38%). This report supports the recommendation of Brunschwig, Daniels, Barber, Bricker, and others that exenteration will cure patients with advanced cervical cancer and may also be used as primary treatment.

It should be noted that in 17 patients the specimen actually proved that the disease was confined to the cervix (Stage II). In 17 additional patients, evidence of spread to the bladder was discovered by laparotomy, indicating the inaccuracies of clinical examination. Thus the therapy for some patients was needlessly radical. There were 11 of 31 patients who had proven bladder involvement with an accumulated five-year survival rate of 35%. The operative mortality from primary exenteration in this report was 10%.

Decker and Ketcham support their choice of radical resection with these observations:

1. "Most patients with Stage III and IV at other institutions are referred to the radiotherapists despite the fact that irradiation cures less than 30 percent of Stage III and less than 10 percent of Stage IV."

2. "The dosage adequate to treat these large tumors for a cure is associated with considerable morbidity, fistula formation, pelvic necrosis, and painful fibrosis, frequently requiring reconstructive surgery to correct the side effects of irradiation therapy."

The second report of Million et al[3] originates from data at M. D. Anderson Hospital and concerns only Stage IV carcinoma of the cervix with bladder invasion. This report defends irradiation treatment by reviewing the outcome of patients with Stage IV cancers limited to the pelvis that could be treated by exenteration but were treated instead mainly by external therapy. Only a relatively small portion of all the patients seen with Stage IV cervical cancer were suited for operation or irradiation. The amount of cancer was usually too large or the metastasis too diffuse and distant to attempt curative treatment. From 1948 to 1963, 284 patients with Stage IV carcinoma were admitted to M. D. Anderson Hospital. Of these, 175 patients (62%), had such advanced disease that even irradiation was not recommended. Of the 109 patients who had bladder invasion, 43 could have been treated surgically, but were treated instead with irradiation. They represent the study group. (These statistics tell us something about why Stage IV has a low cure rate, as quoted by Decker and Ketcham.[1] Many of the patients are untreatable because the disease is widespread, whereas local control of the pelvic disease is often obtained by irradiation.) The 43 patients with Stage IV disease represent 1.7% of all patients seen with cancer of the cervix during these years.

The five-year survival rate of the 43 patients with Stage IV disease due to bladder invasion that were treated by irradiation was 28 percent. Of these patients, 10 developed a vesicovaginal fistula before initiation of irradiation therapy, but none developed fistula during or subsequent to the completion of therapy, thus refuting some fixed beliefs about Stage IV carcinoma of the cervix treated by irradiation. Clinicians have long entertained the fear that irradiation therapy to the patient with bladder invasion would provoke a high incidence of vesico-vaginal fistulae and local persistence in the bladder wall.

In summary, although there is a role for primary exenteration in Stage IV, this is not the only effective treatment. These unfortunate patients have a desperate illness which must be treated intensively by irradiation or by extended surgery. If exenteration is performed, the price to the patient is the loss of urinary continence, seriously impaired sexual function, and perhaps a colostomy. These patients also run a 10 percent risk of early death from the operation. At present, the clinician must decide whether the lesion is resectable by asking the following questions: Is the patient physically suitable for the operation? How well can the patient accommodate the diverted urine and fecal stream? If a positive answer is obtained from this deliberation, the choice of primary exenteration is justified. Spread to the bladder does not, however, distract from employing external irradiation therapy. A 28% cure rate in the group studied by Million and co-workers is noteworthy. Bladder function may be preserved by choosing irradiation therapy because vesicovaginal fistula is rarely induced.

The major force in curing Stages III and IV cancer of the cervix is high-dose irradiation to large areas that often involve the intestine, bladder, and rectum in severe injury. To relieve irradiation-produced intestinal obstruction, bypass anastomosis and resection of the bowel is necessary. The alimentary tract may be shortened, and the patient then becomes a cripple due to poor nutrition. Although less crippling complications may incapacitate the patient for one or more years, she may later recover. These side effects are permissible, if this is the only way that cancer can be cured. It is yet

to be proven, however, whether high-dose levels are essential or necessary for all patients at a given stage. Although some patients with equal cancer populations are curable with small dosage, they are not identifiable before therapy. The radiotherapist must decide whether it is wise to subject patients to the risk of severe complications in an effort to add a small percentage to the cure rate category. We desperately need identification of those cancers more sensitive to a smaller, safer dose level.

New techniques of irradiation are tested by clinical use. Their effectiveness and tolerance are manifested as the patient's post-treatment course is observed. For the radiotherapist there is a longer lag in observing the results of a new treatment plan than for the surgeon. The surgeon gains additional information about the condition of the patient's cancer by exploratory laparotomy, a technique not available to the radiotherapist who must wait for a period of follow-up observation. Further, some of the effects of irradiation are delayed, occurring months or even years later, whereas surgical complications are usually more rapid and acute. There is a greater chance for the radiotherapist to accumulate a large population of patients who have been maltreated before complications begin to appear. Thus, it is essential that radiotherapy plans be modified frequently, and dosage levels advanced cautiously while treating most patients with cancer of the cervix by conventional, proven techniques.

REFERENCES

1. Decker, P. J., and A. S. Ketcham, *Obstet. Gynecol.*, 37, 647–659 (1971).
2. Fletcher, G. H., and F. N. Rutledge, *Am. J. Roentgenol.*, 114, 116–122 (1972).
3. Million. Rodney R., and Gilbert H. Fletcher, *Am. J. Obstet. Gynec.*, 113, (1972).
4. Rutledge, F. N., and G. H. Fletcher, *Am. J. Obstet. Gynec.* 76, 321–334 (1958).

5. Rutledge, F. N., Gilbert H. Fletcher, and Eleanor J. MacDonald, *Am. J. Roentgenol.,* **93,** 607–614 (1965).

6. Smith, J. P., Patrick E. Golden, and Felix Rutledge, *Cancer of the Uterus and Ovary,* Year Book Medical, Chicago, 1966.

7. Smith, J. P., G. E. Randall. J. R. Castro, and R. D. Lindberg, *Am. J. Roentgenol. Radium Ther. Nucl. Med.* **94,** (1972).

8. Sullivan, R. O., and E. Miller, *Cancer* **12,** 1248–1262 (1959).

CHAPTER 5 MANAGEMENT: TREATMENT FAILURES IN CARCINOMA OF THE CERVIX

FELIX RUTLEDGE, M.D.

To avoid the confusion of defining persistent cancer, recurrent cancer, and new growth cancer in the vicinity of previously treated squamous cell carcinoma of the cervix, the title of management of treatment failures will discuss the patient whose treatment was (1) inadequate by present standards, (2) incomplete because of intolerance, (3) unsuccessful because the tumor persisted, (4) inadequate to rid the patient of the disease permanently; therefore treatment had to be repeated because a new disease grew. Some factors that are shared by all of these patients make management difficult. There is limited tissue tolerance because of prior treatment, restricted access to the neoplasia, and the surrounding bladder, rectum, and small intestine are at an increased risk. The spread of neoplasia is similar; methods necessary for diagnosis and localization are similar. There is an equal threat for hemorrhaging, ureteral obstruction, metastasis to vital organs, and final death of the host if secondary treatment fails.

IMPORTANCE OF SUBJECT

The gynecologic oncologist must be concerned with treatment failures for the following reasons:

1. Unless the outcome of treatment is studied conscientiously and inquiringly, the lessons of experience will be missed. Excesses or inadequacies in dosage may be observed during the follow-up period and corrected for future patients. Radiation treatment dosage is often said to be empirical; this statement is true for a newly devised irradiation system, for treatments usually develop by trial and observation. Eventually, a safe and effective therapy evolves. Even when the routine is established, the therapist must never become so confident about his plan for treatment that the search for the cause of treatment failures deteriorates. Old and established routines in treatment still have defects in dosimetry for some patients that can be improved. Treatment has defects when patients develop recurrences within the area field treated. The concerned oncologist is alert for such patients because they are failures to be credited against his management; although most failures are explained by distant metastases, no longer is "cancer" an acceptable explanation for all unsuccessful attempts to cure.

2. The oncologist is obligated to detect recurrences early, while the cancer is most suited for retreatment. Usually the patient fears her cancer will return and entrusts her protection to the physician. She is entitled to a careful surveillance for early diagnosis. This obligation is well recognized: to assist the physician in performing this duty, an office or clinic organization concerned with

posttreatment care is necessary. An effective system for follow-up management is the right of each patient with gynecologic cancer. If the surgeon or the radiotherapist rejects this commitment, it remains his duty to refer the patient elsewhere for care. Although the first treatment is the most successful, retreatment of cancer of the cervix provides additional cures equal to the primary treatment of many cancers, such as those in the lung, stomach, bowel, and large bowel. Therefore, the opportunity for cure by retreatment must not be lost through neglect of follow-up care.

3. Patients with cervical cancer that is not curable still deserve palliative care, for their mental health and well-being improves. Although recurrences may not be suitable for complete eradication, the more offensive part of the growth may be eliminated, pressure effects of the tumor may be relieved, hemorrhage controlled, and pain diminished. Opportunities for tumor regression by chemotherapy are available, although at present the benefits are incomplete and unsustained. For example: a swollen, painful leg may shrink, lung metastasis regress, and obstruction of the tumor masses decrease. Palliative care is an important part of gynecologic oncology, and its accomplishments will prove very satisfying to those physicians who have a compassionate interest in their patients throughout the full course of their disease.

MECHANICS OF TREATMENT FAILURES IN CANCER OF THE CERVIX

A failure to permanently rid the patient of carcinoma of the cervix by treatment may be explained by the following mechanisms: (1) If radical surgery is used, the cancer is incompletely excised and promptly regrows. If irradiation is employed, some of the cancer is beyond the range of the treatment, or the cancer resists destruction and continues to grow. (2) Irradiation produces apparently satisfactory regression, the cancerocidal effects are not complete within the area treated and recidivation ultimately develops. The mechanism responsible for the prolonged interval from primary treatment to late recurrences is poorly understood. In a small number of cases, recidivation occurs late and becomes indistinguishable from the third mechanism. (3) A new genesis of cancer develops within the region treated. The cell type of the new neoplasm is similar to the old. The majority of treatment failures by surgery or irradiation are caused by incomplete eradication of the tumor in the advanced stages and distant metastases in the earlier stages of the disease.

DETERMINANTS OF TREATMENT FAILURE

1. The size and distribution of the neoplastic cell population decide the complexity and success of treatment. A large, bulky tumor adversely affects the action of irradiation therapy (Figure 1). The center of large tumors lacks oxygenation. Anoxia makes cells more resistant to irradiation because the desired cancerocidal ionization by photons needs a physiologic saturation of oxygen. The hypoxic condition near the center of the tumor increases the dose requirements of irradiation 2.5 times the amount that is usually adequate. This problem cannot be solved by increased dosage, for the bladder and intestine would be destroyed. More appropriate treatment given initially will excise large tumor masses before irradiation.

2. The surgeon finds that distribution of the neoplastic cell population is the determinant for radicality of resection. Although surgery is the most efficient method of cure, irradiation has a wider range of application. If the malignant tumor can be removed entirely, with a margin of normal tissue,

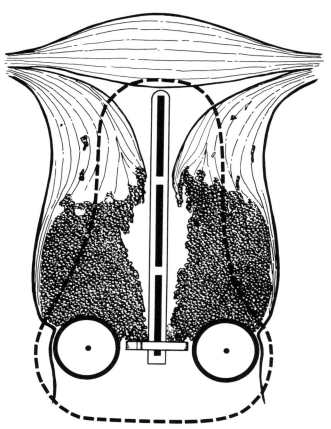

Figure 1 Schematic illustration of a cancer of the cervix growing within the endocervix to form a large, bulky cancer that expands the dimensions of the lower segment of the uterus until the uterus resembles a barrel rather than the usual pear shape. A theoretical radium application is shown, and the composite dosage of irradiation is depicted by the broken line. This isodose line bounds a zone that receives at least 6000 rads, a cancerocidal dose. Cancer noted outside this broken line may not be eradicated by radium therapy. Additional irradiation from external therapy may be used, but the dosage needed carries high risk of intestinal injury; thus a conservative dose would be safer.

then it cannot recur. To accomplish this, the importance of the growth pattern of the tumor must be appreciated: some cancers are prone to local confinement, others are exposed to vaginal examination, and still others infiltrate. Deceptive conditions include a small primary tumor which disseminates widely into many small metastases. Such a case invites incomplete excision and treatment failure.

Cervical cancer is known as an "orderly" disease because it usually spreads outwardly and uniformly from the cervix; occasionally spread is down the vagina and forward toward the bladder, making operation undesirable. Discontinuous metastases beyond the periphery of the tumor (e.g., lymph node metastasis) must be expected for most stages of cancer of the cervix of all growth types. Embolic neoplasia which implants at the dissection site must be avoided. Thus, for similar numbers of cancer cells, the distribution influences the treatment and will influence the selection of surgical or irradiation therapy. The central bulky mass may be the nemesis of the radiotherapist, while small widely dispersed colonies of neoplasia frustrate the surgeon's efforts to be completely effective.

IDENTIFICATION OF RECURRENCES

Careful follow-up of the cervical cancer patient is essential, so that first evidence of recurrent disease can be detected. This is best performed by the physician most involved in the treatment, often the surgeon. Not only must he be a capable surgeon, but he must also be familiar with the natural history of cervical cancer. Knowledge of the common sites and signs of recurrence and when new tumors are most likely to appear will increase his ability.

The symptoms of recurrent cancer resemble those of the primary, but identification of recurrence is more difficult because of changes in the pelvic tissue created by treatment of the condition. Primary treatment by irradiation introduces both acute and chronic tissue changes that can conceal cancer. Generally, one should suspect the patient of harboring recurrent cancer if the cervix and vaginal vault do not heal within six months after irradiation. Nodularity within the vagina points with considerable certainty to recurrent or persistent disease, whereas fibrosis in the pelvic supporting structures may be the result of irradiation or prior operation.

In a study by Morrow[8] at the M. D. Anderson Hospital, of 547 patients with carcinoma of the cervix who developed recurrences after irradiation treatment, the primary cervical lesion and surrounding vagina were healed within six months in only 277 patients; 92 had vaginal vault necrosis at six months, and an additional 41 had significant vaginal mucositis. Nodularity was found by rectovaginal examination in 82 out of 547 patients; while the parametrium was

smooth in 401 patients with recurrence, 27 had distinct pelvic masses. These observations point out the difficulty in detecting recurrences because of the effects of irradiation. Similar confusing findings are present following radical hysterectomy. During the six months after therapy, identification of treatment failures was especially hampered by postoperative effects. Biopsies were often necessary to aid in the clinical examination.

The presence of cancer was established by biopsy of suspected lesions in the vagina, bladder, or inguinal nodes for 20% of the patients in the study; laparotomy was necessary to establish a diagnosis for 20%. Autopsy and a variety of additional tests identified recurrence for 20 percent of the patients; for the other 40 percent diagnosis was not confirmed histologically but was based on clinical impressions.

Tests to screen for recurrent cancer are often worthwhile and should be a part of the routine in the follow-up care of patients. Although vaginal cytology is much less reliable for the detection of recurrence than for finding primary cancer, the test is easily performed and incipient disease is often identified. Irradiation alters the vaginal cells, but these changes need not obscure identification of viable cancer cells. Vaginal biopsy of the suspected area, chest x-ray, and excretory urogram have established the diagnosis most often when the disease is not obvious by visual examination and palpation. For interpretation of the intravenous pyelogram (IVP) there must be a baseline pretreatment study for comparison. This test is made before primary treatment in all patients except those with the earliest stage of the cancer. A routine study of the kidneys after treatment is considered more essential for some patients than for others; therefore we did not make the excretory urogram a routine part of the follow-up examination for the earlier stage lesions that had a normal pretreatment test and no posttreatment urinary tract symptoms.

LOCATION OF RECURRENCES

Central Recurrences

A study of the cause of death and sites of failure in squamous cell carcinoma have been made at intervals at the M. D. Anderson Hospital.[7] We have been especially interested in identifying those patients who develop recurrences within the area treated, for these patients may be saved by improved treatment.

Identification of the site responsible for treatment failure is difficult. Metastasis beyond the pelvis can return to the pelvic region and induce errors. The clinical examination may be indecisive because the pelvic tissues are altered by prior treatment. Irradiation-induced fibrosis may conceal cancer or may be misinterpreted as recurrent cancer. The ability to decide if the primary lesion around the cervix has been cured is made difficult when patients allow the upper vagina to occlude by adhesions. After radium therapy, the cervical canal and the tissues surrounding the external os regularly receive high dosage radiation, and contracture often seals the cervix. Stenosis hampers investigation of the endocervical canal and corpus. Here a cancer may survive, grow, and metastasize beyond the pelvis before being detected. Pelvic wall recurrences are difficult to palpate with accuracy until masses are large and painful. Although the precision for identifying central recurrences and the accuracy by which the investigator can decide which part of the treatment failed may be questioned, these studies are productive for the deficiencies that are discovered.

The cause and incidence of central recurrences in 1341 patients with Stage I and II squamous cell carcinoma of the cervix treated at the M. D. Anderson Hospital between 1948 and 1963 are indicated:[5] 8 of 471 (1.9%) Stage I cases and, 50 of 870 (5.6%) Stage II cases were regrettable treatment failures because they are within the treated area. Some patterns in the clinical characteristics of the cancers were observed to develop central recurrences more often. The treatment plan for these patients was amended by adding surgery to the irradiation therapy.

Regional Recurrences

Incomplete eradication of metastases outward from the cervix and around the pelvic wall produces regional recurrences. These are not found by inspection or palpation of the vagina, and the symptoms are unlike those of central recurrences. Pelvic and back pain, leg edema, and signs of obstructive uropathy are the first indicators. Because detection is delayed, the mechanism of pelvic wall recurrences becomes more complex and less accurate. Located in the intermediate position in the spread pattern pathway between the primary and aortic nodes, regional recurrences must come from either source. Retrograde metastases may be responsible, since positive aortic nodes may produce metastasis to the pelvic wall and be mistakenly attributed to cancer that survived in the treatment field. Although there is ample opportunity for making mistakes in categorizing recurrent sites, these studies are, nevertheless, valuable.

Distant Metastases

Aortic nodes, supraclavicular nodes, lungs, and bone are frequent sites of metastases and are least accessible for treatment. Pulmonary resection of metastases that appear after treatment of cervical cancer may be advisable. Lung metastases that appear after one year or more, if they are single and the only known metastases are most favorable for resection. Although this method contributes little to the total problem of distant metastases since most lung metastases are not suitable for excision, chest x-rays are still advised as part of the follow-up study because there are other means of palliating lung metastases.

METHODS FOR TREATING RECURRENCES

Radical Hysterectomy

The selection of radical hysterectomy for patients with central recurrences is based on the dimensions of the cancer. Radical hysterectomy may be used for the lesion restricted to the immediate vicinity of the cervix and the upper vagina. The margin of safety from fistulization is less when this operation is performed for recurrent cancer than when it is done for the primary disease. There is a high incidence of fistulization after radical hysterectomy because the blood supply of the tissues is impaired by irradiation. There are technical difficulties and increased hazards of operative trauma. Prior irradiation produces tissue contractions which reduce the space between the bladder, the rectum, and the primary lesion of the cervix. Thus the margin of tissue around the specimen that is negative for cancer is smaller.

We have used radical hysterectomy for the treatment of persistent or recurrent cancer following x-ray therapy for 65 patients: of the 47 patients treated five years ago, 26 (55.3%) are free of disease. This success encourages us to use radical hysterectomy for suitable patients, although additional operations to correct fistulization are often necessary. Of the 65 patients treated, 12 had vesicovaginal fistulae, 3 rectovaginal fistulae, and 1 ureterovaginal fistula.

Extended radical hysterectomy, or modified exenteration, is appropriate when recurrences are limited to the area around the cervix with metastasis to the ureter or the bladder. The operation must include a segmental resection of the ureter or removal of a portion of the bladder. Such modifications are a natural development of radical hysterectomy, to make it inclusive although still more conservative than exenteration. These additional resections increase the risk of fistulization. Since we have used this procedure for only 8 patients, we are unable to advocate its adoption.

Pelvic Exenteration

Pelvic exenteration is now accepted as worthwhile therapy for patients with cancer that is either too advanced for conventional treatment or recurrent within the pelvis after irradiation. This procedure, however, is formidable and risky because safety, healing, and recovery are limited. One mistake in management can destroy the patient's chances to benefit. The risk inherent in this procedure can be justified only as a good chance for long-term cancer control. Two basic criteria for using this operation are: the tumor must be totally resectable, and the patient must have an adequate physical reserve for recovery. Otherwise, exenteration should not be used.

ANTERIOR, POSTERIOR, AND TOTAL EXENTERATION

At the M. D. Anderson Hospital we do not believe, as some surgeons do, that total exenteration is always necessary[9] (Figure 2). In their opinion, the bladder, vagina, uterus, and intestines are so intimately related that recurrent cancer involving any of these organs has probably involved the others, although extension may not be apparent.

We have used anterior exenteration when cancer is spreading anteriorly and the rectum is normal. Since cervical cancer spreads anteriorly more often than posteriorly, anterior exenteration is more useful than the posterior procedure. Fewer patients have involvement of the rectum without metastasis to the bladder as well.

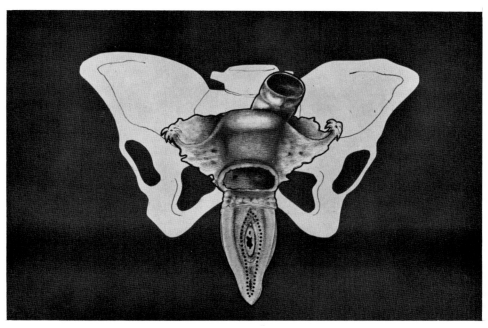

Figure 2 This semidiagramatic view of the total exenteration specimen emphasizes extensive excision of vulva and perineum as well as uterus, vagina, bladder, rectum, and lymph node-containing tissues of the pelvic walls. Some individualization is possible with exenteration. It remains for the surgeon to decide how completely the lower part of the vagina, vulva, and anus need to be removed. Those patients with cancer confined high in the genital tract may have the labia, perineum, and anus conserved. If the cancer margin is high above this level, restoration of the vagina for sexual function is simpler for the surgeon, and the outcome more normal for the patient if the perineum and labia are not excised.

A factor that opposes the use of anterior exenteration, although qualified, is prior high-dose irradiation. If, for example, the sigmoid rectum has sustained a large dose of irradiation, there is less chance that it can be conserved as a functioning intestine. Also, there is always the risk that anterior exenteration will not be adequate resection, thus a cure may be jeopardized because the rectosigmoid segment harbored cancer.

Successful exenteration depends on (1) a wise selection of patients, (2) thorough preoperative study, (3) a perfect plan for resection and reconstruction, (4) a skillfully performed procedure, and, (5) meticulous postoperative care.

SELECTION OF PATIENTS FOR EXENTERATION

Important considerations in choosing patients are: renal reserve, disseminated cancer, age, obesity, systemic disease, previous irradiation, and emotional stability.

Renal reserve. Obviously, renal function must be sufficient to mitigate the strain imposed by pelvic exenteration. Uremia and other disturbances of the first three or four postoperative weeks could be fatal.

Disseminated cancer. Although the usual signs of disseminated cancer are well known, the implication of the pain patterns is less generally appreciated. Distortion and pressure on the large pelvic nerves, veins, urinary tract, and large bowel indicate the size and location of the cancer. Severe pain which courses posteriorly down the leg from the sacrum along the sciatic nerve distribution indicates deep-seated cancer pressing upon the sacral nerve plexes. Cancer located more anteriorly in the pelvis affects the obturator nerve and causes discomfort in the region of the anterior medial upper thigh. Severe leg pain associated with edema points to both venous and lymphatic obstruction caused by massive metastases along the pelvic wall or around the sacral promontory, and indicates inoperability.

Bimanual rectovaginal examination is the most valuable way to determine the resectability of cancer, although this method is by no means infallible. The boundaries of the cancer and fixation in the pelvis are often overestimated because fibrotic tissues may be mistaken for tumor masses.

Age. Although individuals vary, patients who are over 70 usually have some serious physical impediment that will preclude the use of exenteration.

The obese patient's large abdomen causes serious problems even for the most skilled surgeon. The strain on the cardiovascular system imposed by obesity is aggravated by the operation: tumor excision will be less complete, hemorrhage more difficult to control, and anastomosis more likely to be jeopardized for the obese patient. The ileostomy stoma and the colostomy are exposed to greater tension, awkward location, and risk of retraction.

Prior irradiation. The dose and distribution of any prior irradiation is important in selecting patients for exenteration. Those who received a 5000-rad dose or more of external irradiation therapy to the pelvic area, at rates of about 1000 rads/week, have more postoperative complications. High-dose external irradiation applied through large portals injures the abdominal wall and the pelvic organs, including segments of the intestine. These irradiated tissues survive the additional strain poorly. Irradiation also obliterates tissue planes, resulting in a prolonged and bloody operation. Since exenteration is the only treatment for most patients with recurrences after irradiation, patients with these obstacles cannot be excluded automatically. However, prior high-dose irradiation should be recognized as an adverse influence in patient selection.

Emotional factors. A patient who undergoes exenteration needs both maturity and emotional stability to withstand the discomfort and strain of the operation. Some social isolation may tax her emotional stability, and the added personal care necessitated by exenteration will test her maturity. An emotionally unstable person may withdraw from society and may neglect to care for the stomas which, if neglected, threaten her health because the urinary conduit will fail to function as designed.

SPECIAL TESTS FOR SELECTING PATIENTS

Excretory urography. The excretory urogram is the most important preoperative test because the surgeon needs to know the extent of the cancer, how much of the urinary tract must be resected and, most important, the amount of dependable renal reserve.

Lymphangiography. We believe that the lymphangiogram is particularly valuable because the identification of positive nodes is highly accurate. Although false-negative interpretation occurs occasionally, the test is appropriate because the lymphatic channels remain patent and the lymphoid tissue persists even after extensive irradiation.

Other studies. Although the chest examination must be a routine preoperative study, barium enema is not done routinely. Cystoscopy is essential to determine if invasion of the bladder has occurred, because cancer is often in the region of the bladder base.

EVALUATION OF EXENTERATION

Our experience with exenteration spans about 15 years and includes more than 250 operations (Table 1). The majority have been done for recurrent cancer of the cervix following irradiation. A five-year control rate of 28% of recurrent cervical cancer is satisfactory, there are still many unsatisfactory aspects to this experience:

1. Immediate postoperative mortality has been excessive. In the earlier years the threat of death was greatest from hemorrhage with hypovolemia, shock, or renal failure, or the reverse often occurred with excess blood and fluid replacement. Cardiac failure due to

Table 1   Evaluation of Exenteration, M.D. Anderson Hospital

Exenteration, All Types—245	
Anterior	71
Posterior	32
Total	142
Indications	
Recurrences post-irradiation	184
Primary treatment	61
Postoperative complications	
Intestinal obstruction	11
Intestinal fistulae	19
Urinary obstruction	6
Urinary fistulae	14
Pulmonary embolus	3
Coronary occlusion	2
Uremia	4
Severe hemorrhage	5
Hepatitis	3
Acute pyelitis	24
Abscess and septicemia	7

Results—5-year cumulative survival
Various cancer (245 patients)   32%
Recurrent cancer of the cervix (172 patients)   28%

hypervolemia, excess stress, and poor respiratory exchange caused most deaths soon after exenteration. Improvement in intraoperative care, and more skillful immediate postoperative care reduced cardiovascular, pulmonary, and renal system complications. Thus, the mortality during the first postoperative week was reduced.

2. Greater safety in the immediate postoperative period allowed more patients to progress into the later weeks postoperatively when most deaths during recovery period occurred. Longer survival displayed the failure of bowel and urinary tract anastomosis as another weakness of the exenteration operation. Frequently, a urinary or fecal fistula through the perineum or an intestinal obstruction was attributable to the denuded pelvic cavity. This exposed region induced infection, adhesions, and abscess formation; eventually the suture line failed. Urine and fecal contamination of the pelvic cavity aggravated infection around the exposed loops of the small bowel, the ileal conduit and the large pelvic wall blood vessels. Profound hemorrhage occurred in some patients, and in others less profuse but recurrent hemorrhages from these pelvic vessels was troublesome. Secondary abdominal operations with reanastomosis of the intestinal union were necessary to relieve the intestinal obstruction. Revision of the leaking urinary conduit was a similar sequela originating in the pelvic cavity. Secondary abdominal operations to correct these fistulae are especially hazardous, for at this time the patient has a diminished physical reserve: the risk of generalized peritonitis is greater, and often the reconstructive surgery fails to heal.

Efforts to prevent the complication caused by the denuded pelvic cavity led to managing a series of patients by constructing a pelvic floor for the abdominal cavity. This was formed across the abdominal entry to the pelvis. Several techniques were employed. First, a grid of plastic material was used as a "pelvic lid." This was soon abandoned because the material frequently induced the formation of intestinal fistulae, which aggravated the problem. For more physiologic material, a segment of defunctional intestine was selected. An 8-in. segment of sigmoid colon was separated or, if this was not feasible, a similar segment of small bowel was selected. For either, a fan-shaped portion of mesentery to this segment was separated to supply vessels to the bowel segment. The segment ends were closed, then an opening for mucous escape was made in the midsection of the segment. The antimesenteric border of the bowel and the cut margins of its mesentery were sutured along the pelvic brim. The supporting floor prevented the intestines and urinary conduit from descending into the pelvic cavity. The pelvic lid functioned, as planned, to retain the intestine above the pelvis and, except for 2 patients whose pelvic lid collapsed because the attachment failed, the procedure was successful in the remaining 34 patients. This technique was used for patients with total exenteration. Patients who had anterior or posterior exenteration had other tissues available for peritonealization. Although intestinal obstruction and urinary conduit complications decreased markedly by the techniques of pelvic lid construction, postoperative sepsis increased.

The most recent era of patient recovery was notable for death due to septicemia originating in the pelvic cavity. Unusual strains of bacteria, *Serratia marcescens* and Bacteroides, were responsible. For others the more common strains of *Proteus* and *Pseudomonas* were overwhelming. The pelvic lid that had solved the intestinal obstruction problem aggravated the problem of pelvic infection by providing a large, denuded area shaped to pool exudate, an ideal situation for the growth of bacteria. Since conscientious lavage of this region did not prevent sepsis, another procedure was in-

troduced to serve both needs: protection of the bowel and the urinary conduit and obliteration of the pelvic cavity while adding a blood supply course.

Presently, we manage this problem by transferring the omentum to the pelvic cavity (Figure 3). The omentum is detached from the stomach and colon while preserving the left gastroepiploic arterial and venous supply.[1] Ample pedicle for this source is protected. After dividing the multiple small vessels along the greater curvature of the stomach and division of the right gastroepiploic artery, the omentum can be placed

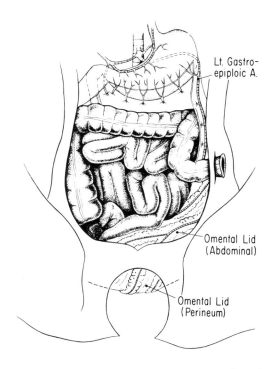

Figure 3 Transfer of the omentum to line the pelvic cavity. This serves as a carpet for the intestines, allowing them to descend and occupy the pelvic cavity. The omental carpet protects the intestines from obstruction while obliterating the space with lessened sepsis from this region. To gain mobility, the right gastroepiploic artery is divided with multiple smaller vessels along the greater curvature of the stomach. The left lateral gutter of the abdomen serves as a passageway to the pelvic cavity.

into the bottom and along the side walls of the pelvic cavity, so that a carpet of vascular, fatty tissue interposes between the intestines and the denuded pelvic walls. This procedure avoids adhesion formation, decreases serum and lymph exudate from the pelvic surface, and provides a new vasculature to aid healing and defend against infection. From the first patient treated in January, 1970, the method has been standard for patients who undergo total exenteration.

Management of the postoperative course has improved. A decline from 12% mortality for earlier years to a current incidence of 7% is creditable, yet safer methods are needed. Exenteration continues to harbor extra hazards. The diverted urinary tract does not always function perfectly, although healing is good. Some patients will harbor resistant chronic urinary tract infection; others may develop a stenosis of the implanted ureter and lose a renal unit. Late complications of the diverted urinary system may mar some of the success of the operation years later.

SUMMARY PELVIC EXENTERATION

Clinical experience has established the pelvic exenteration operation for treating patients with advanced cancer that is unsuitable for conventional treatment or has recurred within the pelvis after irradiation. Pelvic exenteration carries a great risk because the margins for safety and recovery are very limited; thus a single error in management may cause death, result in a fruitless operation, or aggravate the patient's present misery. From the first evaluation for suitability to the completion of the treatment and recovery there are great demands upon the physician's wisdom in identifying the eligible patient, judgment in assessing the physical boundaries of the cancer, diligent investigation for metastasis, skill in the performance of the operation with meticulous and vigilant support of the patient during the postopera-

tive period, and concern for the ultimate outcome. The entire management course is subject to error that leads to increased patient suffering and frustration of the clinician, with a futile dissipation of the energies of the staff, and even to catastrophe.

IRRADIATION TREATMENT OF RECURRENCES

If the patient has not already received a significant amount of irradiation by either radium or external therapy to the pelvic region, she is suitable for irradiation treatment of a recurrence. Irradiation is preferred in these condtions because a wider variety of tumor masses and location in the pelvis are treatable, and are also safer and less crippling than exenteration.

For those patients who have had prior irradiation treatment the amount and distribution of the treatment is important. Tolerance of pelvic organs for additional irradiation must be evaluated very carefully. Since guidelines are vague about the amount that would be considered a significant dose, each patient must be evaluated individually. Some methods of irradiation imply less hazard of exceeding tolerance dosage.

Preoperative radium therapy as a preliminary to radical hysterectomy is a fairly common practice. The dosage fraction is in the range of 25 to 35% of the dose that would be prescribed if irradiation alone were the treatment. Such a patient has enough reserve irradiation tolerance to allow retreatment of her recurrence by irradiation. Recurrence located on the pelvic wall removed from the region of prior intracavitary radium may tolerate a cancerocidal dose of external therapy.

Reirradiation of the pelvic region when the patient has already received a full course of external irradiation is a serious error. To attempt such treatment aggravates the patient's problem. The growth of cancer is not altered by treating again with the diminished amounts required to avoid destroying the tissues that already have a reduced tolerance. Often the irradiation is excessive and sloughs both the bladder and rectum with the formation of fistulae. A progressive necrotic infection, pain, hemorrhage, and growing cancer are common outcomes of such bad judgment.

Treatment Inadequate by Present Standards

Treatment of patients with invasive carcinoma who have had only a simple hysterectomy occurs too often because the simple hysterectomy is inadequate for invasive cancer of the cervix. Hysterectomy may have been the intended treatment for known cancer or, more often, surgery was done for some benign condition and cancer was an unexpected finding. The prevalent impression that such patients have a poor prognosis regardless of what therapy is attempted is erroneous, although there is some logic to such beliefs. The inadequate resection may worsen prognosis because there is a greater risk of local recurrence due to contamination in the operative field with tumor cells. Postoperative irradiation therapy is less successful because the blood vessels to these areas are altered, the uterus as a container for radium is missing, and more distant lymph nodes develop metastases because the pathway of lymphatic drainage is disturbed.

Experience at the M. D. Anderson Hospital shows that patients who have had early stage carcinoma of the cervix and have no gross signs of cancer remaining after hysterectomy have excellent results when given postoperative radiotherapy promptly. Even if there is residual cancer at the apex of the vagina, there is a fair chance of a cure if aggressive radiotherapy is instituted. The prognosis is worsened considerably if treatment is delayed until recurrent carcinoma becomes obvious.

The treatment for these patients combines local vaginal irradiation with total pelvis external x-ray therapy. The methods for local irradiation are: vaginal radium colpostat, transvaginal x-ray therapy, and interstitial radium needles. For the smaller cancers vaginal radium alone accomplished adequate treatment. For the more advanced cancers total pelvic external therapy was the dominant treatment. Since the FIGO staging cannot depict the range of progression of the cervical cancer in such patients, another method uses the operative findings, examination of the uterine specimen, and the pelvic examination postoperatively. Patients are categorized according to the risk and amount of residual cancer present at clinical examination. The following categories are useful for planning treatment:

1. Minimal size cancers that are evident only upon microscopic examination of the specimen.

2 . Grossly evident cancer in the surgical specimen and the negative resection margins.

3. Cancer present at the excision margins of the cervix, but no gross residual cancer evident in the upper vagina or paracervical tissues postoperatively.

4. Grossly evident residual carcinoma or a recurrence of cancer established by clinical examination. These patients, who were further divided into subcategory 4A, received postoperative radiotherapy within six months and subcategory 4B had a delay of more than six months postoperatively before irradiation was begun. Reference to Table 2 shows a parallel increase between amount of cancer and extensity of irradiation. Like carcinoma of the cervix in the intact uterus, as the stage of the disease advances a greater portion of the total irradiation treatment is by external therapy. This necessitates a diminishing dose from the colpostats. The balance of radium and external dosage can be seen in Table 3, the three methods

of delivering irradiation in the left-hand column and the four systems of dosimetry in the four columns at the right.

Material and Methods

Of 148 patients treated at the M. D. Anderson Hospital,[2,5] 27 were Group I, 38 Group II, 15 Group III, 38 Group IV and 30 Group V. Of the 148 patients, 26% received at least 6000 rads whole pelvis; 63% had 5000 or more rads whole pelvis, 76% were given 4000 or more rads whole pelvis, and 22 patients no whole pelvis irradiation. This shows increased emphasis on whole pelvis irradiation for this type of treatment problem.

Results

The outcome of treatment was surprisingly favorable. When Groups I, II, and III were considered together, 71 of 80 (89%) were without evidence of disease at five years. In group IV, 18 of 38 patients (47%) and group V patients 11 of 30 (37%) there was no evidence of disease at five years. The overall survival of 100 out of 148 patients is 68%.

Table 2 Treatment Plan after Simple Hysterectomy for Invasive Cancer of the Cervix

Group Number	Treatment Plan
I	Local irradiation to the vaginal apex with vaginal radium in colpostats.
II	Whole pelvis[a] external x-ray to 3500–4000 rads followed by one 72 hr vaginal radium application or two 48 hr applications, 2 weeks apart.
III	Whole pelvis external x-ray to 5000 rads followed by one 72 hr vaginal radium application.
IV	(1) Whole pelvis alone. (2) Whole pelvis followed by transvaginal x-ray or vaginal radium.
V	(1) Whole pelvis alone. (2) Whole pelvis followed by transvaginal x-ray or vaginal radium.

[a] Whole pelvis x-ray portals are 15×15 cm square.

To evaluate these results the selection of patients for hysterectomy must be kept in mind. A bias toward a more favorable group of patients develops, since inadequate hysterectomy is probably performed for small

Table 3 Dosage Combinations of External X-Ray with Intracavitary or Transvaginal X-Ray after Simple Hysterectomy for Invasive Cancer of the Cervix

External x-ray (tumor dose)[a]	None	3500–4000	5000	6000
Radium colpostats (surface dose)[b]	48 hr–48 hr (8000–9000)	72 hr (5000–6000) or 48 hr–48 hr (7000–8000)	72 hr (5000–6000)	48 hr (4000)
Transvaginal x-ray (given dose)	6000	4000	3000–3500	2500 3000

[a] X-ray dose in rads.

[b] Radium dose in mg/hr.

cancers. The patients in the study were generally younger, which is a favorable factor for cure. Although these patients were treated successfully following inadequate hysterectomy, such treatment is still considered bad practice. To avoid this mistake in patients with abnormal vaginal bleeding apparently benign in origin (e.g., a myomatous uterus), the cause of bleeding should be investigated by dilatation and curettage and endocervical biopsy before operation. Occasionally, however, cancer of the cervix eludes preoperative search. After simple hysterectomy for invasive cancer of the cervix, postoperative irradiation therapy must be given promptly. For some patients the treatment serves as prophylaxis, for others as specific treatment; for each type early treatment is best. This treatment can be simple and safe for the small cancers. For the patients with small cancers that are not treated promptly and allowed to develop clinical evidence of cancer, conditions are more difficult. A pessimistic outlook on the part of the physician should not prevent treatment of patients with gross carcinoma after hysterectomy, for these patients are amenable to successful treatment.

SUMMARY

It would be erroneous to conclude from this study that the best management of carcinoma of the cervix is simple hysterectomy followed by postoperative radiotherapy, because the experiences of others have not been so successful. We continue to view treatment by inadequate hysterectomy as regrettable.[3,4,7]

REFERENCES

1. Adloy, E. S., and H. S. Goldsmith, *Surg. Gynecol. Obstet.*, **135**, 103–107 (1972).

2. Andras, Ellis J., Gilbert Fletcher, and Felix Rutledge, *Am. J. Obstet. Gynecol.* **115**, 647–655 (1973).

3. Barber, H. R., G. V. Pece, and Alexander Brunschwig, *Am. J. Obstet. Gynecol.* **101**, 959–965 (1968).

4. Cosbie, W. G., *Am. J. Obstet. Gynecol.* **85**, 3 (1963).

5. Durrance, F. Y., *Cancer of the Uterus and Ovary,* Year Book Medical Publishers, Chicago, Illinois, 1969.

6. Durrance, Fred Y., G. H. Fletcher, and F. N. Rutledge, *Am. J. Roentgenol.*, **106**, 831–838 (1969).

7. Green, T. H. J., and A. J. Morse, *Obstet. Gynecol.*, **33**, 763–769 (1969).

8. Morrow, Charles, *Recurrent Carcinoma of the Cervix,* M. D. Anderson Hospital, Houston, Texas, 1969.

9. Rutledge, Felix, and B. C. Burns, *Am. J. Obstet. Gynecol.*, **91**, 602–708 (1965).

CARCINOMA OF THE ENDOMETRIUM

CHAPTER 6 ENDOMETRIAL CANCER AND ENDOMETRIAL HYPERPLASIA

RICHARD C. BORONOW, M.D.

Adenocarcinoma of the endometrium is the most common gynecologic cancer. Generally speaking, it is successfully treated, with relatively unsophisticated techniques, yet there is controversy over the best management. Since the majority of these cancers occur in the postmenopausal patient, abnormal bleeding is an early sign and early diagnosis is the rule. Yet it is projected that 3000 to 4000 American women will die of the disease this year.

Endometrial hyperplasia will also be considered in this section. It presents a somewhat confusing picture both from the standpoint of pathologic interpretation and from the clinical implications of this diagnosis.

ENDOMETRIAL ADENOCARCINOMA

Controversies

1. What are the roles of the various diagnostic and screening techniques?
2. Is there a "best" management for endometrial cancer?
3. Is there any value in clinical staging?
4. Do progestins have a role in primary therapy?

The Patient

The majority of patients with endometrial adenocarcinoma (65 to 75%) will be postmenopausal. Most of the remaining patients are in the climacteric years. The disease is uncommon prior to age 40, and very rare prior to the age of 30. Some sort of unclarified endocrinopathy is believed to be operative because so many patients have certain phenotypic characteristics such as obesity, hypertension, diabetes, and a low fertility index. Frequent anovulation is suggested by a past history of irregular uterine bleeding, periods of amenorrhea, and late menarche (Figures 1, 2 and 3).

Patients who should be considered "at risk" for endometrial adenocarcinoma include those with postmenopausal bleeding, patients with the phenotype described above, and those with a history of polyps, endometrial hyperplasia, and endometrial cancer in the family.

Diagnostic Studies

SCREENING

No satisfactory screening method for endometrial cancer in the asymptomatic patient

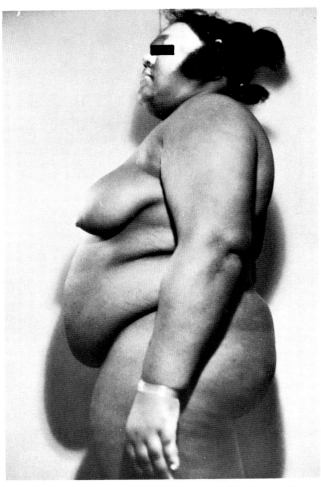

Figure 1 Phenotype of endometrial adenocarcinoma. This 27-year-old obese, nulliparous patient had irregular menses and anovulation and was confirmed to have Stein-Leventhal syndrome.

has been identified. Routine cervical cytology is not satisfactory, routine endometrial biopsy is unrewarding, and there are no solid, supportive data available on the jet washer or other intrauterine screening techniques.[1]

THE SYMPTOMATIC PATIENT

Cytology. Naib[2] reports that even in the presence of known endometrial adenocarcinoma the average cytologic detection rate by the cervical scrape method is only 15%; with vaginal pool and cervical scraping, 40%; with endocervical aspiration and vaginal pool 65%; and with intrauterine and endocervical aspiration and vaginal pool sample, still only 90%.

The jet washer. With an adequate sampling, endometrial cancer is usually found by this technique. Even in Gravlee's initial series, however, only 1084 of 1481 samples were suitable for study.[3] Although current reports are more favorable, the major issue is not evaluation of the symptomatic patient but a screening technique for asymptomatic patients.

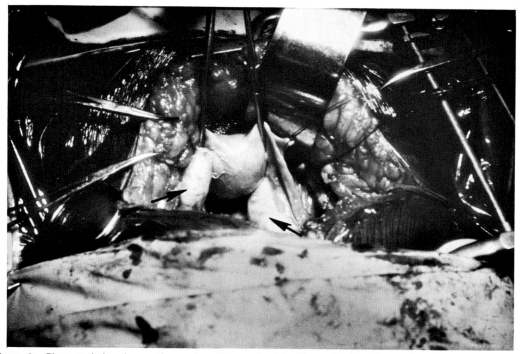

Figure 2 Characteristic sclerocystic ovaries of the patient in Figure 1. Note the moderately enlarged ovaries with smooth, firm cortex.

Endometrial biopsy. If positive, the diagnosis is made. If negative, fractional dilatation and curettage (D & C) is indicated. If this office procedure is done, the cervix and endocervix should be sampled. Hofmeister[4] reported finding endometrial cancer in 124 (0.7%) of 1666 routine office endometrial biopsies done over an 18-year period. However, only 25 (0.14%) of these cancers were unsuspected because of the asymptomatic state of the patient.

Fractional D & C. This is the procedure of choice for diagnosis as well as assessment of cervical involvement (International Stage II). If endometrial cancer is diagnosed by another technique, such as endometrial biopsy or jet washer, endocervical curettage with a Kevorkian curette can also be done on an outpatient basis. The impact on cure rate when corpus cancer invades the cervix is significant (Table 1).

Too often there is failure on the part of the patient or the physician to grasp the significance of postmenopausal bleeding or abnormal climacteric bleeding. Occasionally there is reliance on a normal Pap smear. Occasionally the patient attributes the abnormal bleeding to "change in life" and defers physician counsel. Occasionally the physician prescribes endocrine therapy or simply reassures the patient. And occasionally the abnormal bleeding is dealt with by primary hysterectomy without workup.

Behavior and Spread of Endometrial Cancer

LYMPHATIC DRAINAGE

There is a dual blood supply of the uterus with drainage of the lower uterine segment and cervix through the well-recognized paracervical (parametrial) drainage following the uterine veins and endopelvic fascial support (Figure 4).

The lymphatic drainage of the uterine

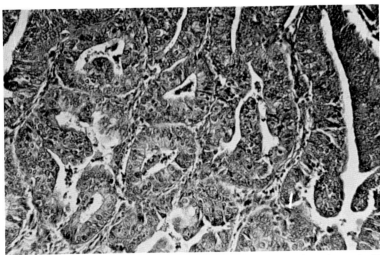

Figure 3 Photomicrograph of well-differentiated adenocarcinoma in the patient shown in Figure 1 (Grade I, FIGO G1).

body is primarily along the course of the ovarian vessels. The lymphatic channels are most evident in the deep myometrial tissue and the subserosal areas in association with larger vessels. Thus metastatic nodes from tumors in this area may be found along the aortic, caval, lumbar, and high common iliac lymph nodes.

Lymphatics, as venous return, anastomose with both systems, and tumors with deep myometrial invasion and lower segment involvement may have both spread patterns. Pelvic node involvement has been reemphasized by the current reports of Lewis et al.,[9] Homesley et al.,[6] and particularly the review by Morrow et al.[10]

The current FIGO staging system for endometrial cancer is given in Table 2.

HISTOLOGIC DIFFERENTIATION

There is a clear correlation between the Broders' grade of histologic differentiation and relative curability, even among Stage 1 tumors (Table 3). The well-differentiated lesions (Figure 3) tend to stay confined to

Table 1   Impact on Cure Rate When Corpus Cancer Involves the Cervix[a]

Clinical Stage	M. D. Anderson Hospital[5] (1948–1963)		Memorial Hospital[6] (1949–1965)	
	Number of Patients	5-Year Survival (%)	Number of Patients	5-Year Survival (%)
Stage I	270	77	539	74
Stage II				
Clinical	19	58	24	54
Biopsy	44	61	68[b]	57

[a] Reprinted, with permission, from reference 7.
[b] Actually Stage I cases with cervical spread determined by pathologist.

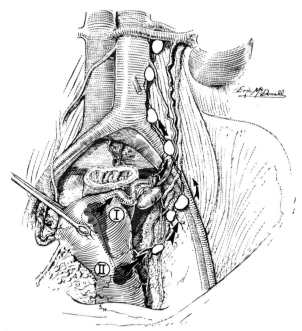

Figure 4 Dual lymphatics of the uterus. Stage I endometrial cancer (I) drains via the infundibulo-pelvic ligament, primarily to nodes of the pelvic brim and retroperitoneal adbominal nodes. Stage II endometrial cancer is extension to involve both corpus and cervix (II) and drains primarily via the paracervical lymphatics to the pelvic nodes. From Boronow, R.C.: Therapeutic considerations in endometrial cancer. *J. Miss. State. Med. Assoc.* **10**: 451, 1969. Reprinted with permission.

the endometrium or superficial myometrium and are highly curable. Those anaplastic tumors (Figure 5) tend to invade the muscle deeply and result in a relatively poor salvage rate even for Stage I. Tumors of an intermediate degree of differentiation (Figure 6) generally show moderate myometrial infiltration and have an intermediate cure rate (Table 4).

OTHER CELL TYPES

In addition to the more common adenocarcinomas of the endometrium, three additional variants are described: A clear-cell (mesonephric) carcinoma occurs rarely, therefore little is known about its biologic behavior. In addition, in a percentage of cases with adenocarcinoma that varies with the vigilance of the pathologist's search, an admixture of adenocarcinomatous elements

and histologically benign squamous metaplasia (or prosoplasia) are found. This lesion is commonly designated as adenoacanthoma (Figure 7). Although some have felt that these lesions represented a more benign cancer, most contemporary opinion suggests a similar stage-for-stage and grade-for-grade salvage with other endometrial adenocarcinomas (Table 5).

Occasionally the admixture is one of malignant glandular and squamous cancer and is designated *adenoepidermoid cancer* by Woodruff and Novak[11] or *adenosquamous cancer* by Ng and associates,[12] Silverberg et al.,[13] and others. Data suggest a more virulent biologic behavior of this mixed malignancy, although there is debate whether the aggressive behavior is due to the malignant squamous component or is caused by the preponderance of poorly differentiated adenomatous components of the tumor.

Table 2   Carcinoma of the Corpus Uteri, FIGO Staging Classification[a]

Stage 0

   Carcinoma in situ. Histological findings suspicious of malignancy. (Cases of Stage 0 should not be included in any therapeutic statistics.)

Stage I

   The carcinoma is confined to the corpus.
      Stage IA: The length of the uterine cavity is 8 cm or less.
      Stage IB: The length of the uterine cavity is >8 cm.
   Stage I cases should be subgrouped with regard to the histological type of the adenocarcinoma as follows;
         G 1: Highly differentiated adenomatous carcinomas.
         G 2: Differentiated adenomatous carcinoma with partly solid areas.
         G 3: Predominantly solid or entirely undifferentiated carcinomas.

Stage II

   The carcinoma has involved the corpus and the cervix.

Stage III

   The carcinoma has extended outside the uterus but not outside the true pelvis.

Stage IV

   The carcinoma has extended outside the true pelvis, or has obviously involved the mucosa of the bladder or rectum. A bullous edema, as such, does not permit allotment of a case to Stage IV.

[a] January, 1971.

PRETREATMENT ASSESSMENT

The purpose of the foregoing is to emphasize that an office endometrial biopsy of endometrial cancer or the same diagnosis obtained with a jet washer is insufficient for optimal treatment planning. A fractional D & C and multiple cervical biopsies should identify involvement of the cervix, with recognition of the second lymphatic spread

Table 3   Distribution and Survival of Stage I Endometrial Adenocarcinoma by FIGO Substages (377 Cases)[a, b]

Stage	Distribution (%)	5-Year Survival (%) Gross	Corrected
IA, Grade 1	5	94	94
IA, Grade 2	23	82	82
IA, Grade 3	11	66	71
IB, Grade 1	11	85	85
IB, Grade 2	38	70	75
IB, Grade 3	12	48	51
Total	100	72	77

[a] Reprinted, with permission, from reference 6.

[b] In Stage I, 377 patients out of 539 patients had sufficient data to substage (70% Stage I patients).

pathway. Pelvic examination under anesthesia may identify submucosal vaginal involvement or parameterial involvement. An understanding of the implications of both the histologic pattern and differentiation may influence therapy.

   The general physical examination, with assessment of neck and groin lymph nodes is mandatory. Chest X-ray is always indicated, an IVP is frequently indicated, and cytoscopy and proctoscopy are necessary in clinically advanced cases.

Therapy and Results

SURVIVAL DATA

In the "Annual Report on the Results of Treatment in Carcinoma of the Uterus, Ovary and Vagina," Volume 15, 1973, salvage rates are now reported by the four-stage FIGO (Table 2) staging system, although not within the substages of Stage I. Stage I five-year survival was 70.0% of 3025 cases treated; with other stages, survivals were 47.4% of Stage II, 28.0% of Stage III, and 4.7% of Stage IV (Table 6). These data represent the experience of 52

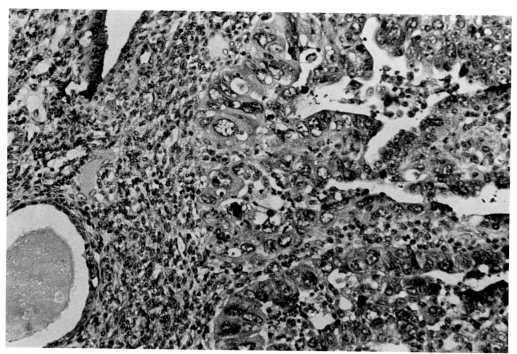

Figure 5 Poorly differentiated adenocarcinoma (Grade 3, or G3, FIGO). Note extreme pleomorphism, with some retention of glandular pattern. While grossly confined to the very suprficial myometrium, there was massive microscopic permeation of the full thickness of the uterine wall.

reporting institutions. Morrow et al.[10] have collected six large and current series (total cases, 2432) and report an average survival of 76% for Stage I; 51% for Stage II; 26% for Stage III; and 8.8% for Stage IV (Table 7).

Of interest in the light of salvage data by clinical stage is the report of del Regato and Chahbazian: an 83% 5-year cure rate in 56 consecutive cases without regard for clinical stage. Their treatment plan is external beam therapy to the entire pelvis[20] and, after an eight-week delay, hysterectomy. They feel that this treatment is suitable for all cases and question the value of staging. This report does not provide any information on the clinical extent of the cases treated. The current FIGO staging system (Table 2) incorporates both histologic differentiation and pretreatment clinical assessment of anatomic spread. We believe best results will be achieved by individualization of treatment utilizing this staging. Before discussing treatment plans for the various stages of cancer, several comments should be made regarding currently employed and available treatment modalities.

RADIATION THERAPY

Since it has long been known that radiation therapy alone could cure some patients with adenocarcinoma of the endometrium confined to the uterus, the biologic effectiveness of the method is well established. The extension of this observation is that preoperative radiation therapy followed by conservative hysterectomy might combine two effective modalities for a somewhat better cure rate than could be achieved with hys-

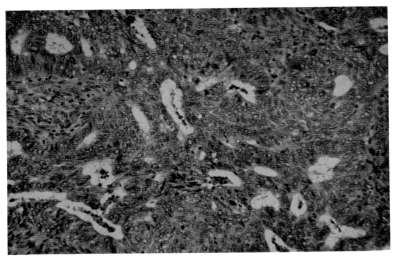

Figure 6 Intermediate degree of differentiation (Grade 2, or G2, FIGO). Glandular pattern and solid areas.

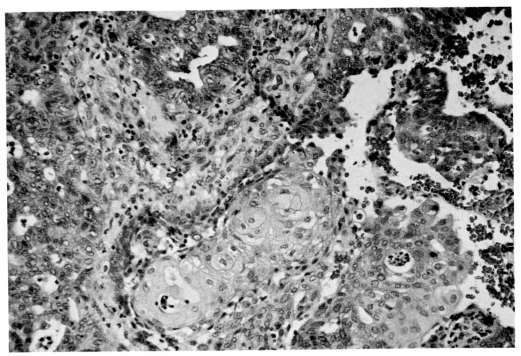

Figure 7 Endometrial adenoacanthoma: predominantly a pattern of poorly differentiated adenocarcinoma with several foci of a differentiated benign squamous component.

Table 4 Survival Related to Depth Invasion and Distribution of Depth Invasion by Histologic Grade of State I Endometrial Adenocarcinoma (539 Cases)[a]

Depth Invasion	Number of Patients	Corrected 5-Year Survival Rates (%)	Histologic Grade			
			G1	G2	G3	Not Recorded
None	100	90	33	31	5	31
Superficial	255	84	18	146	41	60
Deep	93	61	1	48	32	12
Serosal	12	9	—	—	8	4
Parametrial	18	22	1	9	3	5
Not recorded	37	58	2	7	11	17
Radiation therapy only[b]	24	46	1	5	3	15
Total	539	76	56	246	93	144

[a] Reprinted, with permission, from reference 6.
[b] Depth of penetration indeterminate.

Table 5 Comparative Survival of Patients with Stage I Adenocarcinoma and Adenoacanthoma by Modality of Treatment[a]

Modality	Adenocarcinoma		Adenoacanthoma	
	Number of Cases	5-Year Survival (%)	Number of Cases	5-Year Survival (%)
Surgery only	8	75	—	—
Preoperative radium	140	85	34	85
Postoperative radium	4	100	—	—
Postoperative x-ray	2	—	—	—
Pre- and postoperative radiation	3	100	1	100
Radium only	51	53	16	67
Radium and/or x-ray only	3	67	—	—
Preoperative x-ray and radium	4	50	—	—
Postoperative x-ray and radium	2	—	—	—
Preoperative radium and post-operative x-ray	2	—	—	—
Total[b]	219	76	51	79

[a] Reprinted, with permission, from reference 5.
[b] Total: 270 Cases, 77% five-year survival.

Table 6 FIGO Five-Year Survival Rate Calculated for Each of the Four Stages, 1962–1963[a]

	No. of Patients Treated	No. of Patients Alive	Survival Rate (%)
Stage I	3025	2116	70.0
Stage II	595	282	47.4
Stage III	428	120	28.0
Stage IV	149	7	4.7
Total	4197	2525	60.2

[a] Reprinted, with permission, from reference 14.

terectomy alone. However, hard data to prove this contention are lacking.

RADIUM THERAPY

Initially, uterine packing with radium was carried out. It then became apparent that a certain number of tumors recurred in the vaginal vault, and currently most centers utilizing preoperative radium therapy use both intrauterine and intravaginal radium (Figure 8).

EXTERNAL BEAM THERAPY

For more than 30 years there have been vocal proponents of whole pelvis external beam therapy as the preferred method of preoperative radiation therapy. In recent years more voices have been added to this chorus. The premise is that the uterus will be removed and a certain number of patients will develop vaginal as well as other pelvic recurrence; that there may be occult disease in the pelvis, beyond the uterus, that can be treated more effectively by external beam than by radium therapy; and, since the uterus itself will be removed, there is little need for preoperative radium.

SURGERY

It was obvious in earlier decades that patients treated by hysterectomy fared better than those treated by radium alone. Thus, every effort has been made to push operability to its maximum. Currently, conservative hysterectomy is the cornerstone for treatment of endometrial adenocarcinoma when confined to the body of the uterus.

RADICAL HYSTERECTOMY

This technique had its advocates in the past. When applied in a relatively unselective manner, no increase in salvage rate has been evident. Also, the patients are usually older, more obese, and more subject to a variety of medical problems than patients

Table 7 Five-Year Survival for Contemporary Endometrial Adenocarcinoma[a]

	Stage I		Stage II		Stage III		Stage IV		All Stages	
Author	No.	%	No.	%	No.	%	No.	%	No.	%
Wate et al. (1967)[15]	214	78	7	71	30	23	14	0	265	56
Boronow (1969)[5]	270	77	63	60	49	18	15	0	379	64
Kottmeier (1969)[16]	864	71	103	44	135	19	21	19	1123	61
Sall et al. (1970)[17]	243	87	10	50	11	64	43	9	307	68
Shah & Green (1972)[18]	99	72	15	60	5	40	3	33	122	67
Welander et al. (1972)[19]	170	86	7	43	24	58	17	6	218	75
Total	1860	76	205	51	245	26	113	8.8	2432	68
All cases (%)	76.5		8.4		10.4		4.6		100	

[a] Reprinted, with permission from reference 10.

with cervical cancer, and these medical and geriatric considerations increase the risks. When used selectively radical hysterectomy has a role in Stage II cases.

An outline of currently employed treatment plans is included in Table 8. The currently operative treatment plans at the M. D. Anderson Hospital and Tumor Institute are given in Tables 9, 10, 11 and 12.

PROGESTINS

A cooperative study coordinated by Lewis[22] has demonstrated no apparent benefit or harm from progestin given prior to hysterectomy in Stage I disease. Occasionally, a

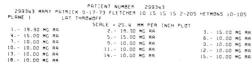

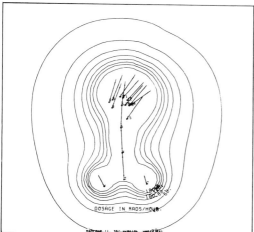

Figure 8 Computer printout of combined Heyman packing in the endometrial cavity with Fletcher-Suit tandem and ovoids in uterus and vaginal fornices. The isodose line of 150 rads/hr approximates the vaginal surface with 2.5 cm diameter vaginal spacers, passes through the proximal paracervical tissues and an area around the corpus that, by extrapolation between the printout and the clinical examination, would correspond to deep myometrium. Thus one leaves the system long enough to deliver a planned dose (i.e., 40 hours, 5000 rads, or 50 hours, 7500 rads, etc.).

patient will be medically unsuitable for hysterectomy or even anesthesia for suitable medium insertion. Under these circumstances high doses of progestin may be of value.

Table 8   A Summary of Contemporary Treatment Plans[a]

Stage I	(1) Uterus normal size for age and parity; and well-differentiated cancer. (FIGO Stage IAG1 and some IBG1).
	a) surgery alone or
	b) preoperative vaginal and uterine radium ([b]) or
	c) preoperative whole pelvis irradiation (c)
	(2) Uterus enlarged or tumor histology less than well differentiated (FIGO Stages IAG2, IAG3, IBG1, IBG2, IBG3).
	a) preoperative vaginal and uterine radium[b] or
	b) preoperative whole pelvis irration[c]
Stage II	(1) Subclinical cervical involvement
	a) uterine and vaginal radium as for Stage I, then hysterectomy or
	b) preoperative whole pelvis irradiation as for Stage I, then hysterectomy or
	c) primary radical hysterectomy and pelvic lymphadenectomy
	(2) Clinical cervical involvement
	a) treat with radium and external beam therapy as cervix cancer, then add conservative hysterectomy or
	b) radium and external beam therapy without hysterectomy or
	c) primary radical hysterectomy and pelvic lymphadenectomy
Stage III	Treat as cervical cancer of comparable clinical findings. Add hysterectomy rarely, only selectively.

[a] Reprinted, with permission, from reference 8.
[b] Vaginal radium, at least 6000 rads surface dose; uterine radium, at least 5000 mg/hr.
[c] 4500–5500 rads midplane dose.

Are There Other Alternatives for Better Primary Therapy?

The vast majority of endometrial cancer cases are diagnosed in the Stage I setting. Most institutions have settled into a standard therapy for Stage I and for other stages. With reasonably satisfactory salvage rates in the Stage I group, it is difficult to identify significant differences from one institution to another. Yet it is clear, even within clinical Stage I disease, that while most patients do well others do poorly. On balance, we may be complacent to accept an overall 75% cure rate. Recently several institutions have shown interest in a more carefully individualized treatment plan (Figure 9). This depends primarily on laparotomy and pathologic findings. This approach may be used effectively in cooperative investigation; until data are collected and studied, however, such plans are not to be recommended for general use.

ENDOMETRIAL HYPERPLASIA

Controversies

1. Is there serious clinical significance to this diagnosis?
2. How should the various types of hyperplasia be treated?

Many features of the histopathologic picture of endometrial hyperplasia have been recognized for decades. In recent years, the clinical implications of endometrial hyperplasia have been subjected to more critical scrutiny, and much data, mainly retrospective, have accumulated.[23-30] Some prospective studies that have emerged are of particular value.[27,31-37]

Certain analogies have been drawn between endometrial hyperplasia and cervical dysplasia. Pathologically both may represent slight to significant distortion and atypia. The course of each may reverse spontaneously or with treatment, may persist unchanged, or progress to a more significant lesion. A number of terminologies have been applied to both.

The histopathologic diagnosis of endometrial hyperplasia is no longer sufficient. There are varying histologic pictures of endometrial hyperplasia, and the type of hyperplasia identified, the age, history, and endocrine status of the patient are all important factors in the evaluation of each case.

What Is It?

The histopathologic picture of endometrial hyperplasia appears to result from sustained, unopposed estrogen stimulation. During the proliferative phase of the ovarian cycle the endometrium is characterized by mitotic activity both in glands and stroma, and these are recognized as the normal precursors of ovulation. If ovulation does not occur and there is no progesterone, the estrogen maintains continued proliferation of the gland and stromal elements. Particularly evident is glandular proliferation with increased numbers of glands, enlargement of glands and pseudostratification of nuclei. It appears that 3 to 6 months of anovulation are necessary to produce pathologic hyperplasia.

Thus from a histologic standpoint there are quantitative and qualitative changes in the glands, and in the absence of structural modifications of individual glands a diagnosis of hyperplasia is rarely permissible. Koss[38] notes two main changes: (1) An increase in the number of cell layers lining glands, two to three, and occasionally more. These cell nuclei may show hyperchromasia and prominent nucleoli. Irregularities of gland shape occasionally are accompanied by papillary proliferation. (2) Marked cystic dilatation of the hyperplastic glands.

It is important not to confuse cystic dilatation of endometrial glands within active nuclei in an atrophic postmenopausal endometrium. This cystic atrophy appears to arise by the same mechanism as cystic dilatation of endocervical glands (nabothian cysts) and is of no pathologic significance.

Table 9 Treatment of Adenocarcinoma of the Endometrium in Technically and Medically Operable Patients[a]

Clinical Situation[b]	Treatment to Uterus	Treatment to Vagina
Small uterus, well-differentiated tumor	Hysterectomy only	Wide vaginal cuff
Enlarged uterus (cavity <8 cm depth), well-differentiated tumor	Radium, one 72 hr tandem or 3,000–3,500 mg/hr with packing Hysterectomy	Colpostats, 7000 rads surface dose in one application
Enlarged uterus (cavity 8–10 cm depth), well-differentiated tumor	Radium, two applications of 2500 mg/hr, 3 wk apart Hysterectomy or 4000 rads whole pelvis irradiation and radium, one Heyman packing 2500 mg/hr and tandem or tandem alone, depending on volume of uterine cavity Hysterectomy	Colpostats, two applications of 4000 rads surface dose in one application after 4000 rads whole pelvis irradiation
Enlarged uterus (cavity greater than 10 cm depth) or anaplastic tumor	4000 rads whole pelvis irradiation and radium, one Heyman packing 2500 mg/hr and tandem or tandem alone, depending on volume of uterine cavity Hysterectomy	Colpostats, 4000 rads surface dose in one application

[a] Reprinted, with permission, from reference 21.
[b] The clinical assessment of uterize size is based on the depth and volume of the uterine cavity and estimation of the size of the fundus by pelvic examination.

Who Gets It?

The same group of patients considered at risk for endometrial adenocarcinoma seems to be those most likely to develop endometrial hyperplasia. It often occurs as women approach the climacteric years and anovulation becomes more frequent. But it may also develop in younger women with sustained anovulation following pregnancy, or anovulation independent of pregnancy, or in conjunction with the Stein-Leventhal sydrome. Or it may develop in conjunction with an estrogen-producing ovarian tumor (granulosa-theca-cell tumor).

What Does It Mean Clinically?

The significant clinical implications of the finding of endometrial hyperplasia depend on the morphologic picture of the hyperplasia, the age of the patient, and other factors previously mentioned. A variety of terms have been applied (Table 13). While an expedient interpretation would suggest that hyperplasia progresses from a cystic variety (Figure 10) through progressively more atypical grades of so-called glandular or adenomatous hyperplasia (Figure 11), through the most atypical (designated by some as carcinoma in situ, Figure 12),

Table 10 Treatment of Adenocarcinoma of the Endometrium in Technically Operable but Medically Inoperable Patients and in Technically Inoperable Patients[a]

Clinical Situation[b]	Treatment to Uterus	Treatment to Vagina
Small uterus, well-differentiated tumor	Tandem (20, 15, and 10 mg) two applications 72 hr each (6000 mg/hr)	Colpostats, two applications 4000 rads surface dose
Enlarged uterus (cavity <8 cm depth), well-differentiated tumor	Heyman packing, two applications 3000 mg/hr or three applications 2500 mg/hr	Colpostats, two applications 4000 rads surface dose
Enlarged uterus (cavity 8–10 cm depth) or anaplastic tumor	External irradiation, 4000 rads whole pelvis Heyman packing or tandem applications, 3500–4000 mg/hr	Colpostats, 4000 rads surface dose
Enlarged uterus (cavity > 10 cm depth) or anaplastic tumor	External irradiation, 4000–6000 rads whole pelvis May add one or two radium applications, depending on response	Colpostats, 4000 rads surface dose if whole pelvis irradiation stopped at 5000 rads
Technically inoperable	External irradiation 4000 rads/4 wk to 6000 rads/6 wk May add radium applications(s) if response to external therapy is satisfactory	Surface dose 2500–4000 rads, depending on amount of external irradiation

[a] Reprinted, with permission, from reference 21.
[b] The clinical assessment of uterine size is based on the depth and volume of the uterine cavtiy and estimation of the size of the fundus by pelvic examination.

Table 11 Adenocarcinoma of the Corpus and Cervix[a]

Clinical Situation	Treatment
Small or normal size uterine cavity	Tandem and colpostats, 72 hr and 48 hr, 2 wk apart Parametrial irradiation Hysterectomy, after 4–6 wk
Enlarged uterine cavity; no extension beyond uterus or cervix	4000 rads whole pelvis irradiation Tandem and colpostats, 72 hr Hysterectomy, after 4-6 wk If medically inoperable, 4000 rads whole pelvis irradiation. Tandem and colpostats, two applications 48 hr each, 3 wk apart. May use Heyman capsules in addition to tandem if uterine cavity is large.
Extension beyond uterus and cervix	4000–6000 rads whole pelvis irradiation. Heyman packing or tandem and colpostats, 3500–4000 mg/hr to uterus, 4000 rads surface dose to vagina

[a] Reprinted, with permission, from reference 21.

and then to invasive adenocarcinoma of the endometrium, this progression is by no means uniform and inevitable. A study by Hark and Sommers[41] of 500 consecutive curettements showed that a single curettage produced relief of irregular uterine bleeding in 70% of women, whether the histologic picture was slight or cystic or adenomatous endometrial hyperplasia: 7% required a second curettage, 16% came to hysterectomy, and none of the cases followed were known to have developed endometrial cancer.

A variety of concurrent, retrospective, and prospective studies have been reported in the literature. In a number of retrospective studies where D & C material from patients who ultimately developed adenocarcinoma of the endometrium was available for study, many patients (61 of 88 cases[30]) were found to have had varying degrees of hyperplasia. Somners[42] believes that cystic hyperplasia is a more remote antecedent and occurs eight to ten years before the development of cancer; that adenomatous hyperplasia is a more recent precursor and is found three to six years before the cancer. The age-incidence data of Gusberg and Kaplan[36] for adenomatous hyperplasia suggests that its peak years are a decade or less before the peak years of endometrial cancer.

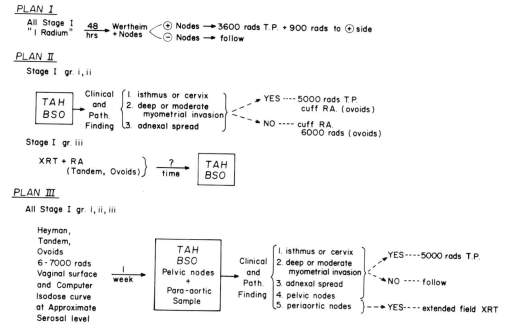

Figure 9 Current pilot study programs for endometrial cancer management. Plan I (Oxford, England): applies radical surgery after preoperative radium and supplements postoperative external beam therapy if posivite nodal metastases are found. Plan II (University of Southern California): employs primary surgery to all but Stage I, Grade III tumors, and bases postoperative external beam therapy upon the findings. Grade III lesions have vaginal radium and external beam therapy postoperatively. Plan III (University of Mississippi): utilizes the theoretical advantages of preoperative radium (see Figure 8) for all cases. Then surgery is carried out within a week to retain histopathologic identity of the irradiated neoplasm. When patients are suitable candidates for nodal surgery, this is done (the parametrium and ureter are undisturbed). Adjunctive external beam therapy is added as noted. Maximum therapeutic and clinical-pathologic data are thus obtained. From Boronow, R. C.: A fresh look at corpus cancer management. *Obstet. Gynecol.* **42**: 448, 1973. Reprinted with permission.

Table 12   Postoperative Irradiation for Adenocarcinoma of the Endometrium[a]

Clinical Situation	Whole Pelvis Irradiation	Vagina
Normal size uterus with well-differentiated, superficial tumor	None	None
Normal size uterus with well-differentiated tumor, limited myometrial invasion	None	Colpostats, 7000 rads surface dose in one application
Enlarged uterus, deep myometrial invasion, anaplastic tumor, residual disease, cervix involvement	5000 rads/5 wk up to 7000 rads[b]/7 wk	Colpostats, 4000 rads surface dose if external irradiation stopped at 5000 rads

[a] Reprinted, with permission, from reference 21.
[b] Reduced fields after 5000 rads.

From available data it appears that endometrial cancer follows cystic hyperplasia in 1 to 2% of cases, and adenomatous hyperplasia in 5 to 15% of cases. Sommers[42] cautions: ". . . while cystic and adenomatous hyperplasia in some women may represent way stations on the route to endometrial carcinoma, in over 85% of these women the endometrium ceases growing at some point and goes no further. After a single curettage the majority are usually incapable of redeveloping either hyperplasia, dysplasia or carcinoma."

Further, the data of Wagner and co-workers[43] challenge any rigid prognostication based on recognized morphologic patterns. Using an indirect method of studying the DNA content of cells in normal tissue relationships (Feulgen-staining for DNA and estimating dye-binding by cytophotometry) they evaluated 16 presumed precursors of endometrial cancer: 6 cystic glandular hyperplasias, 10 adenomatous hyperplasias, and 6 endometrial adenocarcinomas. An aneuploid distribution was found in all of the cancers, and a diploid to tetraploid dis-

Table 13   The Variety of Descriptive Terms for Endometrical Hyperplasia

Source 1[11]	Source 2[29]	Source 3[39]	Source 4[40]	Source 5[35]
Genuine hyperplasia (Swiss-cheese pattern)	Cystic proliferative	Cystic	Cystic	Benign
Proliferative and pseudo-malignant types (include atypical and adenomatous)	Glandular	Adenomatous Grade I	Adenomatous	Atypical, Type 1
	Granular, with atypical epithelial proliferation	Adenomatous Grade II	Anaplasia	Atypical, Type 2
		Adenomatous Grade III (anaplasia and carcinoma in situ)	Carcinoma in situ	Atypical, Type 3

tribution was found in all of the cystic hyperplasias, but the results with the adenomatous hyperplasias varied: 2 were aneuploid and 8 were diploid to tetraploid.

How Does One Treat It?

The first step in therapy will be thorough fractional curettage. This will provide material for diagnosis and will suffice as treatment in many instances.

If the diagnosis is cystic hyperplasia, regardless of the patient age group, observation is probably suitable therapy for most cases. Recurrence of abnormal bleeding, however, demands complete reevaluation.

Adenomatous hyperplasia carries more serious connotations, particularly if the patient is postmenopausal or in the climacteric years or if histologic atypia is evident. This finding in a younger age group also implies some serious risk, as is shown in the work of Chamlin and Taylor[37]: 14% of 97 young women with adenomatous endometrial hyperplasia followed for 1 to 14 years developed cancer.

It is important that these young women either ovulate, are treated by estrogen-progestin medications given cyclically, or have progestin added to the second half of each cycle to oppose the sustained effects of estrogen. One well-accepted management scheme[44] is included in Table 14.

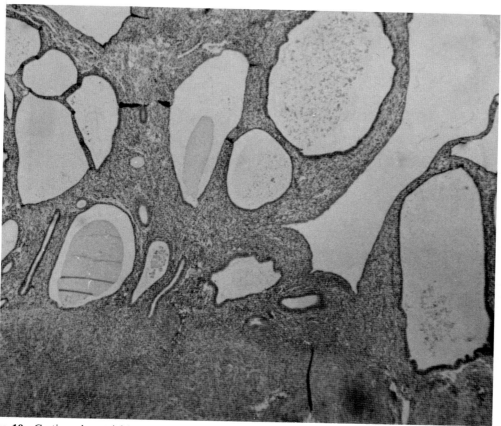

Figure 10 Cystic endometrial hyperplasia.

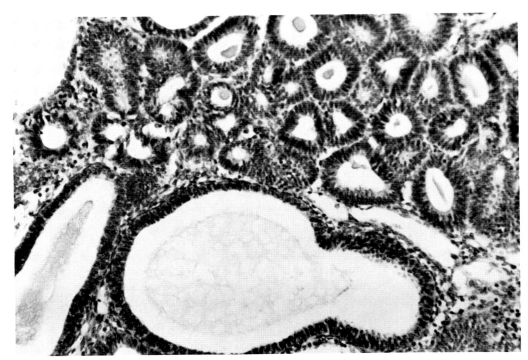

Figure 11 Adenomatous hyperplasia. Crowded glandular pattern with hyperchromatism but preservation of cellular polairty, nuclear uniformity, and minimal atypia.

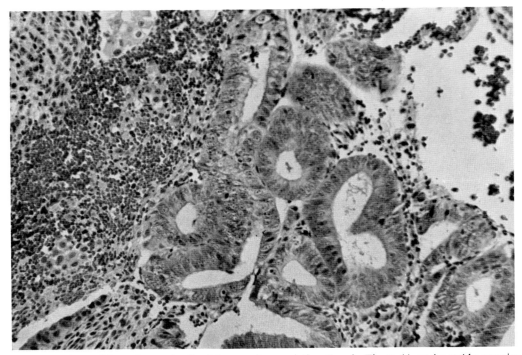

Figure 12 Endometrial carcinoma in situ. More nuclear variation than in Figure 11, and notably prominent nucleoli.

Table 14 Management for Endometrial Hyperplasma and Carcinoma In Situ[a]

Age Group	Treatment Plan
Postpubescent	Estrogen-progestin artificial cycles for 6 months; secure ovulation.
Childbearing	1. Secure ovulation-cortisone, clomiphene, or wedge resection of ovaries, or 2. Estogen-progestin artificial cycles until age 50–52.
Premenopausal	1. Estrogen-progestin artificial cycles until age 50–52. 2. Hysterectomy in uncontrolled cases.
Postmenopausal	1. Hysterectomy. 2. If inoperable, constant in-intramuscular progestins (Depo-Provera or Delalutin) for one year.

[a] Reprinted, with permission, from reference 44.

REFERENCES

1. Anderson, D: Cytologic diagnosis of endometrial carcinoma. *Am. J. Obstet. Gynecol.* In press.
2. Naib, A. M.: *Exfoliative Cytology*, Little, Brown and Company, Boston, 1970.
3. Gravelee, L. C., Jr.: Jet-irrigation method for the diagnosis of endometrial adenocarcinoma. *Obstet. Gynecol.* **34:** 168 (1969).
4. Hofmeister, F. J.: Office endometrial biopsy. Proceedings of the Fifth World Congress of Gynecology and Obstetrics, 1967, p. 683.
5. Boronow, R. C.: Carcinoma of the corpus: Treatment at M. D. Anderson Hospital. In *Cancer of the Uterus and Ovary*, Year Book Publishers, Chicago, 1969.
6. Homesley, H. O., R. C. Boronow, and J. L. Lewis, Jr.: Treatment of adenocarcinoma of the endometrium at Memorial-James Ewing Hospitals, 1949–1965, *Obstet. Gynecol.* In press.
7. Boronow, R. C.: Editorial: A fresh look at corpus cancer management. *Obstet. Gynecol.* **42:** 448 (1973).
8. Boronow, R. C.: Therapeutic considerations in endometrial cancer. *J. Miss. State Med. Assoc.* **10:** 451 (1969).
9. Lewis, B. V., J. A. Stallworthy, and R. Cowdell: Adenocarcinoma of the body of the uterus. *J. Obstet. Gynaecol. Brit. Commonw.* **77:** 343 (1970).
10. Morrow, C. P., P. J. DiSaia, and D. E. Townsend: Current management of endometrial carcinoma. *Obstet. Gynecol.* **42:** 399 (1973).
11. Novak, E. R., and J. D Woodruff: *Novak's Gynecologic and Obstetric Pathology, with Clinical and Endocrine Relations*, 7th edit., W. B. Saunders Company, Philadelphia, 1974.
12 Ng, A. B. P., J. W. Reagan, J. P. Storassli, and W. B. Wentz: Mixed adenosquamous carcinoma of the endometrium. *Am. J. Clin. Pathol.* **59:** 765 (1973).
13. Silverberg, S. B., M. G. Bolin, and L. S. DeGiorgi: Adenoacanthoma and mixed adenosquamous carcinoma of the endometrium: a clinico-pathologic study. *Cancer* **30:** 1307 (1972).
14. Kottmeier, H. L., Ed.: *Annual Report on the Results of Treatment in Carcinoma of the Uterus, Vagina and Ovary*, Vol. 15, International Federation of Gynecology and Obstetrics, Stockholm, Sweden, 1973.
15. Wade, M. E., E. I. Kohorn, and J. M. L. Morris: Adenocarcinoma of the endometrium. *Am. J. Obstet. Gynecol.* **99:** 869 (1967).
16. Kottmeier, H. L.: Individualization of therapy in carcinoma of the corpus. In *Cancer of the Uterus and Ovary*, Chicago, Year Book Medical Publishers, 1969, pp. 102–108.
17. Sall, S., B. Sonnenblick, and M. L. Stone: Factors affecting survival of patients with endometrial carcinoma. *Am. J. Obstet. Gynecol.* **107:** 116 (1970).
18. Shah, C. A., and T. H. Green: Evaluation of current management of endometrial carcinoma. *Obstet. Gynecol* **39:** 500 (1972).
19. Welander, C., M. L. Griem, and M. Newton: Staging and treatment of endometrial carcinoma. *J. Rep. Med.* 8:41 (1972).
20. del Regato, J. A., and C. M. Chahbazian: External pelvic irradiation as a preoperative surgical adjuvant in treatment of carcinoma of the endometrium. *Am. J. Roentgenol* **114:** 106 (1972).
21. Wharton, J. T., J. P. Smith, L. Delclos, and G. H. Fletcher: Irradiation therapy for gynecologic malignancies. In *Davis' Gynecology and Obstetrics*, Harper & Row, Hagerstown, Maryland, 1972.
22. Lewis, G. C., S. H. Nadler, I. D. J. Bros, and N. H. Slack: Adjuvant chemotherapy of cancer of the corpus uteri. *Obstet. Gynecol.* **29:** 797 (1967).

23. Taylor, H. C., Jr.: Endometrial hyperplasia and carcinoma of the body of the uterus. *Am. J. Obstet. Gynecol.* **23:** 309 (1932).

24. Hertig, A. T., and S. C. Sommers: Genesis of endometrial carcinoma: Study of prior biopsies. *Cancer* **2:** 946 (1949).

25. Hertig, A. T., S. C. Sommers, and H. Bengloff: Genesis of endometrial carcinoma; carcinoma in situ. *Cancer* **2:** 964 (1949).

26. Speert, H.: Premalignant phase of endometrial cancer. *Cancer* **5:** 927 (1952).

27. Telinde, R. W., H. W. Jones, and G. A. Galvin: What are the earliest endometrial changes to justify a diagnosis of endometrial cancer? *Am. J. Obstet. Gynecol.* **66:** 953 (1953).

28. Hall, K. V.: Irregular hyperplasia of the endometrium. *Acta Obstet. Gynecol. Scand.* **36:** 306 (1957).

29. Beutler, H. K., M. B. Dockerty, and L. M. Randall: Precancerous lesions of the endometrium. *Am. J. Obstet. Gynecol.* **86:** 433 (1963).

30. Foster, L. N., and R. Montgomery: Endometrial carcinoma; a review of prior biopsies. *Am. J. Clin. Pathol.* **43:** 26 (1965).

31. Payne, E. L.: Clinical significance of endometrial hyperplasia. *Am. J. Obstet. Gynecol.* **34:** 762 (1937).

32. Corscaden, J. A., J. W. Fertig, and S. B. Gusberg: Carcinoma subsequent to radiotherapeutic menopause. *Am. J. Obstet. Gynecol.* **51:** 1 (1946).

33. Kucera, F. Zur histogenese des korpus karzinom. (Histogenesis of carcinoma of the uterine body.) *Zentralbl. Gynakol.* **79:** 347 (1957).

34. Copenhaver, E. H.: Atypical endometrial hyperplasia. *Obstet. Gynecol.* **13:** 264 (1959).

35. Campbell, P. E., and R. A. Barter: The significance of atypical endometrial hyperplasia. *J. Obstet. Gynaecol. Brit. Commonw.* **68:** 668 (1961).

36. Gusberg, S. B., and A. L. Kaplan: Precursors of corpus cancer. *Am. J. Obstet. Gynecol.* **87:** 659 (1963).

37. Chamlin, D. L., and H. B. Taylor: Endometrial hyperplasia in young women. *Obstet. Gynecol.* **36:** 659 (1970).

38. Koss, L. G.: *Diagnostic Cytology and Its Histopathologic Basis,* 2nd Edit., Philadelphia, J. B. Lippincott, 1968.

39. Gusberg, S. B., and D. G. McKay: Malignant lesions of the cervix and corpus uteri. In *Textbook of Obstetrics and Gynecology,* 2nd Edit., Danforth, D. N., Ed., Harper & Row, New York, 1971.

40. Gore, H., and A. T. Hertig: Carcinoma in situ of the endometrium. *Am. J. Obstet. Gynecol.* **94:** 134 (1966).

41. Hark, B., and S. C. Sommers: Endometrial curettage in diagnosis and therapy. *Obstet. Gynecol.* **21:** 636 (1963).

42. Sommers, S. C.: The significance of endometrial hyperplasia and its early diagnosis. In *Gynecologic Oncology,* Barber, H. R. K., and Graber, E. A., Eds., Williams and Wilkins Company, 1970.

43. Wagner, D., R. M. Richart, and J. Y. Terner: Deoxyribonucleic acid content of presumed precursors of endometrial carcinoma. *Cancer* **20:** 2067 (1967).

44. Kistner, R. W.: The effects of progestational agents on hyperplasia and carcinoma in situ of the endometrium. In *Gynecologic Oncology,* Barber, H. R. K., and Graber, E. A. Eds. Williams and Wilkins Company, 1970.

CHAPTER 7

MANAGEMENT OF RECURRENT ENDOMETRIAL CANCER

RICHARD C. BORONOW, M.D.

CONTROVERSIES

1. Surgery vs. radiation therapy for local recurrence.
2. Is there a place for pelvic exenteration?
3. Is one progestin better than another?
4. Are other chemotherapeutic agents of value?

Approximately 90% of patients who will die of endometrical cancer will do so within the first five years posttreatment (Table 1). All recurrences of endometrial cancer pose difficult treatment problems.

Table 1 Cumulative Percentage of Deaths from Cancer at One, Three, and Five Years Among Patients Treated Completely at M. D. Anderson Hospital[a]

Stage	Total Number	Deaths from Cancer Percent Dead (Yr) 1	3	5
I	35	34	83	89
II	11	—	64	82
III	37	49	95	97
IV	12	75	100	100
All cases	95	41	87	93

[a] Reprinted, with permission, from reference 1.

ANATOMIC DATA

Necropsy Experience and Sites of Recurrence

The 1949 autopsy material of Henriksen[2] documented the dual lymphatic spread patterns of endometrial cancer (see Chapter 6, Figure 4). Pelvic drainage, primarily by way of the cardinal ligament, and extrapelvic drainage, by way of the ovarian vessels, tend to produce dissemination that is often reflected both in pelvic and extrapelvic disease. The more recent study of Beck and Latour[3] supports these observations (Table 2).

While these are necropsy data, a somewhat similar pattern is evident when recurrence is first noted. The variety of anatomic sites of an earlier, as well as a more contemporary series of recurrences, are seen in Table 3. As noted in this table, all stages of disease are included and pelvic recurrences predominate.

During the last two decades there has been a decrease in vaginal and central pelvic failure by the increased utilization of pretreatment radiation therapy in Stage I disease. In contemporary experience most clinical recurrence of Stage I disease is extrapelvic. The question of possible further reduction of both pelvic and extrapelvic failures by more

Table 2 Endometrial Cancer Necrospy Data

	Series 1[2]	Series 2[3]
Lymph node involvement	10 cases	36 cases
Mediastinal nodes	—	8.3%
Distant metastases	40%	—
Aortic	40%	61.2%
Common iliac	40%	—[a]
Sacral	30%	—[a]
External iliac	30%	—[a]
Obturator	20%	—[a]
Inguinal	30%	2.8%
Parametrial nodes	10%	—
Parametrium	30%	61.2%
Pelvic nodes	—	58.4%
Distant metastases	64 cases	36 cases
Lungs	30.2%	19.4%
Liver	28.5%	39.0%
Peritoneum	27.0%	66.7% (pelvic)
Ovary	14.2%	47.3% (and tubes)
Bowel, large	9.5%	33.2% (bowel)
Bowel, small	1.5%	
Pleura	7.9%	—
Adrenal	7.9%	2.8%
Bones	7.6%	8.3%
Kidney	—	2.8%
Spleen	—	2.8%

[a] The Series 2 percentage for pelvic nodes includes common iliac, sacral, external iliac, and obdurator involvement, whereas in Series 1 percentages are specifically identified.

customized and, in selected instances, more vigorous primary therapy, was posed rhetorically in the final section of the previous chapter on endometrial cancer.

Influence of Initial Anatomc and Histologic Features

The influence of both anatomic extent of the initial cancer and loss of differentiation of the histologic picture is very real. Finn[4] thoroughly documented this nearly a quarter of a century ago (Tables 4 and 5). One sees unfavorable prognostic features clearly. Conversely, however, the so-called favor-

able prognostic findings do not assure complete success. As noted in these tables, even when confined to the endometrium or superficial myometrium approximately 9% of these lesions recurred, and among the well-differentiated histologic pattern 8% recurred. Table 6 records 124 cases of recurrence studied by Dede, Plentl, and Moore.[5] Well-differentiated lesions accounted for 31.4%, and only superficial myometrial invasion for 23%. Similarly, in the necropsy study of Beck and Latour,[3] 77.8% of the patients studied had deep myometrial invasion or penetration; however 13.9% (5 cases) had only superficial invasion, and

Table 3 Anatomic Sites of Recurrent Endometrial Cancer

	1950 Series[4]	1968 Series[5]
Number of cases	46	124
Number of recurrent sites	102	233
	Percent	Percent
Genital	35	—[a]
Vagina	14	21
Pelvic cavity	11	—[a]
Ovary	3	—[a]
Rectovaginal septum or rectosigmoid	3	7
Cervix or uterus	2	8
Vulva	1	—[a]
Clitoris	1	—[a]
Parametrium	—	20
Other pelvic sites[a]	—	15
Urinary	12	Not specified
Ureter	7	
Bladder	4	
Urethra	1	
Lymph nodes	10	Not specified
Iliac	2	
Aortic	2	
Inguinal	2	
Clavicular	3	
Mediastinal	1	
Abdominal	19	13
Peritoneal	7	
Omentum	3	
Bowel	3	
Liver	4	
Diaphragm	1	
Adrenal	1	
Chest	15	8
Lungs	11	
Pleura	4	
Bone	6	5
Vertebrae	4	
Rib	1	
Cuboid/metatarsals	1	
Surface	5	Not specified
Abdominal wall	4	
Breast	1	
Head and neck	Not specified	2

[a] The percentage for other pelvic sites in the 1968 series includes pelvic cavity, ovary, clitoris, and parametrium recurrences.

Table 4 Influence of Anatomical Extent of Endometrical Carcinoma on Recurrence[4]

Extent	Number	Recurrence	Percent	Average Time from Treatment to Recurrence (years)
Confined to endometrium	111	10	9	2.2
Penetration of superficial myometrium	59	5	8.5	3.6
Penetration of deep myometrium	29	8	27	1.7
Involvement of pelvic organs or nodes	38	8	21	1.1
Extrapelvic involvement	29	18	62	0.5
Total	266	49		

Table 5 Influence of Histological Grade of Endometrial Carcinoma on Recurrence[4]

Grade	Number	Recurrence	Percent	Average Time from Treatment to Recurrence (years)
Differentiated	153	12	8	2.3
Intermediate	52	10	20	2.3
Undifferentiated	61	27	44	1.0
Total	266	49		

8.3% (3 cases) were cancers confined to polyps!

Most investigators have observed that the more anaplastic cancers tend to recur earlier, and these recurrences are more difficult to control than those associated with well-differentiated lesions.

Follow-up Routine

Our method of following patients after treatment involves a thorough system review and careful physical examination each three months for the first two years; each four months for the next two years, at six-month intervals during the fifth year, and yearly thereafter. Pap smears are obtained. The physical examination pays particular attention to neck and groin nodes, careful

palpation for abdominal masses, and a meticulous pelvic examination with attention to the suburethral area, the entire vaginal length, and a rectovaginal examination to

Table 6 Histopathologic Features of Recurrent Endometrial Cancer[5]

	Percent
Histologic differentiation	
Well differentiated	31.4
Poorly differentiated	21.8
Undifferentiated	7.3
Unclassified	34.7
Adenoacanthoma	4.8
Depth of invasion	
Not recorded	38
Superficial	23
Deep	39

carefully assess the vaginal cuff, the paracervical tissues, and the pelvic side-walls. Yearly chest X-rays are obtained, and if there are symptoms and findings that suggest reactive disease, appropriate further diagnostic studies are carried out. Although it is recognized that cancers that recur early tend to have a more virulent biologic course than those that recur late, it still must be considered axiomatic for the clinician that the best second chance is when the recurrent disease is found at the earliest possible moment.

THE PROBLEM OF TREATMENT

The clinical dilemma is illustrated by a fairly comparable experience in the two series shown in Table 3, despite 18 years separating publication dates. In Finn's 46 cases of persistent and recurrent cancer, 27 were not treated: the pelvic disease was considered too advanced in 15 instances, and there was extrapelvic metastasis present in the other 12 cases. Of the 9 patients treated by radiation because their disease was felt to be sufficiently localized (2 in the vaginal vault, 7 with vaginal and pelvic cancer), none were cured. Of 10 patients treated by surgery, 3 had laparotomy only, 2 had palliative surgery, and 5 had definitive surgery; 4 of the latter survived. Thus 4 of 46 (8.7%) patients were salvaged. The more recent experience of Dede et al.[5] is shown graphically in Figure 1. Of 124 patients with recurrence, there were 12 (9.7%) apparent cures.

Thus, although most therapy for recurrent endometrial cancer, just as most therapy of any recurrent cancer, is of a palliative nature, an occasional patient will be a candidate for a curative effort. Selection of secondary therapy depends in large measure upon the location and extent of disease, the training and experience of the clinician, and

the clinical supportive facilities available. Other factors in management of recurrence include whether or not radium or external beam radiation therapy have been previously employed. This is particularly applicable in the case of vaginal or pelvic recurrence. If radiotherapy tissue tolerance has been expended, one must consider surgery or chemotherapy; If tissue tolerance has not been expended, it is appropriate to consider radiotherapy. Finally, any treatment must be individualized for the general condition of the patient.

Pelvic Recurrence

The literature seems preoccupied with the subject of vaginal recurrence. Two reasons are apparent (1) Preoperative radiation therapy will reduce vaginal recurrences, and numerous retrospective and prospective reports were necessary first to postulate this possibility, and then to document it, (2) Isolated vaginal recurrences account for the vast majority of patients whose recurrent endometrial cancer is cured. But with more vigorous primary therapy, the isolated vaginal recurrence—the most curable of recurrences—is becoming more infrequent. Often when vaginal recurrences are observed, there is palpable pelvic recurrence as well and/or clinical or radiographic evidence of dissemination.

In those cases with recurrence clinically confined to the pelvis, the first priority is a careful search for other metastatic disease. If the extensive workup is completed with no evidence of extrapelvic spread, one then considers the following questions:

1. Should surgery or radiation be used for local recurrence?

2. If surgery is selected, how extensive should it be? Should one consider pelvic exenteration?

3. If radiation therapy is used, what kind of treatment plan seems optimal?

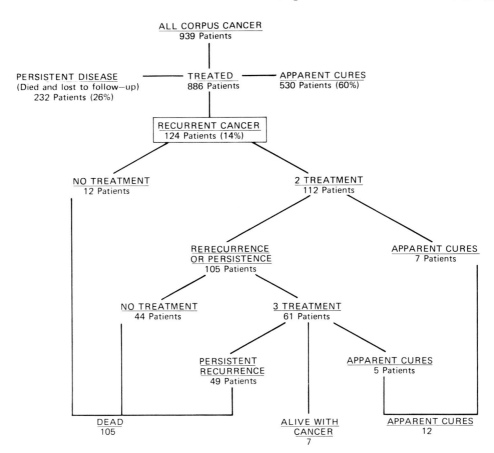

Figure 1 Summary of the morbidity of 124 patients with recurrent endometrial carcinoma. The percentages in brackets refer to treated patients. Apparent cures include patients who died of other causes 5 or more years after therapy, without evidence of disease at autopsy. From Dede, J. A., A. A. Plentl and J. G. Moore: Recurrent endometrial carcinoma. *Surg. Gynecol. Obstet.* **126**: 533 (1968). Reprinted by permission.

APPARENT PURE PELVIC RECURRENCE

Most pelvic recurrence is relatively extensive, and radiation therapy is usually employed. This is precluded, however, if whole pelvis external beam therapy has been used as part of primary treatment (e.g., 4000 or 5000 rads whole pelvis therapy followed by conservative hysterectomy). If it has not, 5000 rads whole pelvis therapy (15 × 15 cm portals), followed by an additional 1000 or 2000 rads to progressively smaller portals (12 cm × 12 cm, 10 cm × 10 cm, or 8 cm × 8 cm) centered

over the bulk of the residual disease may provide some control if the disease is localized. Lymphangiography may be helpful in assessing the pelvic and aortic nodes. Data are not available regarding preirradiation staging laparotomy.

THE ROLE OF PELVIC EXENTERATION

Smaller central disease will occasionally introduce the possibility of surgical resection. Barber and Brunschwig[6] evaluated 36 patients treated by pelvic exenteration, and 13.8% achieved a five-year cure: 14 cases were treated by anterior exenteration and 22 had total exenteration. Of 7 patients operated on within one year of primary treatment, there were no survivors. Of 11 patien (30.6%) who had positive nodes (site not specified), only 1 achieved a five-year cure. Of 4 patietns who had disease involving the small bowel, none survived. There was a complication rate of 61%, a secondary operation rate of 26% (10 patients), and 6 of the 10 patients required more than one additional operation. The associated medical and geriatric problems of patients with endometrial cancer further support the limited role for pelvic exenteration for recurrence of this disease.

The Barber-Brunschwig study does not mention the denominator from which the numerator (36 operations) was drawn; that is, how many patients were explored for exenteration and found nonresectable? Such information would be of interest because extrapelvic spread and pelvic peritoneal spread doom both radical surgery and heavy pelvic irradiation.

Occasionally a sizable bulk of tumor may be resected with preservation, or partial visceral resection and reconstruction, of bladder and rectum, and whole pelvis radiation therapy can follow, provided extrapelvic spread is not found at laparotomy.

Unfortunately in many patients with extensive pelvic recurrence, there is usually metastatic disease in both the pelvic and aortic nodes and definitive treatment is virtually impossible. Occasionally, however, a treatment plan may be customized, with extended field radiation, for example.

APPARENT PURE VAGINAL RECURRENCE

In vaginal recurrence, treatment depends on the extent and location of the recurrence. In the isolated "vaginal cuff" recurrence we generally favor radiation therapy either by needle implant or, if fairly superficial, with vaginal ovoids. Usually this will be supplemented by external beam therapy to the entire field—whole pelvis—of potential metastatic disease. The dose should be brought to the 7000 rad level for the specific volume of gross disease (i.e., 3000 rads with radium and 4000 rads external beam). There may be instances when a lesion is clinically resectable, but if resection is carried out, whole pelvis external beam therapy (4000 to 5000 rads in four to five weeks) should be added to cover the field.

The same considerations apply to metastasis elsewhere in the vagina, but it should be remembered that in locations other than the apex of the vagina, more extensive, although perhaps occult, submucosal, vaginal lymphatic involvement must be anticipated, the entire vaginal cylinder must be treated with an appropriate radium system, and external beam therapy should be added, as previously mentioned.

COMBINED PELVIC AND EXTRAPELVIC RECURRENCE

There are many cases of both pelvic and extrapelvic spread. In selected instances, combinations of available modalities may be used to the patient's benefit. For example, one of our patients with pulmonary metastases and superficial lower vaginal recurrence has remained in complete remission for over three years following vaginal radium and medroxyprogesterone therapy. Another patient with apparently localized recurrence in one rectus muscle had excision (thought to be incomplete) followed by localized external beam radiation and medroxyprogesterone and has been disease-free for four years.

EXTRAPELVIC RECURRENCE

A common manifestation of disseminated endometrial cancer is pulmonary metastasis. Neck and groin nodes may be involved, usually associated with either pulmonary or mediastinal disease in the former, or with parametrial or lateral pelvic wall recurrence in the latter. Liver metastasis and generalized intraabdominal disease are also common.

Three questions arise in considering therapy for disseminated disease:

1. Are there any factors that suggest a more favorable progestin response?
2. Is one progestin better than another?
3. Are other chemotherapeutic agents of value?

Factors of prognostic significance. With regard to the first question, the following factors seem to favor a better clinical response (1) Age: generally younger patients (50 years or under) tend to have a better response rate than older, postmenopausal patients, and the response rate appears to decrease with increasing age, (2) Well-differentiated tumors and moderately differentiated tumors respond better than poorly differentiated tumors. These two factors seem to be interrelated: large series show that younger patients tend to have more well-differentiated or moderately well-differentiated tumors, whereas older patients tend to have a higher percentage of less well-differentiated cancers, (3) The volume of cancer and its location appear to be important factors. Large, fixed solid masses of intraabdominal or pelvic cancer seem to respond unfavorably; conversely, pulmonary metastatic disease shows a generally better response. Liver and osseous lesions show an intermediate response, due perhaps to the better vascularity of these lesions.

Progestin experience. The second question is: is one progestin better than another? Since the first report of Kelley and Baker in 1960,[7] a sizable literature has accumulated reporting on the use of a number of different progestin preparations. The largest experience was accumulated with hydroxyprogesterone caproate (Delalutin) and with medroxyprogesterone acetate (Provera). Optimal dose schedules are elusive from studies in the literature (Table 7). It appears that hydroprogesterone caproate should be

given in a dose of at least 1 g weekly for a minimum of twelve weeks to assess response. Kennedy[16] advises 1 g three times weekly. Kelly[25] says up to 5 g weekly may be needed to control osseous, pelvic, and intraabdominal recurrence. Medroxyprogesterone is usually given 400 mg IM once or twice a week. Most clinicians favor a higher "loading dose" for the first three months of treatment for either agent: If a response is evident, dosages may be reduced for maintenance. Both agents seem equal in value. More recent reports indicate similar efficacy for an oral agent, megestrol acetate (Megase).[23,24]

If one accepts an objective decrease in tumor mass of at least 25%, and this decrease is sustained for at least three months, it would appear from reported experience that approximately 30% of patients will respond. When one excludes those patients dying rapidly of progessive disease and having drugs less than two to three months, the response rate approaches 40%.

A number of dramatic long-term responses have been observed. Additional benefits of progestin therapy are: the agents are essentially nontoxic, often produce a sense of general well-being, an increase in appetite and, frequently, a decrease in pain.

The mechanism of action of progestin is not well established. It may be direct, although some suggest (based hypothetically on the apparent phenotypic, and perhaps genotypic, prototype of the patient with endometrial cancer) that an indirect mechanism is mediated through the pituitary. The histologic changes are compatible with the direct effect, with a secretory conversion, and with changes in both the glands and stroma. The hyperplastic glandular elements mature, become more orderly, and there is a decrease or cessation of mitotic activity; there is progressive flattening, and necrosis. The stroma increases, separates the gland elements, and the back-to-back pattern becomes obliterated. Thus the concept of a

Table 7 Some Representative Reports of Progestins and Advanced Endometrial Cancer

Author(s)	Agents(s)	Dose Range	Number of Patients Treated	Responders No.	Responders %	Duration
Kelley, Baker (1961)[8]	Progesterone Hydroxyprogesterone caproate	150 mg–1000 mg/wk	21	6	29	9 mo–4½ yr
Frick (1965)[9]	Hydroxyprogesterone caproate	1.5–2.0 g/wk	22	4	20	6 mo–3 yr
Anderson (1965)[10]	Medroxyprogesterone acetate	300 mg/day P. O.	20	8	40	3 mo–3½ yr
Masterson, Nelson (1965)[11]	Hydroxyprogesterone caproate	500–1000 mg 3 times/wk	38	7	19	
Kistner, Griffiths, Craig (1965)[12]	Medroxyprogesterone acetate	1–4 g at intervals of 4–12 wk	12	7 (5 with drug only, 2 with drug and XRT)	58	Av., 17 mo Av., 27 mo
Sykes (1966)[13]	Hydroxyprogesterone caproate Medroxyprogesterone acetate	1–1.5 g 2 times/wk	13	5	38	
		400–800 mg/wk IM 400–800 mg P. O./day	11	5	45	
Smith, Rutledge, Soffar (1966)[14]	Medroxyprogesterone acetate Dimethyl-dehydroprogesterone	100 mg–2.7g/wk (most, 250 mg/wk) 40–80 mg/day P. O. (most, 50–60 mg/day)	42	17 (included in above)	40	3–43 mo
Bonte, Dorchmans (1966)[15]	Medroxyprogesterone acetate	0.5–1.0 g/wk, IM or P. O.	26	8	31	8–61 wk
Kennedy (1968)[16]	Hydroxyprogesterone caproate	0.75–3.0 g/wk	41	10	24	Av., 35 mo (6–77 mo)
	Dihydroxyprogesterone acetophenide	0.9 g/wk	34	9	26	Av., 18.5 mo (6–39 mo)

Table 7 (Continued)

Author(s)	Agents(s)	Dose Range	Number of Patients Treated	Responders No.	%	Duration
Briggs, Caldwell, Pitchford (1967)[17]	Progestogens (total)		822	256	31	
	Medroxyprogesterone		103	40	39	
	Hydroxyprogesterone		578	172	30	
	Medrogestone		50	2	4	
	Gestonorone		13	2	15	
Peck, Boyes (1969)[18]	Medroxyprogesterone acetate	0.5–1.0 g/wk IM	23	8	35	
Anderson (1969)[19]	Medroxyprogesterone acetage	2.0 g initially, then 1.0 g/wk IM	68	12 (complete)	18	Av., 53 mo
				13 (partial)	19	Av., 31 mo
Kneale, Evans (1969)[20]	Progestogens		27	13	48	Av., 27 mo (8–53 mo)
	Hydroxyprogesterone caproate	0.5 gm–3 g/wk IM	7	(included in above)		
	Medroxyprogesterone acetate	0.2–1.0 g/wk IM	18	(included in above)		
	Ethynodiol diacetate	10 mg/day IM	2	(included in above)		
Reifenstein (1971)[21]	Hydroxyprogesterone caproate	1.0 g/wk × 4 wk or more	314	22 (complete)	7	These responders lived average of 27 mo longer than nonresponders
				95 (partial)	10	
Malkasian et al. (1971)[22]	Hydroxyprogesterone caproate	0.5–1.0 g/2 times wk. IM	20	5	25	
	Medroxyprogesterone acetate	100 mg/day × 10–14 IM 100 mg 3 ×/wk IM for 6 wk, then 200 mg/mo	25	6	24	

Author	Drug	Dose				Duration
	Dimethyl dehydroprogesterone	100 mg/P.O./day × 7 days then	30	7	23	
		200 mg/P.O./day × 7 days then				
		400 mg/P.O./day × 7 days then				
		800 mg/P.O./day				
Wait (1973)[23]	Megestrol acetate	40–320 mg/P.O./day	81	32	39	Range: 4–72 mo (Av., 7 mo)
Geisler (1973)[24]	Megestrol acetate	40 mg P.O./day	7	1	14	
		80 mg P.O./day	7	3	43	
		160 mg/P.O./day	29	14	48	

Table 8   Treatment Plans for Recurrent Endometrical Cancer

Clinical Setting	Treatment Alternatives
Disseminated recurrence	Progestin therapy occasionally supplemented by local radiation
Bulky pelvic recurrence	External beam therapy
Small central recurrence	External beam therapy vs. Viscera preserving resection followed by external beam therapy vs Exenterative surgery
Vaginal apex recurrence	Radium only vs. Radium plus external beam vs. Exision (with or without supplemental external beam)
Other vaginal recurrences	Radium to entire vagina vs. Radium plus external beam therapy
Other clinically localized but disseminated recurrence (incision, groin, etc.)	Surgical resection plus adjunct of radiation and/or progestin vs. Radiation and/or progestin without surgical resection

direct effect of progestin is consistent with these histologic changes and also with the clinical observations that the more well-differentiated cancers are those most likely to respond and the anaplastic lesions will respond far less frequently.

Other chemotherapy. The third question relates to the efficacy of other chemotherapy. Progestins are the drug of choice, and little evaluative experience has accumulated with other systemic chemotherapy. These agents have usually been employed for patients who have "broken through" original progestin therapy. Since they are often in a deteriorating general condition, the results are extremely difficult to evaluate. Although Cytoxan, Fluorouracil, and Methotrexate have been used occasionally with brief success, the results have generally been disappointing.

The spectrum of clinical settings and therapeutic alternatives discussed in this chapter is summarized in Table 8.

REFERENCES

1. Boronow, R. C.: Carcinoma of the corpus: Treatment at M. D. Anderson Hospital. In *Cancer of the Uterus and Ovary,* Year Book Medical Publishers, Chicago, 1969.

2. Henriksen, E.: The lymphatic spread of carcinoma of the cervix and of the body of the uterus. A study of 420 necropsies. *Am. J. Obstet. Gynecol.* **58:** 924 (1949).

3. Beck, R. P., and J. P. A. Latour: Necropsy reports on 36 cases of endometrial carcinoma. *Am. J. Obstet. Gynecol.* **85:** 307 (1963).

4. Finn, W. F.: Time, site and treatment of recurrences of endometrial carcinoma. *Am. J. Obstet. Gynecol.* **60:** 773 (1950).

5. Dede, J. A., A. A. Plentl, and J. G. Moore: Recurrent endometrial carcinoma. *Surg. Gynecol. Obstet.* **126:** 533 (1968).

6. Barber, H. R. K., and A. Brunschwig: Treatment and results of recurrent cancer of corpus uteri in patients receiving anterior and total exenteration: 1947–1963. *Cancer* **22:** 949 (1968).

7. Kelley, R. M., and W. H. Baker: Progestational agents in the treatment of carcinoma of the endometrium. *Proc. Am. Assoc. Cancer Res.* **3:** 125 (1960).

8. Kelly, R. M., and W. H. Baker: Progestational agents in the treatment of carcinoma of the endometrium. *New. Engl. J. Med.* **264:** 216 (1961).

9. Frick, H. C., II: Progestational drugs in the management of endometrial cancer. *Metabolism.* **14:** 348 (1965).

10. Anderson, D. G.: Management of advanced endometrial adenocarcinoma with medroxyprogesterone acetate. *Am. J. Obstet. Gynecol.* **92:** 87 (1965).

11. Masterson, J. G., and J. H. Nelson, Jr.: The role of chemotherapy in the treatment of gynecologic malignancy. *Am. J. Obstet. Gynecol.* **93:** 1102 (1965).

12. Kistner, R. W., C. T. Griffiths, and J. M. Craig: Use of progestational agents in the management of endometrial cancer. *Cancer* **18:** 1563 (1965).

13. Sykes, M. P.: Management of endometrial cancer. *Med. Clin. North Am.* **50:** 833 (1966).

14. Smith, J. P., F. Rutledge, and S. W. Soffar. Progestins in the treatment of patients with endometrial adenocarcinoma. *Am. J. Obstet. Gynecol.* **94:** 977 (1966).

15. Bonte, J., and A. Dorchmans: Treatment of adenocarcinoma of the uterus with medroxyprogesterone. *Gynecol. Obstet.* **65:** 179 (1966).

16. Kennedy, B. J.: Progestins in the treatment of carcinoma of the endometrium. *Surg. Gynecol. Obstet.* **127:** 103 (1968).

17. Briggs, M. H., A. D. S. Caldwell, and A. G. Pitchford: Sex hormones in female cancer. *Lancet* **2:** 100 (1967).

18. Peck, J. G., and D. A. Boyes: Treatment of advanced endomerial carcinoma with a progestational agent. *Am. J. Obstet. Gynecol.* **103:** 90 (1969).

19. Anderson, D. G.: Progestogen brings remissions. *J. Am. Med. Assoc.* **209:** 1020 (1969).

20. Kneale, B., and J. Evans: Progestogen therapy for advanced carcinoma of the endometrium. *Med. J. Aust.* **2:** 1101 (1969).

21. Reifenstein, E. C., Jr.: Hydroxyprogesterone caproate therapy in advanced endometrial carcinoma. *Cancer* **27:** 485 (1971).

22. Malkasian, G. D., Jr., D. G. Decker, E. Mussey, and C. E. Johnson: Progestogen therapy of recurrent endometrial carcinoma. *Am. J. Obstet. Gynecol.* **110:** 15 (1971).

23. Wait, R. B.: Megestrol acetate in the management of advanced endometrial carcinoma. *Obstet. Gynecol.* **41:** 129 (1973).

24. Geisler, H. E.: The use of megestrol acetate in the treatment of advanced malignant lesions of the endometrium. *Gynecol. Oncol.* **1:** 340 (1973).

25. Kelley, R. M.: Hormonal and chemotherapeutic management of carcinoma of the endometrium. In *Gynecological Oncology,* H. R. K. Barber and E. A. Graber, Eds., The Williams and Wilkins Company, Baltimore, 1970.

CHAPTER 8 SARCOMAS OF THE UTERUS

J. TAYLOR WHARTON, M.D.

The diagnois of uterine sarcoma implies a grave prognosis. Since sarcomas of the uterus are rare, it is difficult for most gynecologists to accumulate a significant amount of experience in managing this disease. Therefore it is best that treatment be administered under the supervision of a gynecologic oncologist.

Until recently, the only available treatment for uterine sarcomas has been surgical excision, which is effective only in neoplasms confined to the uterus. Today, however, advances in chemotherapy and radiation therapy have made these modalities worthy of therapeutic trial, either singly or in combination. With this combined approach, even relatively advanced uterine sarcomas can now be treated.

CLASSIFICATION

The classification of uterine sarcomas used at The M. D. Anderson Hospital is based on a combination of histogenetic and clinical considerations (Table 1). In the former sense, these neoplasms may be divided into three large groups: (1) those arising from the myometrium, (2) those arsing from the endometrium and (3) those arising from nonspecific connective tissue elements such as blood vessels, nerves and their coverings, and fibrous or adipose tissue. The first category consists, in a practical sense, mainly of leiomyosarcoma and its clinically variant presentations. Endometrial sarcomas are subdivided as suggested by Ober,[7] a concept which clarifies the relationship among these complex tumors. Table 2 gives the basic terminology. A modification of Ober's classification to include leiomyosarcomas and endometrial stromal sarcoma in the same category has been suggested by Kempson and Bari.[6] Since myometrial leiomyosarcoma presents different problems from endo-

Table 1   Classification of Uterine Sarcoma[4]

A. Myometrial origin
    1. Leiomyosarcoma
    2. Leiomyoblastoma

B. Endometrial or endometrial stromal origin
    1. Pure homologous type
       (a) Endometrial stromal sarcoma
       (b) Endolymphatic stromal myosis
    2. Pure heterologous type
       (a) Rhabdomyosarcoma
       (b) Chrondrosarcoma
       (c) Others
    3. Mixed homologous type
       (a) Carcinosarcoma
    4. Mixed heterologous type
       (a) Mixed mesodermal sarcoma[a]

C. 1. "Accidental sarcoma" (i.e., angiosarcoma, neurofibrosarcoma, etc.)

[a]Mixed mesodermal sarcoma is a general term and may be used to refer to any tumor with heterologous components, either alone or mixed with homologous elements.

Table 2   Uterine Sarcomas: Basic Terminology

1. Pure: composed of one cell type.
2. Mixed: composed of more than one cell type.
3. Homologous: contains tissue elements indigenous to the uterus.
4. Heterologous: contains elements foreign to the uterus e.g., cartilage, striated muscle, or bone).

metrial stromal sarcoma, we prefer to regard it as separate.

The "accidental" sarcomas of the uterus are not different from histologically similar neoplasms arising in other structures and will not be considered here. Reticuloendothelial neoplasms categorized among the mesenchymal tumors by some investigators, are, in our opinion, a separate group of lesions unrelated to the neoplasms under discussion.

LEIOMYOSARCOMA

Since leiomyosarcoma is the most common sarcoma of the uterus, there is a good chance that every gynecologist will at some time be required to treat a patient with this neoplasm. The diagnosis is frequently made by histologic examination of the specimen from an operation for suspected uterine fibroids. Occasionally, invasion of the adjacent pelvic structures or metastasis to the upper abdomen leaves little doubt about the malignant nature of the tumor discovered.

Clinical Features

The most frequent sign of leiomyosarcoma is profuse vaginal bleeding. Pelvic pain if present, is the result of rapid enlargement of the tumor. In many respects, the clinical setting is indistinguishable from that produced by benign uterine tumors. A rapid increase in uterine size may be the only clue that a sarcoma is present.

Preoperative diagnosis may be made by dilation and curettage or endometrail biopsy if the tumor is submucosal. More often, however, it is intramural or subserosal, and diagnosis by curettage is improbable. Occasionally a leiomyosarcoma may form a fleshy mass which protrudes through the cervix and can be biopsied.

Pathology

Leiomyosarcomas may be grossly indistinguishable from leiomyomas. Although the more undifferentiated examples may be soft and lack the characteristic whorllike pattern of myomas, these features are not diagnostic. Metastatic lesions are usually nodular, soft or firm, and have pseudocapsules, but they may also form soft, friable masses which lack capsules, invade diffusely, and blend with adjacent structures.

The histologic evaluation of uterine smooth muscle tumors is difficult. A majority of leiomyosarcomas have microscopic features such as cellularity, anisokaryosis, hyperchromatism, and abnormal mitoses, which leaves little doubt about their malignant potential. Frequently, however, one encounters a smooth muscle tumor which, though benign in appearance, contains a central focus of atypical cells. To predict the behavior of such a tumor may prove impossible, despite the most painstaking examination.

Several attempts have been made to formulate a set of predictive histologic criteria for this group of tumors. The most reliable of these is the enumeration of mitoses as proposed by Taylor and Norris.[9] In the series reported by these authors lesions with fewer than 10 mitoses in 10 high-power fields (HPF) were found to be benign regardless of the degree of cellular atypia, whereas tumors with 10 or more mitoses in 10 (HPF) recurred or metastasized in 31 of 36 patients. Kempson and Bari, however, reported that 5 of 6 patients whose tumors had a mitotic rate of 5 to 9/10 HPF either died of tumor or developed metastases.[6] Silverberg's experience is similar, and includes a patient with fewer than 5 mitoses/ 10 HPF who died of tumor.[8] Our own observations lead to the conclusion that although mitotic rate is an important factor in the histologic grading of leiomyosarcomas and the presence of 10 or more/10 MPF connotes an overwhelmingly high probability of recurrence of metatasis, mitotic rate alone is not an infallible prognostic criterion. Actually, it seems that histologic grading based on any criterion or combination of criteria is applicable only to groups of patients and is of limited value when applied to an individual.

Whether or not leiomyosarcoma can arise from preexisting benign leiomyoma has been a subject of prolonged debate.[1] If such malignant degeneration occurs, it must be, considering the frequency of leiomyoma, an extremely rare event. Certainly, the prevention of malignancy cannot be regarded as a valid indication for surgical extirpation of the myomatous uterus.

When cellularity or cellular abnormality is limited to a part of an otherwise histologically benign mass, special care in interpretation is needed. Anoxia and other degenerative influences may produce bizarre nuclear changes in benign myomas, recognizable by the total absence of intranuclear details and the presence of accompanying cytoplasmic degeneration. Such retrogressive changes should not be interpreted as evidence of malignancy. When well-preserved cells with definite malignant characteristics form part of a myomatous tumor it is important to determine the location and extent of the atypical portion. When the malignant part of the mass is central and completely surrounded by benign tissue, recurrence and metastasis are infrequent no matter what the histologic grade may be. When, however, the malignant cells extend beyond the limits of the myoma, or when there is an irregular infiltrating margin, the expected behavior is that of any other leiomyosarcoma of equivalent grade.

There are two clinicopathologic variants of uterine leiomyosarcoma that deserve special mention. The first of these is the benign metastasizing leiomyoma. This self-contradictory term has been applied to those rare patients who usually develop single or multiple pulmonary metastases 5 years or more after hysterectomy for benign leiomyoma. In some instances, review of the uterine tumor reveals evidence of low-grade malignancy overlooked on initial examination. In the majority of cases, however, both the primary and the metastatic lesions are completely lacking in malignant features and appear to be entirely benign leiomyomas. It is our opinion that such lesions should be regarded as extremely low-grade leiomyosarcomas whose extremely indolent, malignant behavior is not detectable morphologically. When the pulmonary lesion is single, segmental resection often results in prolonged control.

A second and somewhat similar lesion is intravenous leiomyomatosis. Here, the veins draining a myomatous uterus are filled with columns of histologically benign leiomyomatous tissue, often extending as far as the pelvic walls. Simple hysterectomy, of course, results in transection of the tumor-filled vessels. Occasionally, when the presence of this lesion is recognized preoperatively and is adequately encompassed by the surgical procedure, recurrence is unusual. When, intravascular tumor is left behind, however, local recurrence and occasionally metastasis to the upper abdomen or lungs should be anticipated. Ordinarily the period between the initial operation and clinical recurrence is a matter of many years. Because of its behavior, intravascular leiomyomatosis, like benign metastasizing leiomyoma, is best regarded as a special type of low-grade leiomyosarcoma.

Treatment

Surgical excision offers the best chance for cure of leiomyosarcoma. Total abdominal hysterectomy and bilateral salpingo-oophorectomy is the operation of choice. The adnexa should be removed if the presence of malignancy is recognized at the time of surgery or if the diagnosis has been made preoperatively. If the diagnosis is made postoperatively, then reexploration and removal of the adnexa is not recommended.

Preoperative radiotherapy should be used when possible (Table 3). There is little evidence that radical hysterectomy or pelvic lymphadenectomy improves results. Since radiation and chemotherapy, either alone or in combination, may be effective in controlling advanced disease, it is wise to remove as much tumor as possible. Postoperative therapy is most efficient when residual disease is minimal.

We do not advise additional therapy when a small, well-circumscribed sarcoma with a low or intermediate mitotic index is discovered in the postoperative specimen. However, in the case of a uterus densely adherent to the pelvic wall or adjacent structures that probably indicates extrauterine extension, further therapy, usually radiation alone, is worthy of consideration. Additional therapy is also indicated when the sarcoma is active (greater than 10 mitoses/10 HPF), even if the lesion is apparently confined to the uterus.

The treatment of recurrent or metastatic leiomyosarcoma confined to the pelvis and/or abdomen is surgical excision followed by radiation alone or in combination with chemotherapy. Table 4 gives the treatment plan now in use. This approach is quite aggressive, and fatal complications have resulted. Extreme caution is mandatory, and therapy should be supervised by a physician experienced in gynecologic oncology.

Patients with distant metastases receive chemotherapy. The chemotherapy regimen routinely used for gynecologic sarcomas at

Table 3   Sarcomas of the Uterus: Guide to Radiation Therapy, The M. D. Anderson Hospital

Clinical Situation	Treatment to Uterus	Treatment to Vagina
(a) Preoperative[a]	4000 rads whole pelvis and radium, one Heyman packing 2500 mg/hr and/or tandem alone, depending on volume of uterine cavity	Colpostats, 4000 rads surface dose in one application
(b) Postoperative	5000 rads whole pelvis 15 × 15 cm field	Colpostats, 3000 rads surface dose in one application
	or	
	reduce field, if 6000–7000 rads required due to large volume residual tumor	None
(c) Inoperable—advanced disease or medical problem	4000–5000 rads whole pelvis plus one or two Heyman packings and/or tandem alone, depending on cavity size and tumor volume	Colpostats, 4000 rads surface dose
	or	
	7000 rads whole pelvis alone with reduction of field size after 5000 rads	

[a]A total abdominal hysterectomy and bilateral salpingo-oophorectomy is performed 6 weeks after completing radiation therapy.

Table 4   Uterine Sarcomas, The M. D. Anderson Hospital

Leiomyosarcoma	
Spread beyond uterus	
Aggressive combination[a]	Standard combination
Irradiation	Irradiation
Whole abdomen, by moving strip (2600 rads) Pelvic boost, anterior and posterior portals (2000 rads)	Whole pelvis, anterior and posterior portals (5000 rads)
Chemotherapy	Chemotherapy
Vincristine 1.5 mg/M² BSA q. wk × 10–12 wks.[b] Actinomycin D .5 mg/day × 5 days when irradiation starts.[d] AC[c] for 2 years following irradiation.	Vincristine 1.5 mg/M² BSA × 10–12 wks.[b] AC[c] for 2 years following irradiation.

[a] May produce very severe bone marrow depression.
[b] May produce severe neurotoxicity requiring dose reduction (max dose 2.5 mg/wk).
[c] AC = Actinomycin D and Cytoxan IV daily for 5 days every month for two years starting one month after completion of radiation therapy.
[d] Augments toxicity when given prior to irradiation and reserved for patients with mixed mesodermal sarcomas.

the University of Texas, M. D. Anderson Hospital is shown in Table 5. Adriamycin in combination with other agents, as described by Gottlieb et al.,[5] has also produced favorable responses in patients with sarcomas.

Table 5   Chemotherapy for Uterine Sarcomas: VAC Regimen,[a] The M. D. Anderson Hospital

Vincristine: 1–1.5 mg/M² BSA[b]/wk IV for 12 consecutive weeks

Cytoxan: 5–7 mg/kg/day IV × 5; repeat each month for 2 years

Actinomycin D: .5 mg/day IV × 5; repeat each month for 2 years

[a] May produce severe bone marrow depression and neurotoxicity.
[b] Body surface area.

ENDOMETRIAL STROMAL SARCOMA

Endometrial stromal sarcoma and its variant, endolymphatic stromal myosis, comprise the pure homologous type of endometrial sarcoma. Because it is histologically distinctive and clinically somewhat different from the other members of this group, it is appropriate to discuss it separately. A bewildering variety of names have been applied to this lesion, among them stromal adenomyosis, stromal nodules, and stromatous endometriosis. Although there is strong evidence that hemangiopericytoma of the uterus rarely occurs, it is probable that many of the tumors reported under this designation are actually endometrial stromal sarcomas.

Clinical Features

Endometrial stromal sarcoma occurs from adolescence to senility. Although most patients are perimenopausal, about one third are postmenopausal. Irregular bleeding is the most common and often the only symptom. Abdominal or pelvic pain is present in a minority of patients. Pelvic examination usually reveals a diffusely or nodularly enlarged uterus which, in advanced cases, may be fixed to other pelvic structures or to the pelvic walls. Since many of these tumors protrude into the endometrial cavity, currettage or endometrial biopsy is often diagnostic.

Pathology

There is great variability in both gross and microscopic appearance. The tumor may form a soft mass, with extensive hemorrhage and necrosis. The mass may be well or poorly circumscribed, may involve the myometrium alone or both endometrium and myometrium, with protrusion into the endometrial cavity. The endolymphatic stromal myosis variant may produce only a focal or diffuse thickening of the myometrium, or there may be grossly visible cords of tumor within the myometrial and parametrial vessels.

Histologically, endometrial stromal sarcomas are composed of small, plump oval cells with scanty cytoplasm resembling the cells of endometrial stroma. The degree of anaplasia varies widely. In some tumors the cells appear almost normal, whereas in others the nuclei are hyperchromatic or vesicular, larger than normal, and show frequent mitoses. Occasionally, in examples with little anaplasia, there may be clusters of benign epithelial cells.

Prognosis depends upon two factors: degree of circumscription, and anaplasia as revealed by the mitotic index. Most often, a well-circumscribed tumor is composed of cells showing little anaplasia. Occasionally, however, bland-appearing stromal cells may be found infiltrating myometrium or filling myometrial vessels. Such lesions, although less aggressive than overtly malignant examples, typically produce late recurrence or metastasis.

Treatment

Total abdominal hysterectomy and bilateral salpingo-oophorectomy is the recommended treatment for endometrial stromal sarcoma. We prefer to use preoperative radiotherapy (Table 3). These sarcomas can frequently be diagnosed by endometrial sampling, which provides an opportunity for preoperative irradiation more often than is the case with leiomyosarcomas.

Recurrent or metastatic sarcomas can be managed in much the same way as leiomyosarcomas (Table 4). Therapy is individualized and perhaps less intense for certain patients.

There is evidence that some of these tumors may be hormone-dependent or responsive.[2] Progesterone therapy (Depo-Provera, 250 mg/wkIM) may be given for a trial period prior to the use of cytotoxic agents for metastatic disease.

MIXED MESODERMAL SARCOMA

The remaining types of endometrial sarcoma we group together colloquially (and rather illogically) under the term mixed mesodermal sarcoma. Histologically, these tumors are composed of a mixture of stromal sarcoma and carcinoma, or contain heterologous sarcomatous elements alone or in combination with stromal sarcoma or carcinoma. Although the term applied to these tumors is less than satisfactory, it groups together a complex of related neoplasms with similar clinical behavior and avoids the objectionable and imprecise term, "carcinosarcoma."

Clinical Features

Mixed mesodermal sarcomas are extremely malignant and spread early to regional lymph nodes and adjacent viscera. Although the spread pattern is similar to adenocarcinoma of the endometrium, it is more aggressive. Vascular invasion is common, and lung, liver, and bone metastases occur. Several reported cases in the literature suggest that prior uterine radiation therapy may play an etiologic role in the development of this tumor.

Diagnosis is usually established by dilation and curettage or endometrial biopsy in a postmenopausal bleeding patient with an enlarged uterus. The uterine cavity usually contains a necrotic, polypoid friable tumor which may protrude beyond the external os.

Pathology

As implied earlier, the histology of this group of tumors seems bewildering and complex and includes pure heterologous sarcomas, most often rhabdomyosarcomas, and leiomyosarcomas. Mixtures of these plus endometrial stromal sarcoma with carcinoma, or complex mixtures containing a multiplicity of carcinomatous and sarcomatous elements of various types are also encountered. The carcinomatous component may be either endometrial type of an adenocarcinoma, squamous carcinoma, or rarely, papillary carcinoma. Several specimens we have studied suggest that these tumors may have multiple sites of origin within the uterus. Metastases may contain any of the components of the primary tumor or may themselves be mixed. In our experience, attempts to evaluate prognosis on the basis of histology have not produced meaningful results.

Treatment

Various treatment modalities and combinations have been used in the treatment of patients with mixed mesodermal sarcoma. Reports in the literature show that control is not obtained by simple hysterectomy or irradiation alone. Extended hysterectomy or irradiation plus operation should produce the best results.

From March, 1944 to December, 1969, 101 patients with mixed mesodermal sarcoma of the uterus were seen at the M. D. Anderson Hospital;[3] are available for analysis of treatment techniques. The more recent treatment plan includes whole pelvis x-ray therapy and intracavitary radium followed by hysterectomy 4 to 6 weeks after irradiation (Table 3). We prefer the combination of irradiation and hysterectomy to either irradiation or hysterectomy alone. Although attention has been called to the frequency of distant metastasis from this disease, in our experience recurrences are as prone to develop in the pelvis or lower abdomen.

Table 6 shows the results based on the treatment method. Those patients treated with preoperative irradiation followed by an extrafascial hysterectomy had a better survival and lower incidence of local recurrence. In our series, 73% of deaths occurred within thirteen months of diagnosis, and 88% within twenty-four months of diagnosis. Since almost all recurrences or distant metastases occurred within the first two years, some assessment of treatment results can be made from patients followed less than the conventional five years. The extent of the disease at the initiation of therapy significantly influences prognosis (Table 7).

Chemotherapy for distant metastases is difficult and generally disappointing. We have not obtained responses with proges-

Table 6 Mixed Mesodermal Sarcoma Results Based on Treatment Method, The M. D. Anderson Hospital[3]

Treatment	Number of Patients	NED[a] (2 yr)	Local Control
Hysterectomy alone	5	2	2
Hysterectomy plus postoperative XRT	7	4	5
Preoperative radium plus hysterectomy	12	7	10
Preoperative XRT plus radium plus hysterectomy	5	3	4
XRT only	5	2	2
Total	34	18 (53%)	23 (68%)

[a] No evidence of disease.

Table 7 Mixed Mesodermal Sarcoma Results Based on Extent of the Disease, The M. D. Anderson Hospital[3]

Extent of Disease	Number of Patients	NED[a] (2 yr)	Local Control (pelvis)
Group I Corpus alone	34	18/34 (53%)	23/34 (68%)
Group II Cervix, vagina and/or parametrium	35	3/35 (8.5%)	10/35 (29%)
Group III Outside pelvis	25	0/25 (0%)	5/25 (20%)

[a] No evidence of disease.

terone derivatives. Combination chemo-therapy (Table 5) offers the best chance for palliation.

REFERENCES

1. Christopherson, W. M., E. O. Williamson, and L. A. Graz, *Cancer, 29,* No. 6, 1512.
2. Baggish, M., and D. Woodruff, *Obstet. Gynec., 40,* No. 4, 4487 (1972).
3. DiSaia, Phillip J., et al., *Am. J. Roentgenol. Radium.*
4. Gallager, H. Stephen, *The M. D. Anderson Hospital, Houston, Texas*
5. Gottlieb, J., et al., *Cancer Chemother. Rep.* **58,** 265.
6. Kempson, R. L. and W. Bari, *Hum. Pathol.,* **3,** 331–349 (1970).
7. Ober, W. B., *Ann. N. Y. Acad. Sci.,* **75,** 568 (1959).
8. Silverberg, S. G., *Obstet. Gynec.,* **38,** 613–628 (Oct. 1971).
9. Taylor, H. B., and H. J. Norris, *Arch. Pathol.* **82,** 40–44 (July 1966).

CHAPTER 9 GESTATIONAL TROPHOBLASTIC DISEASE

RICHARD C. BORONOW, M.D.

CURRENT CONTROVERSIES

1. Prophylactic treatment of hydatidiform mole.
2. Drug of choice, and single drug vs. alternate drug therapy.
3. Place for multiple drug therapy and multiple modality therapy.
4. Role of surgery.
5. Should these diseases be treated in cancer centers?

Gestational trophoblastic neoplasms represent a fascinating, rare family of tumors that has captured the interest of clinicians for many years, and of investigators especially during the last several decades:

Clinical Variability

Although there are benign and malignant forms, even the histologically benign form may ultimately assume a fatal course either by invasion and dissemination in a histologically benign configuration (invasive mole), or by apparent conversion to the histologically malignant variant (choriocarcinoma).

Chemotherapeutic Investigation

Choriocarcinoma, historically a fatal disease of young women (within 1 to 2 years in the vast majority of cases), was the first malignant tumor shown to be chemotherapeutically curable. That observation in the mid-1950s led to enormous laboratory and clinical studies in the broad field of cancer chemotherapy.

Immunologic Investigation

As pregnancy is a homograft that appears to defy rejection (unless labor is immunologically triggered), so choriocarcinoma with its mixed genetic background is a malignant homograft that is not rejected, but progresses to kill the host in most instances.

DEFINITIONS OLD AND NEW

The Descriptions of James Ewing[1]

HYDATID MOLE

Although hydatid mole, also called hydatidiform mole, or H. mole, is the most common variant of gestational trophoblastic neoplasia, it occurs approximately in only 1 in 2000 pregnancies in North America, the frequency varies worldwide and is reportedly 10 times more common in Mexico and the Far East (Table 1). It has the gross characteristic of multiple grapelike vesicles filling and distending the uterus. Histologically the vesicles are composed of swollen, hydrophilic, avascular villi with peripheral nests of syncytiotrophoblastic or cytotrophoblastic elements. Although histologic study of this trophoblast, assessing the degree of hyper-

Table 1   Incidence of Hydatidiform Mole[2]

Country	Incidence	Author
United States	1/2,000 pregnancies 1/1,699 deliveries 1/2,093 pregnancies	Hertig & Mansell[3] Brewer & Gerbie[4]
Great Britain	1/835 pregnancies	Das[5]
Australia	1/695 pregnancies	Beischer & Fortune[6]
France	1/500 pregnancies	Brindeau, et al.[7]
Mexico	1/200 pregnancies	Marquez-Monter et al.[8]
Philippines	1/173 pregnancies	Acosta-Sison[9]
Taiwan	1/120 pregnancies	Wei & Ouyang[10]

plasia and/or anaplasia, provides some basis for predicting a benign or malignant course for the mole, this correlation is not absolute and all patients must be followed by gonadotropin titers. The lack of absolute precision in morphologic prediction is reflected in the modification of Hertig and Mansell's classification shown in Table 2.

The clinical picture is clearly defined: the initial amenorrhea and subjective symptoms of pregnancy intervene, followed by intermittent, then more sustained spotting and bleeding; and the uterine growth rate in no less than 50% of cases exceeds expected growth for the period of amenorrhea. In some instances the nausea and vomiting are accentuated to hyperemesis gravidarum. Occasionally toxemia of pregnancy develops. Rarely the codevelopment of a normal fetus occurs (Figure 1).

Table 2   Hydatidiform Mole Classification[11]

Group	Name	Histologic Criteria
I	Benign	None to slight hyperplasia of the trophoblast
II	Probably benign	Slight to moderate hyperplasia
III	Possibly benign	Hyperplasia with slight anaplasia
IV	Possibly malignant	Moderate anaplasia with hyperplasia
V	Probably malignant	Marked anaplasia with hyperplasia
VI	Malignant	Exuberant trophoblastic growth (variable mitotic activity) with marked anaplasia and often evidence of endometrial invasion.

Suggested New Classification[3]

New Grade	New Name	Old Group	Old Name
1	Apparently benign	Group I	Benign
2	Potentially malignant	Group II	Probably benign
		Group III	Possibly benign
		Group IV	Possibly malignant
3	Apparently malignant	Group V	Probably malignant
		Group VI	Malignant

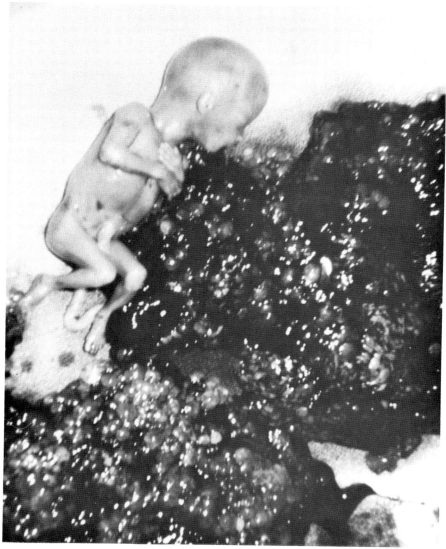

Figure 1 The rare association of viable intrauterine pregnancy with hydatidiform mole. University of Miss. Medical Center #237609.

If the diagnosis is not established by the time uterine growth reaches 18 to 20 weeks size, the absence of the objective signs of pregnancy—skeletal parts, fetal heart, objective motion of the fetus—greatly increase the index of suspicion. The human chorionic gonadotropin (HCG) titer is usually above that expected for the corresponding gesta-tional age, higher than is seen in normal pregnancy. This, however, is not diagnostic; serial titers coupled with the balance of clin-ical and laboratory assessment are necessary (Table 3). The passage of a grapelike vesicle is considered diagnostic.

Currently, termination is generally carried out with suction curettage with the addition

Table 3   Presumptive Diagnosis of Molar Pregnancy[2]

Clinical

    Vaginal bleeding
    Lower abdominal pain
    Uterine size larger than gestational dates
    Absent fetal heart tones
    Early toxemia
    Uterus probes easily

Laboratory

    HCG greater than 500,000 IU/l
    Absent fetal heart by ECG
    Absent fetal heart by electrical amplification
    Ultrasound sonogram of uterus

Radiographic

    Pelvic roentgenogram
    Pelvic arteriography
    Amniography

of a liberal oxytocin infusion. The roles of prophylactic chemotherapy and of surgery will also be discussed later. Approximately 80% of H. moles will have an uneventful outcome. In one large report 81.5% of cases had a benign course, 16% progressed to invasive mole, and 2.5% to choriocarcinoma.[3]

CHORIOADENOMA DESTRUENS

This is the second variant of trophoblastic neoplasia and is also called destructive mole, invasive mole, or malignant mole. This entity implies invasion by a mole into or through the myometrium, with or without metastases. The metastases must contain hydatidiform villi. This variant develops in approximately 16% of H. moles. Invasion into or through the wall of the uterus may cause significant, even fatal, hemorrhage compounded by infection and sepsis. Mortality rates of 4 to 17%, with an average of about 14% in earlier series, have been reported.[12] Postevacuation bleeding is likely to persist or develop soon. Even before the advent of other symptoms, a persistently elevated gonadotropin titer will be present. Histologically, *Chorioadenoma destruens* is

identical to H. mole; one can only make the diagnosis of invasive mole by virtue of its invasive location. It may also be diagnosed when "deported" to other areas such as lung, or to a more accessible location for biopsy such as the vagina. One should be cautioned that biopsy of these highly vascular deposits may be associated with major blood loss. Such metastases of histologically benign tissue properly underscore the aggressive and potentially lethal quality of this neoplasm.

CHORIOCARCINOMA (CHORIOEPITHELIOMA)

Although approximately 2.5% of H. mole progresses to choriocarcinoma (conversely, choriocarcinoma is preceded by H. mole in about 50% of cases), this neoplasm may be preceded by any gestational event: it may follow abortion, ectopic pregnancy, or normal intrauterine pregnancy. In Hertig's data, choriocarcinoma was preceded by pregnancy in 22.5% of cases, or 1:160,000 normal after molar evacuation the clinician is alerted, but postpartal or postabortal suspicion is greatly diminished. Retained products or subinvolution will be suspected. These cases are most treacherous, because they are least suspected; widespread dissemination may be present before the diagnosis is made. Magrath and associates have stressed the medical presentations (pulmonary, CNS, GI tract symptoms) of choriocarcinoma.[13] Odell and co-workers have reviewed the various endocrine aspects (including occasional thyrotrophic activity) of trophoblastic neoplasms.[14]

Histologically the lesion is composed of hyperplastic and anaplastic syncytial and cytotrophoblastic elements. Villus formation is absent (Figure 2). Some cases of choriocarcinoma remain localized in the uterus for some time. More often the disease disseminates (Table 4), early in its course. In fact disseminated choriocarcinoma with a histologically negative uterus is a common finding.

Table 4 Metastases in Trophoblastic Disease

A. Necropsy Data in 263 Cases of Choriocarcinoma[3,15]

Organ	Number of Cases	Percent of Cases
Lung	158	60
Vagina	105	40
Brain	46	17
Liver	43	16
Kidney	34	13
Uterine wall	28	10
Spleen	24	9
Intestine	24	9
Broad ligament	19	7
Ovary	16	6
Lymph node	16	6
Pelvis	15	5
Cervix uteri	11	4
Pancreas	5	2
Skin and subcutaneous tissue, thyroid gland, and heart	4	1
Fallopian tube, adrenal, bladder, omentum, diaphragm, and bone marrow	3	1
Spinal cord, abdominal wall, breast, mediastinum, menentery, femur, and rib	1	1

B. Clinical Data in 38 Patients with Metastatic Trophoblastic Disease (MTD)[16]

Site	Number of Cases	Percent of Cases
A. Solitary foci	26	
Lung	19	
Vagina	1	
Brain	0	
Liver	2	
Pelvis	4	
B. Multiple foci	12	
Vagina	2	
Brain	5	
Liver	4	
Pelvis	6	
C. Combined (Groups A and B)	38	
Lung	19	50
Vagina	3	8
Brain	5	13
Liver	6	16
Pelvis	10	26

Other Features

THECA-LUTEIN CYSTS

Palpable unilateral or bilateral adnexal enlargement, occasionally quite sizable, occurs in patients with gestational trophoblastic neoplasms (Figure 3). Pathologically this represents multiple theca-lutein cysts, presumably secondary to HCG stimulation. The reason for their presence in only about one-third of cases is unknown. Unless there is a rare adnexal accident such as torsion, these ovaries may be followed expectantly; they are benign, and involute within several months of successful chemotherapeutic treatment.

CHROMOSOME PATTERN

A summary of cytogenetic studies reveals that approximately 80 to 90% of H. moles are sex-chromatin positive (XX). Triploidy occurs in about 13%. The significance of these observations is still unclear.[6,17,18]

New Clinical Definitions

With the advent of chemotherapeutic management of gestational trophoblastic neoplasms and with management based primarily on the presence or absence of HCG, precise histologic identification of these lesions is not always possible. Specifically,

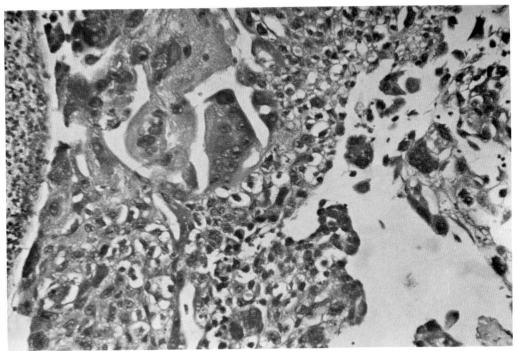

Figure 2 Choriocarcinoma. Syncytiotrophoblast in upper left and anaplastic cytotrophoblast in lower left and center of field.

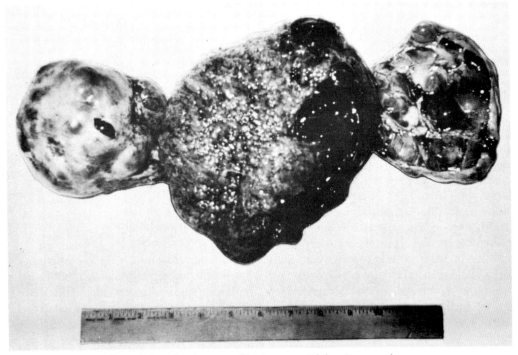

Figure 3 Bilateral theca-lutein cysts with uterus containing 4 mo. molar pregnancy.

even with a positive HCG titer and a positive pelvic arteriogram, curettings frequently fail to confirm the true histology of the invasive trophoblastic disease in the wall of the uterus (either invasive mole or choriocarcinoma). If uterine conservation is planned, and the management is by chemotherapy, one must settle for a diagnosis of nonmetastatic trophoblastic disease (NMTD). In the same fashion, given circulating HCG and evidence of metastatic disease in lung, liver or brain, treatment is with chemotherapy and/or radiation therapy: one acknowledges he is treating metastatic trophoblastic disease (MTD). Again, precise histologic definition is not always possible. The chest lesion may represent deported trophoblast of invasive mole or choriocarcinoma; brain and liver metastases more usually represent choriocarcinoma (see Table 5 and Therapeutic Methods). As has been repeatedly observed however, both from necropsy material and from cases in which there is pretreatment histologic confirmation of choriocarcinoma, these cases require more vigorous treatment regardless of whether they are MTD or NMTD. Thus the clinical response under therapy will

Table 5 Therapeutic Classification for Gestational Trophoblastic Disease[16]

1. Molar pregnancy
   a) Preevacuation
   b) Postevacuation (within 8 weeks)

2. Persistent or retained mole (after 8 weeks)

3. Nonmetastatic trophoblastic disease (NMTD)
   a) No histologic evidence of choriocarcinoma
   b) Choriocarcinoma

4. Metastatic trophoblastic disease (MTD)
   a) No histologic evidence of choriocarcinoma
   b) Choriocarcinoma (low risk)
   c) Choriocarcinoma (high risk)

Categories 3a, 3b, 4a, 4b, and 4c are based on available pathologic material.

often suggest the true histologic identity of the disease.

DIAGNOSTIC METHODS

Histology

The passage of a grapelike villus and histologic study of this material and that obtained by evacuation of the uterus have been discussed. Currettings will often miss trophoblast that has invaded the uterine wall (either invasive mole or choriocarcinoma).

Human Chorionic Gonadotropin

This is the most important diagnostic test for these diseases. The presence of HCG in the nonpregnant patient indicates trophoblastic disease. Either biologically or immunologically, HCG appears to cross-react with luteinizing hormone (LH), and so a normal HCG titer is in the order of approximately 20 to 30 IU (the pituitary level of LH). Titers of this hormone are essential in the follow-up management of H. mole and in the follow-up and treatment of trophoblastic neoplasia. Independently, Delfs[19] and Brewer[20] (Table 6) demonstrated that while the HCG titer usually will return to normal within a week or two of evacuation of H. mole, it should be normal by eight weeks postevacuation or, in most instances, the patient should be treated. This is based on their data that without treatment the patient is at an approximate 50% risk of developing either invasive mole or choriocarcinoma. Of course, if the titer plateaus or rises before eight weeks the patient is at greater risk. Although this eight-week follow-up is standard practice in the United States, however, it should be noted that 50% of these patients will ultimately return to normal. On this basis Bagshawe[22] recommends careful, continued follow-up with weekly titers beyond eight weeks, provided the titer continues to decline. In studing the first two col-

Table 6   Follow-up of Hydatidiform Mole by HCG Titers

	Delfs[19] (1959)	Brewer[20] (1961)	Brewer[21] (1968)
Total molar pregnancies, postevacuation	119	161	51
No. positive titer, 30 days	44	90	35
Percent positive titer, 30 days	37	60	68.6
No. positive titer, 60 days	26	59	15
Percent positive titer, 60 days	21.8	36.7	29.4
No. hysterectomies after 60 days	11	29	none
Invasive mole in specimen	6	16	
Choriocarcinoma in specimen	5	13	
No. patients treated after 60 days[a]	11	29	11
Percent surgery	9.2	18	
Percent chemotherapy			21.6
No. deaths from disease	2	0	0
No. patients not treated after 60 days[b]	15	30	4
No. complications	0	0	0
No. days for normal titer	70–250	75–180	70–142

[a] Usually titers were declining but high, or steady and high, or rising; occasionally there were clinical indications.

[b] Usually titers were falling steadily and sufficiently low to justify follow-up.

umns of Table 6 it becomes apparent that not all patients were treated at eight weeks, and critical assessment of the titers was employed. The third column also reflects this. Thus although a time factor has been shown to be significant, all these authors assess each case in a critical, individual manner. A similar experience is reflected in the recent data of Goldstein (Figure 4).

It is essential to recognize that commercially available biologic pregnancy tests are ordinarily positive in the 3000 to 10,000 IU range and commercially available immunologic tests are sensitive only to the 650 to 750 IU range, although concentration techniques can improve them slightly. In following a patient after the mole has been evacuated, these tests are useful only as long as the titer is positive. Once it becomes negative, testing with a more sensitive method (bioassay or radioimmunoassay) is mandatory. It is well known that disseminated choriocarcinoma can be present with HCG levels below the sensitivity of the commercial tests.

Some centers are studying beta-subunit measurements of HCG. This fraction is not present on the LH molecule and should therefore allow precise HCG determinations to a level of zero. It appears that further study and clinical correlation with this radioimmunoassay are needed before it will replace current methods.

Chest X-Ray

Choriocarcinoma may metastasize to the chest with three different radiographic patterns (1) the so-called cannonball metastases, (2) miliary nodules, (3) lymphatic and vascular prominence. Invasive mole may also metastasize to the lungs, usually manifesting as one of the latter two forms of spread. H. mole has occasionally been reported to metastasize to the chest, but

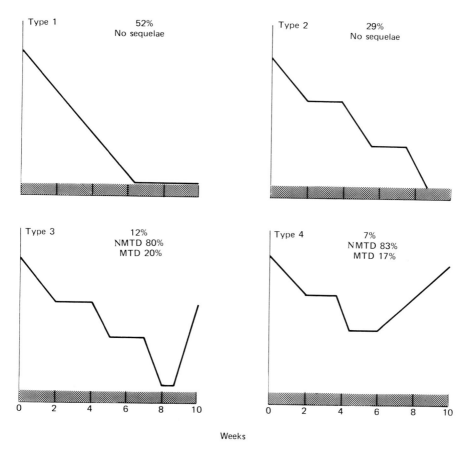

Figure 4   Types of HCG regression curves following molar pregnancy. Four types of gonadotropin regression slopes observed following evacuation in 116 untreated patients with molar pregnancy. Complications were limited to patients with Type 3 and Type 4 patterns. Percentages indicate relative frequency of nonmetastatic trophoblastic disease (NMTD) and metastatic trophoblastic disease (MTD) in each group. From Goldstein, D. P.: The chemotherapy of gestational trophoblastic disease. *JAMA* **220**: 209 (1972). Reprinted with permission.

most observers feel that any form of metastasis, even benign metastasis representing deportation, carries a more malignant connotation and should move the designation of the disease beyond that of H. mole and into the category of MTD. Occasionally deportation can produce heart strain and embolic symptoms. This has been noted symptomatically and occasionally radiographically after evacuation of the mole by curettage. A few cases of embolic death from histologically benign disease have been reported.

Pelvic Arteriography

Percutaneous femoral arteriography as a diagnostic tool in trophoblast disease is relatively new in this country. Myometrial invasion of trophoblastic neoplasia produces hypervascularity with increased tortuosity and increased numbers of vessels, early arteriovenous shunting with venous pooling and evidence of "lakes," and often early filling of the ovarian vein on the involved side (Figure 5. Although these findings are characteristic of trophoblastic neoplasia in the

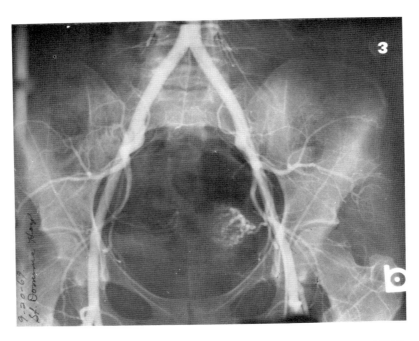

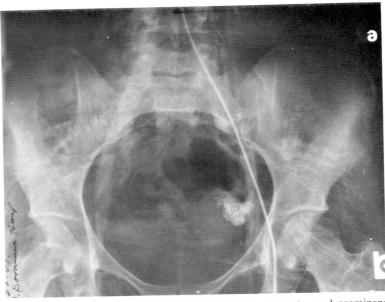

Figure 5 (a) Record 1.0 sec from start of injection demonstrates asymmetry and prominence of left uterine artery with similarly enlarged and prominent spiral arteries in uterus. (b) Figure 5a is arterial, whereas Figure 5b (0.5 sec later) shows early venous filling as well as persistence of the arterial phase. This suggests arteriovenous fistula. (c) Record (0.5 sec later) is 2.0 sec from injection and shows further venous phase. (d) demonstrates a residual venous (4.5 sec after injection) as well as evidence of a dilated ovarian vein on the left (arrow). This arteriogram was taken with a Sanchez-Perez Serialograph. Angioconray (40 ml) was infused, using a Cordis Pressure Injector (600 psi) and 2 exposures/sec were obtained, the first starting the instant injection began. From Boronow, R. C.: Pelvic arteriography after chemotherapy of malignant trophoblastic disease. *Obstet. Gynecol.* **36**: 675 (1970). Reprinted with permission.

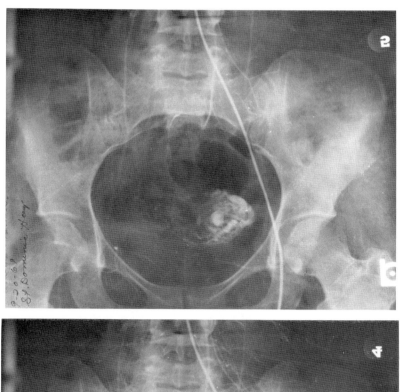

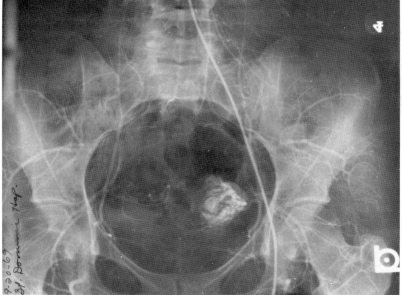

Figure 5 (*continued*)

uterus, they may also be associated with metastatic deposits in the pelvis.

Amniography

The amniotic tap will be dry, and this finding in itself is presumptive evidence of H. mole. Injection of radiopaque material produces a characteristic "honeycombed" or "moth-eaten" pattern compatible with the multiple grapelike vesicular structures within the uterine cavity (Figure 6), and is diagnostic for molar pregnancy.

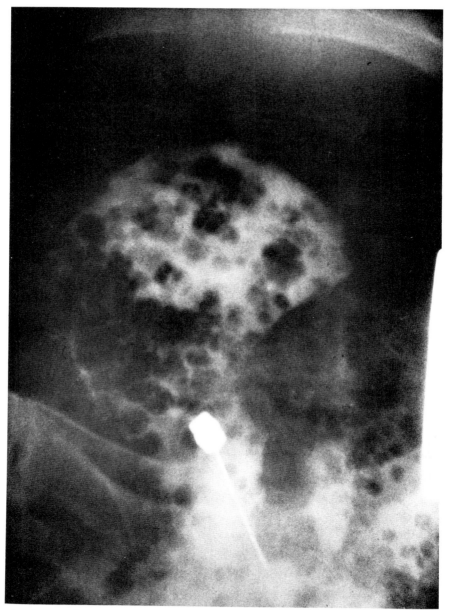

Figure 6 Amniogram demonstrating the characteristic "honeycombed" pattern or "moth-eaten" pattern of the multiple vesicles of hydatidiform mole.

Sonography

Two-dimensional ultrasonograms demonstrate the enlarged uterus with diffusely distributed multiple echoes compatible with the multiple villi at high sensitivity; at lowest sensitivity there are almost no intrauterine echoes. Characteristically absent are the usually discernible intrauterine structures such as the placenta and the fetal head (Figure 7).

Other Studies

Liver function studies and liver scan as well as neurologic examination, visualization of

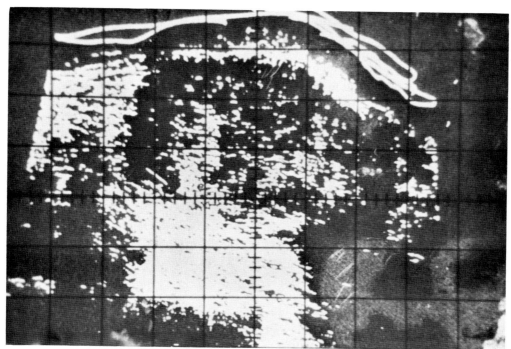

Figure 7 Longitudinal high-intensity sonogram demonstration pattern of hydatidiform mole with diffuse multiple echoes of villi and absent identifiable placenta and fetal head. Linear, anterior abdominal wall at top and sacral promonotory at bottom of picture.

ocular fundi, EEG, and brain scan are essential baseline determinations in assessing the metastatic or nonmetastatic nature of the disease.

THERAPEUTIC METHODS

Surgery

Prior to the advent of chemotherapy, surgery played the major therapeutic role. Today the uterus can usually be preserved if continuation of reproductive capacity is desired. Reproduction following chemotherapy appears unimpaired both quantitatively and qualitatively.[23] The molar pregnancy was often terminated by hysterectomy when childbearing was no longer an issue. Nevertheless, there were occasional reported instances of disseminated choriocarcinoma

that developed at a later date. For the most part, however, this treatment was definitive. For invasive mole or for choriocarcinoma without evidence of metastasis, hysterectomy was performed. The precise histologic definition of the lesion could be established only after resection of the uterus. Data from the Albert Mathieu Chorioepithelioma Registry[24] suggest that only about 40% of patients with apparently localized choriocarcinoma were cured by hysterectomy. This is in stark contrast to a salvage rate of at least 75% of patients with metastatic disease now treated by chemotherapy.

Hysterectomy is currently used as follows: for benign mole, it will frequently be performed when further reproduction is not desired. Nevertheless, one must still follow the patient with HCG titers or treat with chemotherapy at hysterectomy, usually operating on the third day of a five-day course of drug as recommended by Lewis.[25] Since follow-up with HCG titers is mandatory whether or not chemotherapy is used, this author prefers to withhold chemotherapy until clearly indicated. Hysterectomy may also be indicated in management in the event of hemorrhage or sepsis from uterine or pelvic tumor, or in instances where residual pelvic disease appears to be becoming drug-fast.

Prophylactic Therapy of Moles

Goldstein has championed the prophylactic treatment of H. mole at the time of evacuation.[29] His results have been excellent and others have adopted this therapeutic point of view. Conversely, Brewer has demonstrated that it is safe to follow the patients with declining titers to the eight-week post-evacuation period (or less as indicated), and treat only those patients whose titers have not returned to normal; if not normal at 8 weeks some patients will still not be treated, provided the titer level and slope of decline suggest the safety of further follow-up.[21] Both methods treat the titer. Prophylactic treatment appears effective in preventing persistent local neoplasm or dissemination of the trophoblastic neoplasm. The latter method identifies and treats only those specifically at risk, whereas the former will treat the 80% of patients who have a benign course regardless of what is done. We do not treat prophylactically.

Chemotherapy

In the mid-1950s with the demonstration of the curability of disseminated choriocarcinoma by chemotherapy, a new chapter in the management of this disease was written. The first successful agent was Methotrexate. Actinomycin D has proved equally valuable, less toxic, and has become the drug of choice at many centers.[26] Apart from its increased toxicity, Methotrexate does not seem to cross the blood-brain barrier as effectively as Actinomycin D, and should not be used

where there is evidence of liver disease since it is particularly hepatotoxic. The usual dose of Actinomycin averages 0.4 to 0.5 mg/day IV for most patients (9 to 13 μg/kg/day) for five days. The drug is a severe vesicant, so that a free-flowing infusion is mandatory. The usual dose of Methotrexate is 20 to 25 mg/day (0.3 to 0.4 mg/kg/day) for five days, and can conveniently be given orally, intramuscularly, or intravenously. Some prefer the IV route both for a higher pulsed serum level and apparently lower toxicity, although the intramuscular route is most commonly used. Drug courses should be repeated as rapidly as toxicity clears, with an average "window" of about seven days from the day of the last dose of one course to the first dose of the next course. If a single drug is used and the tumor seems to be developing resistance (less than the generally anticipated tenfold drop in titer after each course), one can switch to the other agent (sequential therapy) with good results.[27] (see Table 7 and Dynamic Management). Based on the slightly different toxicity of these two agents, Smith has treated a large series of cases with alternate courses of Actinomycin D and Methotrexate (alternate-sequential therapy), with excellent results, and treatment time is shorter.[2]

Radiation

When brain metastases and/or liver metastases are demonstrated, whole brain and/or whole liver radiation to the level of 2000 rads, usually in 10 consecutive treatment days, appears to have definite value.[30] Since this dose approaches hepatotoxic levels, liver function studies must be monitored daily. The brain tolerates this dosage level well. Radiation therapy is administered simultaneously with chemotherapy.

Infusion Therapy

Some treatment centers report good results with direct arterial infusion of chemotherapeutic agents into the liver and occasionally

Table 7   Two Management Methods for Non-Metastatic Trophoblastic Disease and Metastatic Trophoblastic Disease in Low Risk or Good Prognosis Categories

A. Single Agent Method of Hammond[28]

1. Repetitive 5-day courses: Methotrexaet 15–25 mg/day IM or Actinomycin D 10–13 μg/kg/day IV.

   a. Consider hysterectomy during first course of chemotherapy if further reproduced is not desired.

   b. Minimum interval between courses: 7 days.

   c. Maximum interval between courses: 14 days (unless laboratory values are too low).

   d. Oral contraception for pituitary suppression.

2. Repeat 5-day courses of the same drug until:

   a. HCG titer drops to normal pituitary range—cease therapy.

   b. HCG titer "plateaus" are elevated—change to alternate drug.

   c. HCG titer rises tenfold—change to alternate drug.

   d. New metastases appear—change to alternate drug.

3. Monitor oncolytic effect by weekly HCG titers, chest X-rays, and pelvic examinations.

4. Treatment safety factors (done daily during therapy, less frequently between courses)— do not start, continue, or resume a dose of medication if:

a. White blood count is less than 3000/mm³

b. Polymorphonuclear leukocytes are less than 1500 mm³

c. Platelets are less than 100,000/mm³

d. There are significant elevations of BUN, SGOT, or SGPT.

5. Treatment is terminated when HCG titer is within normal pituitary ranges. Three consecutive, normal weekly HCG titers to diagnose remission.

6. Follow-up:

   a. HCG titers monthly every 6 months, bimonthly every 6 months, then every 6 months thereafter.

   b. Physical and pelvic examinations, chest X-rays, and blood survey every 3 months for 1 year, every 6 months thereafter.

   c. No pregnancy for 1 year.

B. Alternate Sequential Therapy of Smith[2]

Drug	Dosage
Methotrexate	15–30 mg/day IV for 5 days
Actinomycin D	0.5 mg/day IV for 5 days

The drugs are given sequentially and alternately as soon as the oral and hematological toxicity from the preceding drug has subsided.

the uterus, for primary or secondary management in resistant cases.

Prognosis by Categories of Trophoblastic Disease

Among cases of nonmetastatic trophoblastic disease, a 100% salvage rate is expected. In low risk or good prognosis forms of metastatic disease, one can anticipate a salvage rate approaching 100% today.[2,16,28,32] Single-drug therapy is usually adequate.

Clinical experience suggests that if the disease is antedated by the obstetrical event by greater than four months and/or if the HCG titer is above 100,000 IU, the salvage rate is significantly adversely affected. It is also recognized that patients with cerebral and hepatic metastasis also showed particularly unfavorable salvage rates (20 to 25%). In addition, patients with metastatic disease, initially in the good prognosis category, who show progression or become resistant to single-drug therapy move into the poor prognosis category. These patients should be treated with three-drug therapy (Actinomycin D, Methotrexate, and Chlorambucil or Cytoxan) in conjunction with whole brain radiation if cerebral metastases are present, and either intraarterial hepatic infusion or radiation therapy to the liver if significant liver disease is present (Table 8). Remarkably, salvage among these cases with high risk or poor prognosis disease is now reported in the order of 70 to 85%.[28,32] These results continue to improve as greater experience is gained, since mortality among the high risk cases was, in the past, fairly

equally divided between deaths from this disease and deaths from treatment toxicity.

Most centers will treat all categories of patients one course beyond the first normal titer. Three consecutive weekly normal titers suggest 90% control of the disease. Regular follow-up titers are indicated for a minimum of one year (usually monthly for six months and bimonthly for the next six months). If the uterus is still in place, oral contraceptives are indicated to prevent pregnancy and to control a false-positive titer that might occur during an LH surge. Three consecutive monthly negative titers suggest 98% control of the disease.[33]

Table 8 Two Management Methods for Metastatic Trophoblastic Disease in High Risk or Poor Prognosis Categories

A. Three-Drug Program of Hammond[31]
  Use: For selected patients with poor prognosis.
    1. Initial therapy
       a. Admission HCG titers 100,000 IU/24 hr.
       b. Duration of disease in excess of 4 months
       c. Cerebral or hepatic metastases
    2. Subsequent therapy
       Only in other patients after developing disease resistant to single-agent treatment and adjunctive chemotherapy.
  Drug Plan
    1. Three drugs given simultaneously each day for 5 days:
       a. Methotrexate—15 mg/day/IM
       b. Actinomycin D—0.5 mg IV/day
       c. Chlorambucil 10 mg day/po
    2. Unusual safety criteria for toxicity
    3. Repetitive courses with minimum interval of 10 days between each
  Complications
    1. Major morbidity (severe marrow suppression)
    2. Mortality 10–15%

Adjuncts
    1. Organ radiation to liver and/or brain as indicated
       a. 2000 rads
       b. Delivered in 10–14 days
    2. Intraarterial infusion selectively to liver or uterus

B. Three-Drug Program of Smith[2]
  Use: Only for poor prognosis patients not demonstrating entirely satisfactory response to alternate-sequential therapy (Table 7B).

  Drug Plan
    1. Three drugs given simultaneously each day for 5 days:
       a. Actinomycin D—0.5 mg day/IV
       b. Methotrexate—10 to 15 mg day/IV
       c. Cytoxan—150 to 250 mg day/IV
    2. The 5-day courses of treatment are repeated as soon as the oral and hematological toxicity from the preceding treatment has subsided.

DYNAMIC MANAGEMENT

The substance of the former section may be reviewed in conjunction with Table 5, *Therapeutic Classification for Gestational Trophoblastic Disease,* used at the New England Trophoblastic Disease Center. In this classification we have discussed our views regarding termination and the post-evacuation follow-up for the first eight weeks.

For Group 2 with an elevated HCG titer with or without symptoms, one should conduct a metastatic survey as described herein and then employ single-agent chemotherapy or the alternate-sequential schedule as outlined in Table 7. If further childbearing is not desired, hysterectomy can be carried out on the third day of the first course of drug. In surgical cases and nonsurgical cases, subsequent drug is indicated by the response of the HCG titer.

Group 3 is managed essentially in the same way. Curettage in the first course of chemotherapy may or may not confirm choriocarcinoma. Goldstein differentiates between Groups 2 and 3 by the degree of myometrial invasion demonstrated by pelvic arteriography or curettage or both. In Group 4, curettings may or may not reveal choriocarcinoma, or biopsy of an identifiable metastasis may provide the final histologic picture. In any event, the full workup as previously described is carried out for Group 4 and 4b, and chemotherapy as outlined in Table 7.

For Group 4c, the high risk group (liver and/or brain metastasis, HCG titer over 100,000 IU, and duration of four or more months from the obsterical event), should be treated with three-drug therapy and, if indicated, adjunctive radiation, as described in Table 8.

This author believes that all patients in Groups 2, 3 and 4 are best managed in treatment centers. The grim results of sub-optimal care have been reviewed.[2]

IMMUNOLOGIC INVESTIGATION

The interesting investigative data that have accumulated on the subject of the fetus as a homograft, the variety of studies attempting to explain the successful growth and dissemination of choriocarcinoma (as a homograft), and the occasional documented cases of spontaneous regression are beyond the scope of this discussion. Two recent reports with sizable bibliographies[33,34] review in part some of the current activities on this topic.

REFERENCES

1. Ewing, J.: Chorioma. *Surg. Gynecol. Obstet.* **10:** 366 (1910).

2. Smith, J. P.: Trophoblastic disease: diagnosis and management. In *Endocrine and Nonendocrine Hormone-Producing Tumors,* Year Book Medical Publishers, Chicago, 1973.

3. Hertig, A. T., and H. Mansell: Hydatidiform Mole and Choriocarcinoma. In *Tumors of the Female Sex Organs, Atlas of Tumor Pathology.* Armed Forces Institute of Pathology, Washington, D.C. 1956.

4. Brewer, J. I., and A. B. Gerbie: Early development of choriocarcinoma. In *Choriocarcinoma; Transactions of a Conference of the International Union Against Cancer,* Holland, J. F., Hreshchyshyn, M. M. Berlin, Germany, Springer-Verlag, 1967.

5. Das, P. C.: Hydatidiform mole: a statistical and clinical study. *J. Obstet. Gynecol. Brit. Commonw.* **45:** 265 (1938).

6. Beischer, N. A., and D. W. Fortune: Significance of chromatin patterns in cases of hydatidiform mole with associated fetus. *Am. J. Obstet. Gynecol.* **100:** 276 (1968).

7. Brindeau, A., A. Hinglais, and M. Hinglais: La mole hydatidiform. Bulletin de la Federation des societes de gynecologie et d'obstetrique de tange, Francaise **4:** 3 (1952).

8. Marquez-Monter, H., G. Alfara de la Vega, M. Robles, A. Bolio-Cicero: Epidemiology

and pathology of hydatidiform mole in the General Hospital of Mexico: a study of 104 cases. *Am. J. Obstet. Gynecol.* **85:** 856 (1963).

9. Acosta-Sison, H.: The chance of malignancy in a repeated hydatidiform mole. *Am. J. Obstet. Gynecol.* **78:** 876 (1959).

10. Wei, P., and P. C. Ouyang: Trophoblastic disease in Taiwan: a review of 157 cases in a 10-year period. *Am. J. Obstet. Gynecol.* **85:** 844 (1963).

11. Hertig, A. T., and W. H. Sheldon: Hydatidiform mole: a pathological clinical correlation of 200 cases. *Am. J. Obstet. Gynecol.* **53:** 1 (1947).

12. Greene, R. R.: Chorioadenoma destruens. *Ann. N.Y. Acad. Sci.* **80:** 143 (1959).

13. Magrath, I. T., P. R. Golding, and K. D. Bagshawe: Medical presentations of choriocarcinoma. *Brit. Med. J.* **2:** 633, 1971.

14. Odell, W. D., R. Hertz, M. B. Lipsett, G. T. Ross, and C. B. Hammond: Endocrine aspects of trophoblastic neoplasms. *Clin. Obstet. Gynecol.* **10:** 290 (1967).

15. Park, W. W., and J. C. Lee: Choriocarcinoma: A general review with an analysis of 516 cases. *Arch. Pathol.* **49:** 205 (1950).

16. Goldstein, D. P.: The chemotherapy of gestational trophoblastic disease. *JAMA* **220:** 209 (1972).

17. Carr, D. H.: Cytogenics and the pathology of hydatidiform degeneration. *Obstet. Gynecol.* **33:** 333 (1969).

18. Baggish, M. S., J. D. Woodruff, S. H. Tow, and H. W. Jones, Jr.: Sex chromatin pattern in hydatidiform mole. *Am. J. Obstet. Gynecol.* **102:** 363 (1968).

19. Delfs, E.: Chorionic gonadotropin determination in patients with hydatidiform mole and choriocarcinoma. *Ann. N. Y. Acad. Sci.* **80:** 125 (1959).

20. Brewer, J. I.: *Textbook of Gynecology,* 3rd edit. The Williams and Wilkins Company, Baltimore, 1961.

21. Brewer, J. I., E. E. Torok, A. Webster, and R. E. Dolkart: Hydatidiform mole. A followup regimen for identification of invasive mole and choriocarcinoma and for selection of patients for treatment. *Am. J. Obstet. Gynecol.* **101:** 557 (1968).

22. Bagshawe, K. D., P. R. Golding, and A. H. Orr: Choriocarcinoma after hydatidiform mole. Studies related to effectiveness of followup practice after hydatidiform mole. *Brit. Med. J.* **3:** 733 (1969).

23. Pastorfide, G. B., and D. P. Goldstein: Pregnancy after hydatidiform mole. *Obstet. Gynecol.* **42:** 67 (1973).

24. Brewer, J. I., R. T. Smith, and G. B. Pratt: Choriocarcinoma. Absolute 5 year survival rates of 122 patients treated by hysterectomy. *Am. J. Obstet. Gynecol.* **85:** 841 (1963).

25. Lewis, J., Jr.: Chemotherapy and surgery in the treatment of gestational trophoblastic neoplasms. *Surg. Clin. North Am.* **49:** 371 (1969).

26. Goldstein, D. P., P. Winig, and R. L. Shirley: Actinomycin D as initial therapy of gestational trophoblastic disease. *Obstet. Gynecol.* **39:** 341 (1972).

27. Ross, G. T., D. P. Goldstein, R. Hertz, M. B. Lipsett, and W. D. Odell: Sequential use of methotrexate and actinomycin D in the treatment of metastatic choriocarcinoma and related trophoblastic diseases in women. *Am. J. Obstet. Gynecol.* **93:** 223 (1965).

28. Hammond, C. B., L. G. Borchert, L. Tyrey, W. T. Creasman, and R. T. Parker: Treatment of metastatic trophoblastic disease: good and poor prognosis. *Am. J. Obstet. Gynecol.* **115:** 451 (1973).

29. Goldstein, D. P.: Five years' experience with the prevention of trophoblastic tumors by the prophylactic use of chemotherapy in patients with molar pregnancy. *Clin. Obstet. Gynecol.* **13:** 945 (1971).

30. Brace, K. C.: The role of irradiation in the treatment of metastatic trophoblastic disease. *Radiology* **91:** 540 (1968).

31. Hammond, C. B., and R. T. Parker: Diagnosis and treatment of trophoblastic disease: A report from the Southern Regional Center. *Obstet. Gynecol.* **35:** 132 (1970).

32. W. B. Jones, and J. L. Lewis: Treatment of gestational trophoblastic disease. *Am. J. Obstet. Gynecol.* **120:** 14 (1974).

33. Lewis, J. L., Jr.: Chemotherapy of gestational choriocarcinoma. *Cancer* **30:** 1517 (1972).

34. Li, M. C.: Trophoblastic disease: natural history, diagnosis, and treatment. *Ann Int. Med.* **74:** 102 (1971).

CARCINOMA OF THE OVARY

CHAPTER 10 OVARIAN CANCER

RICHARD C. BORONOW, M.D.

The scourge of ovarian cancer looms ever greater on the American scene (Table 1). Although it represents the third most frequent gynecologic malignancy, it is now the number one killer. For the first time in the annals of recorded U.S. medical statistics, it has passed cervical cancer as the mortality leader among gynecologic cancers, and only colon, breast, and lung cancers kill more American women each year.

Clinical progress is subtle at best. Pap smears are of no value in detection. Primary therapy in selected instances has improved somewhat, but the overall impact of this therapy on morbidity and mortality is not statistically significant.

Research progress is also limited. The major visible thrust is among pathologists working for clarification of existing tumors and terminology and for a universally acceptable classification. The FIGO classification of the more common epithelial neoplasms is recorded in Table 2. The new WHO Classification is shown in Table 3.

The comparative incidence of ovarian cancers at operation is recorded in Table 4.

Retrospective clinicopathologic studies show that understanding of the biologic behavior of some of these neoplasms is being better defined, and in reports from several treatment centers Phase II and III chemotherapy trials suggest potential areas of real progress, particularly with some of the rarer tumors (see Chapter 13). These are valuable in terms of prognosis and carry therapeutic implications. To date, virologic investigation has been unrewarding. Some effort has been made to study cul-de-sac cytology, and these studies are continuing. However, the current clinical data are not promising. There is today a flurry of activity with a variety of immunologic investigations being undertaken with the hope of a screening, diagnostic serologic test to be based on the identification and purification of one or several specific ovarian cancer-associated antigens. This must be regarded as hopeful at best at this time.

EPIDEMIOLOGY

Little firm, human epidemiologic data are available on ovarian cancer. Critical studies are few and quantitatively limited. Wynder and associates[4] have critically studied the experience at Memorial Hospital in New York. Few available studies evaluate the individual ovarian malignancies, but rather

Table 1 Estimated Gynecologic Cancer Deaths and New Cases (1975)[1]

Site	Estimated New Cases	Estimated Deaths
Cervix (invasive)	19,000	7,800
Corpus	27,000	3,300
Ovary	17,000	10,800
Other female genital	4,600	1,000

Table 2   Histologic Classification of the Common Primary Epithelial Tumors of the Ovary (FIGO)[2]

I. Serous cystomas
   (a) Serous benign cystadenoma.
   (b) Serous cystadenomas with proliferating activity of the epithelial cells and nuclear abnormalities, but no infiltrative destructive growth (low potential malignancy).
   (c) Serous cystadenocarcinomas.

II. Mucinous cystomas
   (a) Mucinous benign cystadenomas.
   (b) Mucinous cystadenomas with proliferating activity of the epithelial cells and nuclear abnormalities, but no infiltrative destructive growth (low potential malignancy).

III. Endometrioid tumors (similar to adenocarcinomas in the endometrium)
   (a) Endometrioid benign cysts.
   (b) Endometrioid tumors with proliferating activity of the epithelial cells and nuclear abnormalities, but no infiltrative destructive growth (low potential malignancy).

IV. Mesonephric tumors
   (a) Benign mesonephric tumors.
   (b) Mesonephric tumors with proliferating activity of the epithelial cells and nuclear abnormalities, but no infiltrative destructive growth (low potential malignancy).
   (c) Mesonephric cystadenocarcinomas.

V. Concomitant carcinoma, unclassified carcinoma (tumors which cannot be allotted to one of the groups I, II, III, or IV).

group them as one entity: ovarian cancer. Berg and Baylor[5] express dissatisfaction at the classification confusion encountered in their review of 10,000 cases of ovarian cancer, and applaud the classification efforts of Sully (Table 3). Fathalla,[6] in a detailed review based on 169 references, discusses available epidemiologic data on human

Table 3   World Health Organization Histological Classification of Ovarian Tumors[3a]

I. Common 'Epithelial'' Tumors
   A. Serour Tumors
      1. Benign
         (a) cystadenoma and papillary cystadenoma
         (b) surface papilloma
         (c) adenofibroma and cystadenofibroma
      2. Of borderline malignancy (carcinoma of low malignant potential)
         (a) cystadenoma and papillary cystadenoma
         (b) surface papilloma
         (c) adenofibroma and cystadenofibroma
      3. Malignant
         (a) adeonocarcinoma, papillary adenocarcinoma, and papillary cystadenocarcinoma
         (b) surfade papillary carcinoma
         (c) malignant adenofibroma and cystadenofibroma
   B. Mucinous Tumours
      1. Benign
         (a) cystadenoma
         (b) adenofibroma and cystadenofibroma
      2. Of borderline malignancy (carcinoma of low malignant potential)
         (a) cystadenoma
         (b) adenofibroma and cystadenofibroma
      3. Malignant
         (a) adeoncarcinoma and cystadenocarcinoma
         (b) malignant adenofibroma and cystadenofibroma
   C. Endometrioid Tumors
      1. Benign
         (a) adenoma and cystadenoma

Table 3 **(continued)**

(b) adenofibroma and cysta-denofibroma

2. Of borderline malignancy (carcinoma of low malignant potential)

   (a) adenoma and cystadenoma

   (b) adenofibroma and cysta-denofibroma

3. Malignant

   (a) carcinoma

     (i) adenocarcinoma

     (ii) adenoacanthoma

     (iii) malignant adenofibroma

   (b) endometrioid stromal sarcomas

   (c) mesodermal (müllerian) mixed tumors, homologous, and heterologous

D. Clear Cell (Mesonephroid) Tumors

1. Benign: adenofibroma

2. Of borderline malignancy (carcinomas of low malignant potential)

3. Malignant: carcinoma and adenocarcinoma

E. Brenner Tumors

1. Benign

2. Of borderline malignancy (proliferating)

3. Malignant

F. Mixed Epithelial Tumors

1. Benign

2. Of borderline malignancy

3. Malignant

G. Undifferentiated Carcinoma

H. Unclassified Epithelial Tumors

II. Sex Cord Stromal Tumors

A. Granulosa-Stromal Tumors

1. Granulosa cell tumor

2. Tumors in the thecoma-fibroma group

   (a) thecoma

   (b) fibroma

   (c) unclassified

B. Androblastomas: Sertoli-Leydig Cell Tumors

1. Well differentiated

   (a) tubular androblastoma; Sertoli cell tumor (tubular adenoma of Pick)

   (b) tubular androblastoma with lipid storage; Sertoli cell tumor with lipid storage (folliculome lipidique of Lecene)

   (c) Sertoli-Leydig cell tumor (tubular adenoma with Leydig cells)

   (d) Leydig cell tumor; hilus cell tumor

2. Of intermediate differentiation

3. Poorly differentiated (sarcomatoid)

4. With heterologous elements

C. Gynadroblastoma

D. Unclassified

III. Lipid (Lipoid) Cell Tumors

IV. Germ Cell Tumors

A. Dysgerminoma

B. Endodermal Sinus Tumor

C. Embryonal Carcinoma

D. Polyembryoma

E. Choriocracinoma

F. Teratomas

1. Immature

2. Mature

   (a) solid

Table 3 (continued)

      (b) cystic

        (i) dermoid cyst (mature cystic teratoma)

        (ii) dermoid cyst with malignant transformation

   3. Monodermal and highly specialized

      (a) struma ovarii

      (b) carcinoid

      (c) struma ovarii and carcinoid

      (d) others

  G. Mixed Forms

V. Gonadoblastoma

  A. Pure

  B. Mixed With Dysgerminoma Or Other Form Of Germ Cell Tumor

VI. Soft Tissue Tumors Not Specific To Ovary

VII. Unclassified Tumors

VIII. Secondary (Metastatic) Tumors

IX. Tumor-Like Conditions

  A. Pregnancy Luteoma

  B. Hyperplasia Of Ovarian Stroma and Hyperthecosis

  C. Massive Oedema

  D. Solitary Follicle Cyst and Corpus Luteum Cyst

  E. Multiple Follicle Cysts (Polycystic Ovaries)

  F. Multiple Luteinized Follicle Cysts and/or Corpora Lutea

  G. Endometriosis

  H. Surface-Epithelial Inclusion Cysts (Germinal Inclusion Cysts)

  I. Simple Cysts

  J. Inflammatory Lesions

  K. Parovarian Cysts

Tabe 4 Comparative Incidence[a] of Ovarian Cancers at peration[3]

Type	Percent
Serous borderline tumor	10–15
Serous carcinoma	25–35
Mucinous borderline tumor	5–10
Mucinous carcinoma	5–10
Endometrioid borderline tumor	1–2
Endometrioid carcinoma	15–20
Clear cell carcinoma	4–6
Undifferentiated carcinomas and adenocarcinomas otherwise unclassifiable	5–10
Dysgerminoma	1–2
Embryonal teratoma	1–2
Malignant tumors in dermoid cysts	1–2
Granulosa cell tumor	5–10
Metastatic carcinomas	4–8
Others	1–2

[a] The percentages are estimates based on the author's experience and various sources in the literature. They do not apply to ovarian cancers in the Orient, where the incidence of the common carcinomas is lower, but that of malignant germ cell tumors is at least relatively higher.

ovarian cancer, spontaneous ovarian tumors in animals, and experimental ovarian tumors.

Support for the concept that ovarian cancer is an environmental and/or cultural disease is derived from observations on high- and low-incidence populations (Table 5). The incidence rate per hundred thousand per year in the United States ranges from 10 to 13, whereas in Japan the rate is 2.2. Since both countries probably have comparable diagnostic and therapeutic capabilities this discrepancy needs further study. Whatever the factors, it is remarkable that there is an increased risk of developing ovarian cancer in the first generation of Japanese immigrants in the United States, and that these immigrant populations ultimately develop ovarian cancer at a rate approaching that of their host country. Socioeconomic factors have been indicted: the highest incidence in this country appears in the upper

Table 5 International Incidence Rates for Selected Ovarian Cancers[5,7]

| Registry | Incidence of All Ovarian Cancer[a] | Incidence of Specific Types[a,b] | | | | No. Cases in Histology Series |
		Adeno-carcinomas[c]	Granulosa Cell Cancer	Dysger-minoma	Malignant Teratoma	
Sweden	14.4	11.8	1.2	0.14	0.17	3060
Alameda County, California (white)	12.6	10.6	0.3	—	0.22	286
Southwest region, England	12.2	7.0	0.6	0.20	0.07	846
Nevada	11.7	8.2	0.8	0.07	0.25	190
Connecticut	11.3[d]	13.2	0.7	0.30	0.21	915
Birmingham, England	10.8	7.9	0.3	0.05	0.16	1235
Liverpool, England	10.4	7.9	0.2	0.08	0.04	773
Alameda County, California (black)	10.4	9.9	0.5	—	0.69	27
Oxford, England	10.1	6.6	0.2	0.17	0.02	464
El Paso, Texas (non-Latin)	9.8	6.7	0.8	—	0.11	48
Bulawayo, Rhodesia (African)	9.7	9.2	—	—	—	5
Cali, Colombia	9.2	6.5	1.1	0.19	0.10	88
Vas, Hungary	9.0	2.3	0.1	0.92	0.10	57
El Paso, Texas (Latin)	8.8	5.2	0.2	0.19	0.20	30
Scotland	8.8	4.4	0.3	0.06	0.04	1206
Slovenia	8.6	5.5	0.2	0.10	0.02	335
Jamaica	8.3	4.9	0.3	0.13	0.32	47
Rural Poland	7.8	3.1	0.5	0.04	—	19
Miskolc, Hungary	7.7	5.1	0.2	0.20	—	33
Natal, South Africa (African)	6.4	3.1	0.6	—	0.20	23
Cracow, Poland	6.3	3.4	0.2	0.14	0.25	118
Bombay, India	6.1	1.7	0.1	0.06	—	103
Szaboles-Szatmar, Hungary	5.6	2.3	0.2	0.07	—	59
Katowice, Poland	5.5	1.9	—	—	—	52
Natal, South Africa (Indian)	3.3	1.2	—	—	0.45	6

[a] Rate per 100,000, age standardized to world population.
[b] Microscopically confirmed cases only.
[c] Includes all cystadenocarcinomas—mucinous, serous, and unspecified.
[d] Time period different for this incidence rate.

classes. This observation has been questioned because of differences in available medical care. Wynder and associates suggest that a dietary factor may be operative.

Although some families show a history of ovarian cancer, and isolated reports of ovarian cancers in twins have occurred, there is no solid evidence of genetic predisposition.[6,8,9] A number of studies indicated a positive correlation between ovarian cancer and infertility or lowered fertility in nuns and other single women.[6,10]

Malignant transformation of endometriosis has been documented, but it is rare.

The higher incidence rates in the United States among immigrant populations and previously identified groups of women in this country, and in chronically stressed animals (Table 6) introduce psychosomatic cofactors which are almost impossible to quantitate

Table 6   Ovarian Tumors in Domestic Animals[6,11]

Tumor Type	Canine	Equine	Bovine	Ovine	Porcine	Feline	Total
Adenocarcinoma, cystadenocarcinoma cystadenoma	40	1	8	0	1	2	52
Granulosa cell tumor	28	2	44	5	0	0	79
Dysgerminoma	6	0	0	0	0	0	6
Teratoma	2	4	0	0	0	0	6
Others	3	1	0	0	0	0	4
Total ovarian neoplasms	79	8	52	5	1	2	147
Total all neoplasms	5854	464	1371	129	167	174	8159

and are generally greeted with rejection or cautious skepticism by most of the medical community. Southam[12] states: "That the psyche might exert a significant influence on the etiology or the pathogenesis of malignant neoplastic disease seems entirely reasonable to me; in fact it seems probable. But I know of no solid evidence for the existence of such effect. . . . Until reasonable mechanisms for such an influence are elucidated, or until influence of the psyche on neoplasia is more certainly demonstrated, I prefer to remain skeptical, but not negativistic."

Although the etiology of ovarian cancer is unknown, epidemiology is beginning to develop data; currently, however, no conclusions can be reached.

ANATOMIC SPREAD AND STAGING

The most common ovarian cancers are the epithelial cancers (Tables 2, 3, 4). While there is a tendency for capsular involvement and breakthrough of any of the ovarian tumors, this is particularly true of the epithelial cancers. The serous variety is classically associated with papillary excrescences on the surface (Figure 1). Thus, the majority of ovarian cancers are found with spread beyond the ovary, involving pelvic or abdominal viscera and peritoneal surfaces. Vascular compartment invasion (lymphatic

and hematogenous) does occur, but is less appreciated because the surface spread of ovarian cancer dominates the clinical picture. Also, some tumors appear to arise bilaterally more than others (Table 7).

Table 7   Bilaterality in Ovarian Cancer[3]

Type	Bilaterality (%)	
	Total Cases	Stage I Cases
Serous carcinoma	67	33
Mucinous carcinoma	20	10
Endometrioid carcinoma	33	13
Clear cell carcinoma (mesonephroma)	10	
Undifferentiated, unclassified adenocarcinoma	54	
Dysgerminoma	5–12	
Teratoma	10–15	
Granulosa cell	5	

The Spread of Ovarian Cancer

All four classical methods of cancer spread apply to ovarian cancer. These include spread by the lymphatics, by the bloodstream, by local extension, and by surface seeding. Hematogenous metastasis and lymphatic metastasis are of less importance in most ovarian cancers than in many other

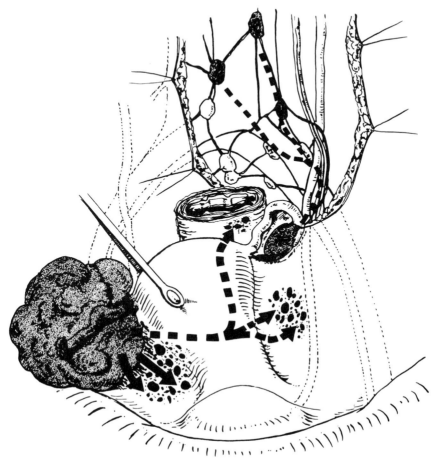

Figure 1 Local extension by contiguity (solid arrow) and peritoneal seeding (dashed arrow) are the major methods of spread of ovarian cancer, and dominate the clinical picture. Lymphatic spread (smaller dashed line) also occurs.

more common malignancies because the other mechanisms of spread usually occur more often and earlier, produce the major symptoms, and even provide the mechanism for death in the majority of cases. Nevertheless lymphatic involvement does occur, although the quantitative and qualitative aspects of this spread have not been adequately defined either in primary therapy or other aspects of subsequent therapy including "second look" operations.

LOCAL EXTENSION

This involves contiguous structures such as the tube, uterus, bladder, rectosigmoid, and other pelvic peritoneum. The degree of local extension determines the resectability of the ovarian lesion. If contiguous structures are heavily involved, simple removal of the primary lesion cannot be expected to accomplish much. Adjunctive chemotherapy and/ or radiotherapy will be necessary for hope of long-term survival. Nevertheless bulk-reductive surgery is of value[13] and should be as vigorous as the skill of the surgeon allows with relative safety.

PERITONEAL SEEDING

This is the major mechanism for dissemination of ovarian cancer. It should be emphasized that in the case of an entirely encapsulated ovarian cancer there is some hope that it has not spread beyond the pelvis; if there are papillary excrescences on the surface, however, there is the probability of seeding and a pattern of spread that is usually incurable. Once the capsule is broken the slightest, malignant cells may be freely shed —surgically or by growth of the tumor—to the peritoneal surface and thus disseminate the disease. Adjunctive therapy must be used in these instances if there is to be any reasonable hope for salvage. Data collected on cases clinically confined to the ovary (Stage 1) are seen in Table 8. This material by Webb and associates on the unfavorable outcome in cases with surface excrescences on the ovary, occult capsular involvement as suggested by adhesions of the ovarian tumor with contiguous structures, and rupture of the mass at surgical resection, provides support for the thesis of peritoneal seeding.

Table 8   Variations in Epithelial Ovarian Stage I Cancer Survival[14]

Finding	Five-Year Survival (%)
Intracystic	90
Extracystic	68
Adherent	50
Ruptured	58

Clinical Staging

The currently employed FIGO staging classification, adopted in October, 1974, is recorded in Table 9, and is based on the clinical findings at clinical examination and surgical exploration.

No classification of ovarian cancer is ideal because of the multiplicity of cell types involved, and their great variation and natural history; the FIGO listing is no exception. It is essential to use it, however, to assess and

Table 9   FIGO Stage Grouping for Primary Carcinoma of the Ovary Based on Findings at Clinical Examination and Surgical Exploration[2a]

Based on findings at clinical examination and surgical exploration. The final histology (and cytology when required) after surgery is to be considered in the staging.

Stage I	Growth limited to the ovaries.
Stage IA	Growth limited to one ovary; no ascites. (i) No tumor on the external surface; capsule intact. (ii) Tumor present on the external surface or/ and capsule ruptured.
Stage IB	Growth limited to *both* ovaries; no ascites. (i) No tumor on the external surface; capsule intact. (ii) Tumor present on the external surface or/and capsule (s) ruptured.
Stage IC	Tumor either Stage IA or Stage IB, but with ascites[a] present or positive peritoneal washings.
Stage II	Growth involving one or both ovaries with pelvic extension.
Stage IIA	Extension and/or metastases to the uterus and/or tubes.
Stage IIB	Extension to other pelvic tissues.
Stage IIC	Tumor either Stage IIA or Stage IIB, but with ascites[a] present or positive peritoneal washings
Stage III	Growth involving one or both ovaries with intraperitoneal metastases outside the pelvis and/or positive retroperitoneal nodes.

Table 9 (continued)

	Tumor limited to the true pelvis with histologically proven malignant extension to small bowel or omentum.
Stage IV	Growth involving one or both ovaries with distant metastases. If pleural effusion is present there must be positive cytology to allot a case to Stage IV. Parenchymal liver metastases equals Stage IV.
Special category.	Unexplored cases are thought to be ovarian carcinoma.

ᵃAscites is peritoneal effusion that in the opinion of the surgeon is pathological and/or clearly exceeds normal amounts.

compare our results. Preferably it should be supplemented by an exact record of cell type and histologic grade of malignancy, not only for comparing treatment and results, but more signficantly for planning appropriate primary and secondary therapy. It is no longer acceptable to lump all ovarian malignancies into a single category.

DIAGNOSTIC CONSIDERATIONS

Only rarely are there early signs and symptoms, and there are no currently available screening detection methods of suitable validity. Thus detection and diagnosis should be considered under two categories (1) the individual tumors themselves and (2) currently available detection methods.

Behavior of Ovarian Tumors

EPITHELIAL TUMORS

At least 60 to 70% of ovarian cancer is represented by the more common epithelial tumors (Tables 2, 3, 4). Treacherously, these epithelial tumors develop in a silent fashion. A pelvic/abdominal mass, the presence of ascites, pelvic pressure, abdominal distention, and an often vague history of progressive gastrointestinal tract symptoms such as increased flatulence, eructation, obstipation and the like are often the presenting symptoms and findings (Table 10). Thus these "early" signs and symptoms are usually Stage II and Stage III malignancies when confirmed by laparotomy. The prognosis is very unfavorable.

The serous cancers are the most common. They have generally been regarded as the most lethal of the epithelial cancers. Recent work has reviewed salvage in the epithelial cancers by histologic grading, by clinical staging, and by both variables. Decker and associates[16] found low-grade serous lesions (Grades 1 and 2) and high-grade lesions (Grades 3 and 4) almost equally distributed (236 to 256), but the low-grade lesions were usually found in the early stages and the high-grade lesions in the later stages. A significant difference was found in their study of the mucinous cancers: 144 of a total of 155 tumors were low grade, and only 36 showed an advanced clinical stage. Thus these interrelated factors (histologic grade and clinical stage) probably explain the discrepancy in the overall salvage rates quoted for serous and mucinous ovarian cancers. Indeed, both as composite groups and when broken down into stages the survival graphs of tumors by histologic differentiation could be virtually superimposed (Stage I data, Table 11). Stage for stage, the salvage rate for the so-called borderline lesion (category b in Table 2) is even more favorable[2,17] (Table 13).

The peak ages of ovarian epithelial cancer are in the fifth and sixth decades with the vast majority of cases occurring between 35 and 75 (Figure 2). Scully[3] notes that 7 to 8% of epithelial ovarian cancers occur under age 35.

Table 10 Complaints Reported by Patients Found to Have Ovarian Cancer[10]

Symptoms	Taylor's Series[15]		Schueller's Series[10]	
	Patients	Percent of Series	Patients	Percent of Series
Abdominal distention	43	36.0	185	35.9
Chronic low abdominal pain	29	24.0	160	31.0
Postmenopausal bleeding	15	12.0	41	8.0
Acute low abdominal pain	12	10.0	14	3.0
Metrorrhagia	5	4.0	42	8.0
Inguinal node enlargement	4	3.0	6	1.2
Menorrhagia	4	3.0	3	
Weight loss	2		32	6.0
Menometrorrhagia	2		0	
No symptoms	2		17	
Rectal fullness	1		9	
Rectal bleeding	1		2	
Unknown	2		5	
Total number of patients	122		516	

Table 11 Stage I Ovarian Epithelial Cancer Survival by Grade[16]

		Number	5-Year Survival (%)
Serous	Grade 1	62	87
	Grade 2	29	51
	Grades 3, 4	39	54
Mucinous	Grade 1	84	89
	Grade 2	14	73
	Grades 3, 4	2	—

This author believes that because of these data and our inadequate therapeutic tools for ovarian cancer, if hysterectomy is indicated, ovaries too should be removed in any woman 35 years or older.[18]

Representative examples of ovarian epithelial cancer are seen in Figures 3–7.

SEX CORD STROMAL TUMORS

In the past, particularly in the USA, these were called sex cord mesenchyme tumors.

Morris and Scully[22] apply this term to all tumors originating ultimately from the sex cords, mesenchyme, or both, of the embryonic ovary. They prefer this term to others such as "mesenchymoma" and "gonadal stromal tumor" that are based on the controversial assumption that the sex cords and their derivatives originate from the mesenchyme rather than the coelomic epithelium.

Granulosa cell tumor. The most important of this group is the granulosa cell tumor which accounts for 5 to 10% of ovarian neoplasms. In most instances because of their estrogen production there may be symptoms of end-organ stimulation. Thus relatively early bona fide symptoms may be present. Although the majority of these tumors occur in the menstrual years, and may be associated with menstrual irregularity that demands careful pelvic exam and further evaluation, others occur in the postmenopausal group and, less commonly, in the premenarchal group. Among these patients, evidence of breast stimulation and uterine bleeding prompt careful investiga-

Table 12   Survival for Obviously Malignant Carcinomas[2]

Clinical Stage	Serous Carcinoma No. of Cases			Mucinous Carcinoma No. of Cases			Endometrioid and Mesonephric Carcinoma No. of Cases			Unclassified Carcinoma No. of Cases		
	Treated	Alive 5 yr	%	Treated	Alive 5 yr	%	Treated	Alive 5 yr	%	Treated	Alive 5 yr	%
IA	212	116	54.7	104	76	73.1	102	64	62.7	65	37	56.9
IB, IIA	138	50	36.2	51	22	43.1	78	41	52.6	28	11	39.3
IIB	209	52	24.9	50	21	42.0	120	58	48.3	67	10	14.9
III	414	26	6.3	76	12	15.8	134	10	7.5	200	9	4.5
IV	137	4	2.9	24	0		35	0		76	3	3.9
Total	1110	248	22.3	305	131	43.0	469	173	36.9	436	70	16.1

Table 13   Survival for Cases of So-Called Low Potential Malignancy, All Types[2]

Clinical Stage	No. of Cases		
	Treated	Alive 5 yr	%
IA	188	157	83.5
IB, IIA	90	62	68.9
IIB	71	46	64.8
III	76	33	43.4
IV	26	5	19.2
Total	451	303	67.2

tion. These tumors are bilateral in about 5% of cases. Overall salvage is reasonably good. This is especially true if the histologic pattern is well differentiated (follicular or trabecular) rather than poorly differentiated (sarcomatoid). Delayed (beyond five years) recurrence is relatively common.

GERM CELL TUMORS

Malignant germ cell tumors are usually encountered in children and young adults; thus a pelvic mass in this population clearly suggests a malignant ovary. In rare instances of pure or mixed ovarian choriocarcinoma, elevation of human chorionic gonadotropin (HCG) with a positive pregnancy test will be found.

Dysgerminoma. This tumor accounts for 1 to 2% of ovarian cancer: 50% of the cases occur in young women under 20 years of age and another 25% in those between 20 and 29.[5] Bilaterality is reported to be from 5 to 12%.[3] Histologically identical to seminoma, these tumors are radiosensitive. It is the most common of germ cell malignancies.

Endodermal sinus tumors. Endodermal sinus tumors are uncommon, histologically characteristic tumors that may be pure or mixed. Their behavior is highly aggressive. Although it was uniformly fatal in the past, aggressive combination chemotherapy achieves apparent cures in some of these patients today.

Teratomas. Berg and Baylor[5] noted a bimodal age distribution. About 50% of the cases occurred in women under 30 years of age, 6% in the decade from 30 to 39, then an increase in occurrence with a mode of about 57. Experience in the United States,

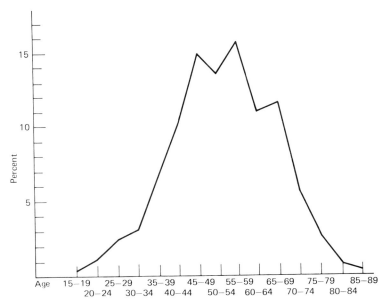

Figure 2 New York State data demonstrating the sharp rise in ovarian cancer after age 35. The peak age groups are dominated by epithelial cancer and, under 35, by germ cell tumor. From Randall, C. L., and Schueller E. F.: Malignant lesions of the fallopian tubes and ovaries. In *Textbok of Obstetrics and Gynecology*, 2nd edit. D. N. Danforth, Ed. Harper and Row, New York, N.Y., 1971). Reprinted with permission.

however, suggests that these tumors are rare in patients over 40.[3,19] The rare mixed mesodermal tumor of the ovary is now included in the WHO classification in the Epithelial Tumor group. In the past many have designated them as teratomas, which may explain this discrepancy. The Berg and Baylor report also mentions a significantly greater number of black women with these tumors.

GONADOBLASTOMA

These rare tumors may be pure or associated with dysgerminoma, rarely with choriocarcinoma. In the pure form they do not metastasize. They arise in abnormal testes and also in the dysgenetic ovary. They are usually found in phenotypic females who are virilized to some extent. They are almost always chromatin negative and have a *Y* chromosome. They may also develop in phenotypic males. Because they are at least premalignant, and since the patient's gonads are useless organs, they should be removed.[3,20,21]

METASTATIC CANCER

This is not simply an academic consideration. Metastatic disease must always be considered when an ovarian mass (or masses) is discovered.[23] Munnell and Taylor[24] reported that 20% of all ovarian cancers were found to be metastatic. In another large series, including autopsy material, Gallager[25] noted that the incidence of ovarian metastases actually exceeded that of primary carcinoma. Santesson and Kottmeier[26] reported 6% of ovarian cancers encountered by the surgeon exploring a pelvic/abdominal mass were metastatic. Although the most frequent primary lesions are in the breast, colon, stomach, and endometrium, cancers from virtually every primary site have been reported to spread to the ovaries. Thus the possibility of metastatic disease must always be considered in critical preoperative evaluation of the patient with a pelvic mass.

Detection Methods

As stressed in the foregoing, signs and symptoms of ovarian cancer are elusive. The

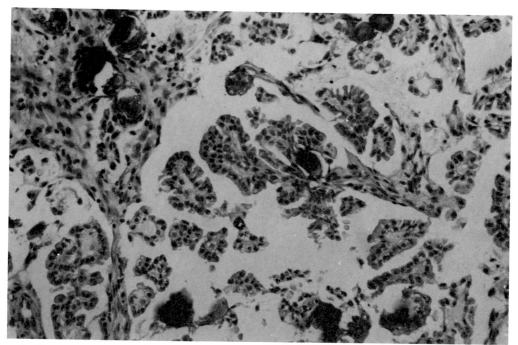

Figure 3 Serous carcinoma, well differentiated. Note psammoma bodies throughout field, with fair uniformity of proliferating cells in many areas as single layers.

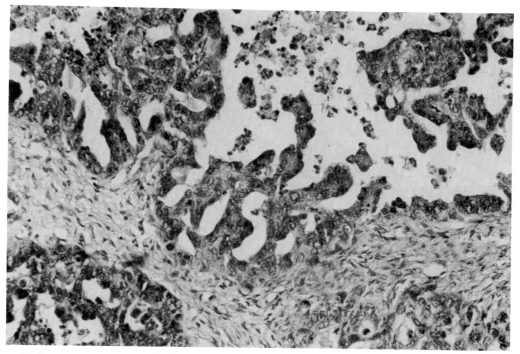

Figure 4 Serous carcinoma, poorly differentiated. There is some retention of papillary pattern, but marked cellular pleomorphism.

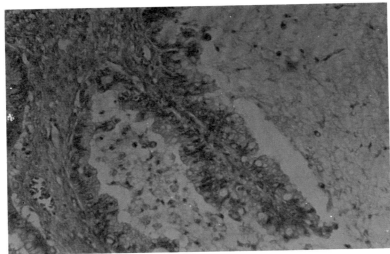

Figure 5 Mucinous carcinoma, well differentiated. Papillary formation with some pallisading can be seen.

physical findings are the usual method of detection. In most instances laparotomy is needed to confirm both early and advanced disease. An understanding of the individual tumors in terms of age distribution, possible endocrine function and the like are impor-

tant in evaluating pelvic masses among all age groups. Clearly, a pelvic mass found in an adolescent or in a premenarchal child suggests malignancy and warrants further study. Finally, as has been emphasized recently by Barber and Graber,[27] the presence

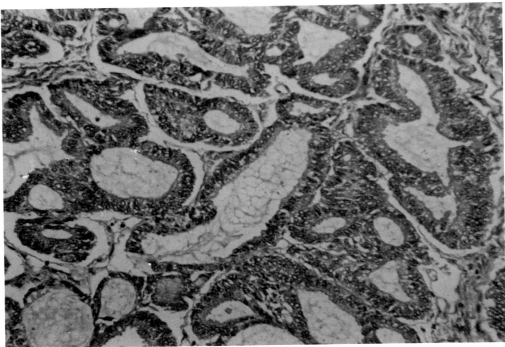

Figure 6 Endometrioid carcinoma. Glandular pattern with tall lining cells, similar to endometrial cancer.

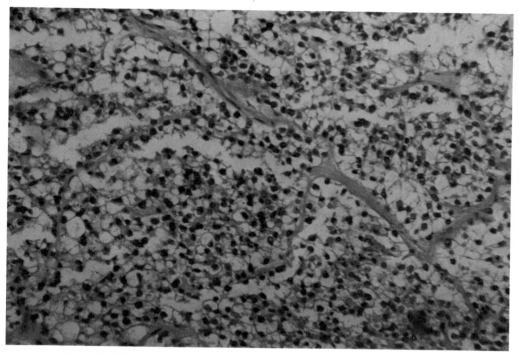

Figure 7 Mesonephric carcinoma. This clear-cell cancer presents a solid pattern.

of an adnexal mass of almost any size in the postmenopausal patient should raise suspicion of neoplasm. As these authors have pointed out, the postmenopausal ovary should be atrophic, less than several centimeters in greatest diameter, and virtually nonpalpable in the office (Figure 8).

CUL-DE-SAC ASPIRATION

There is no early detection of ovarian cancer for practical purposes. The cul-de-sac tap for cytologic study is championed by some.[28,29] Its disadvantages include (1) Technical problems and interpretive differentiation of ovarian and mesothelial cells,[29] (2) The clear implications that if malignant cells have been shed freely into the cul-de-sac they are also likely to be shed freely elsewhere, and that while the diagnosis may be early, the cancer is not, (3) A consensus among practicing gynecologists that if routine culdocentesis were done as a part of each office visit, their practices would soon

dwindle to nothing, since the procedure is a very uncomfortable experience for most patients.

Data are, however, being gathered, and perhaps culdocentesis and cytologic study of washings obtained may have a place when D & C is done on the age group at risk.

IMMUNOLOGIC STUDIES

In recent years, the recognition of tissue-specific and tumor-associated antigens, and the interest in the carcinoembryonic antigen (CEA) initially reported with colon cancers, have caused much investigation to be directed at the antigenicity of ovarian neoplasms in the hope that serologic screening tests may be devised. The specificity of these antigens remains elusive. CEA, a variety of fetal proteins, and other antigens are now discovered in association with a variety of cancers including ovarian cancers.[30,31,32] Thus despite the great effort being made at this time, hope rather than clinically appli-

Normal ovary
Premenopausal
3.5 x 2 x 1.5 cm

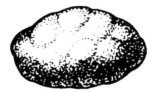

Early menopause
(1 - 2 years)
2 x 1.5 x 0.5 cm

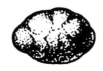

Late menopause
(2 - 5 years)
1.5 x 0.75 x 0.5 cm

Figure 8   From Barber, H. R. K., and E. A. Graber: The PMPO syndrome (post menopausal palpable ovary syndrome). *Obstet. Gynecol* **38**: 921 (1971). Reprinted with permission.

cable data surrounds current immunologic study and speculation. Tumors are antigenic. Yet even the precise identification of ovarian tumor antigens, still an investigative effort with diverse preliminary results,[33,34,35] remains far from being clinically applicable to the asymptomatic patient.

PROGNOSTIC FACTORS

Certain general prognostic factors are evident. The clinical extent (clinical stage) of the disease is the most significant (Table 12). In addition, we now have documentation of the less favorable prognosis with lesser degrees of histologic differentiation, corrected by stage of disease, for the epithelial tumors in particular (Tables 11, 13). Thirdly, precise histologic identification and an understanding of the biologic behavior of the full spectrum of ovarian malignancy is essential.

From the standpoint of radiation therapy, the dysgerminoma is particularly radiosensi-

tive. The more common epithelial tumors appear to have an intermediate degree of radiosensitivity, largely influenced perhaps by a volume-dose relationship. Scant data are available on the radiosensitivity of granulosa-theca tumors, although some of these tumors seem to respond. The malignant teratomas do not appear to be at all radiosensitive.

With chemotherapy, only the epithelial tumors show some degree of response to the conventionally employed alkylating agents. Currently, Phase II studies demonstrate the potental benefit of other new agents. Multiple drug programs are the only hope for advanced germ cell tumors. Also, preliminary trials suggest the value of combinations for the epithelial tumor.

The prognostic significance of capsular involvement by gross breakthrough, adhesions to other strutures, and rupture at the time of removal have been discussed. Ascites with malignant cells or peritoneal washings positive for malignant cells, even in the absence of ascites, is similarly ominous.

In a Stage IA clinical setting, appreciation of a variety of these prognostic factors becomes important in the young patient whose reproductive capacity is at stake. Modifications of so-called standard therapy may occasionally be acceptable when the lesion is intracystic (encapsulated) and the contralateral ovary is grossly normal; when the tumor is a well-differentiated germ cell or gonadal stromal tumor or a Grade 1 epithelial tumor; when a sizable wedge of the apparently normal contralateral ovary is removed for study and is negative, and when a solid doctor-patient relationship exists. Most clinicians and pathologists are relieved that this clinical setting is not frequent!

Table 7 classifies the data collected by Scully, which indicates the probability of bilaterality in Stage I disease for the three more common tumors, and the apparent total bilaterality for most of the other tumors.

REFERENCES

1. American Cancer Society: *Cancer Facts and Figures,* New York, 1975.

2. Kottmeier, H. L., Ed.: *Annual Report on the Results of Treatment in Carcinoma of the Uterus, Vagina and Ovary,* Vol. 15, International Federation of Gynecology and Obstetrics, Stockholm, 1973.

2a. International Federation of Gynecology and Obstetrics, Stockholm, 1974.

3. Scully, R. E.: Recent progress in ovarian cancer. *Hum. Pathol.* **1:** 73 (1970).

3a. Scully, R. E., S. F. Serov, and L. H. Sobin, Eds.): *Histological Typing of Ovarian Tumors,* World Health Organization, Geneva, 1973.

4. Wynder, E. L., H. Dodo, and H. R. K. Barber: Epidemiology of cancer of the ovary. *Cancer* **23:** 352 (1969).

5. Berg, J. W., and S. M. Baylor: The epidemiologic pathology of ovarian cancer. *Human Pathol.* **4:** 537 (1973).

6. Fathalla, M. F.: Factors in the causation and incidence of ovarian cancer. *Obstet. Gynecol. Surv.* **27:** 751 (1972).

7. Doll, R., C. Muir, and J. Waterhouse, Eds.: *Cancer Incidence in Five Continents,* Vol. II, International Union Against Cancer, Berlin, 1970.

8. Li, F. P., A. H. Rapaport, J. F. Fraumeni, and R. D. Jensen: Familial ovarian carcinoma, JAMA **214:** (1970).

9. McCrann, D. J., D. J. Marchant, and W. A. Bardawil: Ovarian carcinoma in three teenage siblings. *Obstet. Gynecol.* **43:** 132 (1974).

10. Randall, C. L., and E. F. Schueller: Malignant lesions of the fallopian tubes and ovaries. In Danforth, D. N., Ed., *Textbook of Obstetrics and Gynecology,* 2nd edit., Harper & Row, New York, 1971.

11. Smith, H. A., and T. C. Jones: *Veterinary Pathology,* 3rd edit., Lea & Febiger, Philadelphia, 1966.

12. Southam, C. M.: Emotions, immunology and cancer: how might the psyche influence neoplasia? In Second Conference on Psychophysiological Aspects of Cancer *Ann. N.Y. Acad. Sci.* **164:** 473 (1969).

13. Hreshchyshyn, N. M.: Single-drug therapy in ovarian cancer: factors influencing response. *Gynecol. Oncol.* **1:** 220 (1973).

14. Webb, M. J., D. G. Decker, E. Mussey, and T. J. Williams: Factors influencing survival in stage I ovarian cancer. *Am. J. Obstet. Gynecol.* **116:** 222 (1973).

15. Taylor, H. C., Jr.: Studies in the clinical and biological evolution of adenocarcinoma of the ovary. *J. Obstet. Gynaecol. Brit. Commonw.* **66:** 827 (1959).

16. Decker, D. G., E. Mussey, T. J. Williams, and W. F. Taylor: Grading of Gynecologic malignancy: epithelial ovarian cancer. In Proceedings of the Seventh National Cancer Conference, J. B. Lippincott Company, Philadelphia, 1973.

17. Julian, C., and J. D. Woodruff: The biologic behavior of low-grade papillary serous carcinoma of the ovary. *Obstet. Gynecol.* **40:** 860 (1972).

18. Gibbs, E. K.: Suggested prophylasis for ovarian cancer. *Am. J. Obstet. Gynecol.* **111:** 756 (1971).

19. Norris, H. J., and R. D. Jensen: Relative frequency of ovarian neoplasms in children and adolescents. *Cancer* **30:** 713 (1972).

20. Shellhas, H. F., J. M. Trujillo, F. N. Rutledge, and A. Cork: Germ cell tumors as-

sociated with XY gonadal dysgenesis. *Am. J. Obstet. Gynecol.* **109:** 1197 (1971).

21. Gallager, H. S., and R. P. Lewis: Sequential gonadoblastoma and choriocarcinoma. *Obstet. Gynecol.* **41:** 123 (1973).

22. Morris, J. M., and R. E. Scully: *Endocrine Pathology of the Ovary,* C. V. Mosby Company, St. Louis, 1958.

23. Boronow, R. C., and D. N. Danforth: Surgical treatment of cancer of the ovary. *J. Int. Fed. Gynecol. Obstet.* **4:** 253 (1966).

24. Munnell, E. W., and H. C. Taylor: Ovarian carcinoma: a review of 200 primary and 51 secondary cases. *Am. J. Obstet. Gynecol.* **58:** 943 (1949).

25. Gallager, H. S.: Differential diagnosis of primary and metastatic ovarian cancers. In *Carcinoma of the Uterine Cervix, Endometrium and Ovary,* Year Book Publishers, Chicago, 1962.

26. Santesson, L., and H. L. Kottmeier: General classification of ovarian tumors. In *Ovarian Cancer,* Gentil, F., and Jungueira, A. C., Eds., *UICC Monograph Ser.,* Vol. II, Springer-Verlag, New York, 1968.

27. Barber, H. R. K., and E. A. Graber: The PMPO syndrome (post menopausal palpable ovary syndrome). *Obstet. Gynecol.* **38:** 921 (1971).

28. Graham, R.: Diagnosis of ovarian carcinoma by cul de sac aspiration. In *Ovarian Cancer,*

Gentil, F., and Junqueira, A. C., Eds., UICC Monograph Ser., Vol. II, Springer-Verlag, New York, 1968.

29. McGowan, L., and B. Bunnag: A morphologic classification of peritoneal fluid cytology in women. *Int. J. Gynaecol. Obstet.* **11:** 173 (1973).

30. Wilkinson, E. J., E. G. Friedrich, and T. A. Hasty: Alphafetoprotein and endodermal sinus tumor of the ovary. *Am. J. Obstet. Gynecol.* **116:** 711 (1973).

31. Gerfo, P. L., J. Krupey, and H. J. Hansen: Demonstration of an antigen common to several varieties of neoplasia. *New. Engl. J. Med.* **285:** 138 (1971).

32. DiSaia, P. J., B. J. Haverback, B. J. Dyce, and C. P. Morrow: Cacrinoembryonic antigen in patients with gynecological malignancies. *Am. J. Obstet. Gynecol.* **121:** 159 (1975).

33. Levi, M. M., S. Keller, and I. Mandl: Antigenicity of a papillary serous cystadenocarcinoma tissue homogenate and its fractions. *Am. J. Obstet. Gynecol.* **105:** 856 (1969).

34. Gall, S. A., J. Walling, and J. Pearl: Demonstration of tumor-associated antigens in human gynecologic malignancies. *Am. J. Obstet. Gynecol.* **115:** 387 (1973).

35. Ioachim, H. O., B. Dorsett, M. Sabbath, B. O. Anderson, and H. R. K. Barber: Antigenic and morphologic properties of ovarian carcinoma. *Gynecol. Oncol.* **1:** 130 (1973).

CHAPTER 11 PRINCIPLES OF SURGICAL AND IRRADIATION TREATMENT FOR CARCINOMA OF THE OVARY

J. TAYLOR WHARTON, M.D.

Ovarian carcinoma of müllerian origin is a leading cause of death from gynecologic malignancy. These cancers may be discovered by any surgeon who performs laparotomies. Survival rates are low and have not improved appreciably over the last two decades. Perhaps the trend could be reversed if presently available treatment knowledge was uniformly applied to every patient with ovarian cancer. This could be accomplished if the principles of management were understood by all physicians responsible for the care of these patients.

The information obtained at the initial laparotomy is vital to successful therapy planning. The operating surgeon must determine the exact extent of the cancer, obtain adequate tissue for documentation of histologic type and differentiation, and estimate the volume of unresectable cancer remaining in the abdomen. This information is necessary for optimal therapy planning. This chapter will discuss the basic principles of surgical management and apply the information to an overall treatment plan.

SURGICAL TREATMENT

Total abdominal hysterectomy and bilateral salpingo-oophorectomy is the standard treatment. Hysterectomy is necessary because metastases to the uterus are common; it also eliminates a useless organ that may make posttherapy pelvic evaluation difficult and/or cause additional complications. Since epithelial cancers frequently occur in both ovaries, failure to remove them both risks a recurrence even though one ovary may appear normal. An exception to this rule may be practiced for the patient with a well-differentiated Stage IA mucinous carcinoma. A conservative approach may be permissible for a young patient to whom fertility is especially important. The surgeon should realize, however, that such treatment is a compromise, and that it would be wise to remove the other ovary and uterus following completion of the patients reproductive career. During the interval, regular postoperative examinations should detect enlargement of the remaining ovary in time to institute an effective second operation.

Radicality of Operation

Some gynecologists advocate omentectomy as routine surgery. In our opinion, it remains unproven that total omentectomy improves survival when the omentum appears normal. Even though excision of the acces-

177

sible part of the omentum is simple, the benefit of partial omentectomy to reduce recurrences is also doubtful. Since total omentectomy is a difficult and potentially hazardous procedure, we recommend it only when the omentum contains cancer.

Resection and anastomosis of a portion of the intestine is recommended if removal of the metastatic site clears the abdomen of all known cancer. A radical intestinal resection with excision of multiple segments can be associated with a prolonged recovery period, leading to debilitation and delaying postoperative treatment.

The surgical effort should be aggressive since the surgeon frequently finds conditions that seem impossible. Persistent dissection frees the adherent cancer and the bulk of the tumor can be removed.

SPREAD PATTERN

Ovarian cancer is a disease of the entire abdominal cavity. Once it has spread beyond the ovary there is a tendency for the cancer to involve multiple sites in the pelvis and abdomen. Multiple mechanisms for metastasis must be available. Direct extension is readily understood since the cancer penetrates the capsule and invades adjacent tissue. Cancer cells that are free in the peritoneal cavity have a tendency to implant. Areas such as the peritoneum lateral to the colon attachments and beneath the diaphragm are particularly important. When the patient is supine, the subdiaphragmatic regions represent dependent areas and perhaps gravity augments spread to these areas. Often multiple small nodules found on the surface of the dome of the liver or on the peritoneum covering the diaphram represent the only clinical evidence of metastasis to the abdominal cavity. Care should be exercised when palpating the lateral and inferior aspect of the liver surface because excessive manipulation can result in injury.

Lymphatic metastasis also seems to play a major role, and superficial involvement of the peritoneum may be diffuse. Retroperitoneal lymph node metastasis may also occur. The lymphatics that drain the ovary follow the ovarian veins. The left ovarian vein joins the left renal vein and the right vein empties into the vena cava. Therefore, the precaval and paraaortic nodes may represent first chain nodes in patients with metastatic ovarian cancer.

Peritoneal and pelvic cytology may also reveal clusters of malignant cells in an otherwise normal appearing abdomen. Specimens are obtained by lavaging the areas lateral to the ascending and decending colon and also the pelvis with isotonic saline. The solution is then promptly sent to the cytology laboratory for processing.

THERAPY SELECTION

Epithelial ovarian tumors respond in a similar manner to both radiation and chemotherapy. Careful treatment selection is essential if the full potential of either modality is to be realized. By determining the exact extent of metastasis and volume of residual disease, the surgeon supplies the necessary information for this selection.

Radiation therapy will be ineffective if even the smallest implants are present on or above the liver or on the peritoneum covering the kidneys. This occurs because both organs are very sensitive to radiation, and irreversible damage will result at doses below the levels required to control tumor implants.[13] Therefore, the liver and kidneys are shielded with lead during radiation therapy, although this protection also provides a pootential sanctuary for tumor cells.

Tumor volume also influences radiation therapy. This can be demonstrated by examining data for squamous carcinomas (Table 1). The larger the volume of tumor treated, the higher the dose of radiation required. Small aggregates or implants are well controlled with lower doses, which are also safe for normal tissue. A similar volume/dose relationship exists for epithelial

Table 1 Dose-Tumor Volume Relationships for Approximately 90% Control in Squamous Cell Carcinomas of the Upper Respiratory and Digestive Tracts[4]

Tumor Size	Radiation Dose (rads)
Microscopic aggregate	5000
< 2 cm	6000
2–4 cm	6800
4–6 cm	7310
> 6 cm	7890

cancers of the ovary. Therefore if the physician elects to use radiation therapy, the volume of tumor treated must be small so that a cancerocidal dose can be given without exceeding normal tissue tolerance.

Clinical experience in treating ovarian cancer strongly supports the preceding statements. The survival rate decreases as the size of the tumor implants increase. Based on this experience, it is less desirable to treat patients with radiation when the tumor volume exceeds 2 cm in greatest diameter.[3]

Patients with clinically recognizable ascites are poor candidates for radiation therapy. Ascites should aid the dissemination of free cells within the peritoneal cavity, allowing some to be protected by the lead shielding covering the liver and kidney. Since ascites also poses technical problems for radiotherapists because the volume of the abdomen may change from day to day, the

Table 2 Radiation Therapy: Criteria for Patient Selection, The M. D. Anderson Hospital

1. Residual tumor masses 2 cm or less in diameter.
2. No evidence of clinically recognizable ascites.
3. No evidence of metastatic deposits on the peritoneum of the liver and kidneys.
4. No history of prior abdominal radiation.
5. No evidence of distant metastasis.

requirements for irradiation therapy are rigid. Table 2 summarizes the essential information.

RADIATION THERAPY

General Aspects

Radiotherapy has been used for some time as an adjunct to surgery as primary therapy for nonresectable disease, and for palliation in advanced cases. Since the majority of patients with all stages of ovarian cancer need some type of additional treatment postoperatively, irradiation is often chosen. There is no agreement among radiotherapists about the need for whole abdominal postoperative irradiation in patients with Stages I and II cancer, nor is there a standard system of dose rate or treatment fields for use when whole abdominal irradiation is warranted. The general concensus in most of the major institutions that have accumulated considerable experience is that patients selected for irradiation therapy should receive treatment to the entire abdomen plus irradiation to the pelvis. This broad treatment plan is based on the concept that ovarian cancer is a disease of the entire abdomen, since cells that escape from the primary ovarian tumor circulate throughout the entire abdominal cavity. Obviously these cells cannot be reached if treatment is directed to the pelvis only.

Since patients with Stage I cancer have a recurrence incidence of 25%, operation alone is not dependable. The value of irradiation therapy for these patients is a subject of considerable controversy. Almost all authors reporting large numbers of treated patients stress that the nonrandomized nature of their studies prejudices their results and they emphasize the need for controlled series. The classic study by Munnell[9] reported 194 cases of Stage IA ovarian cancer and noted a better survival rate with surgery alone. Here the surgeons felt that some form of additional therapy was necessary in spite of the staging in the group that received radiotherapy, and therefore a direct comparison between the treated and untreated patients was not possible.

A review of the literature on Stage II disease suggests that radiotherapy is clearly beneficial for patients whose disease is confined to the true pelvis but not surgically resectable. Delclos and Quinlan,[2] Hanks and Bagshaw,[5] and Rubin and associates[10] have reported favorable results with surgery plus radiotherapy in Stage II disease.

When extension outside the true pelvis occurs, in Stages III and IV, the results of radiotherapy are poor. Five-year survival rates approximate 15% regardless of the method chosen. Mean survival is usually less than one year. Although ovarian carcinoma is radiosensitive, the major difficulty in applying radiotherapy is in encompassing the whole tumor with effective doses that do not exceed patient tolerance.

Abdominal irradiation can be associated with significant toxicity. Hanks and Bagshaw provide considerable information about toxicity in a series of 129 patients in all stages of disease treated with whole abdominal irradiation.[5]

Types of Radiation

External irradiation with a linear accelerator, cobalt unit, or betatron delivers a high dose into the depths of the tumor and is best used as postoperative therapy for ovarian cancer. Isotopes only penetrate a few millimeters into the tumor and can only treat cancers as free cells within the peritoneal cavity or as a very small surface implant.

EXTERNAL IRRADIATION

Different irradiation treatment techniques are used at individual centers. Large portals may be applied, and a dose of 3000 rads over four to five weeks can be delivered to the whole abdomen with an additional 1000 or 2000 rads to the pelvis. Pelvic irradiation with extended fields to cover the common iliac and lower paraaortic nodes has also been employed. Some radiotherapists irradiate the lower abdomen, usually giving the patient 5000 rads over a five-week period. Other techniques such as combination chemotherapy and irradiation therapy are currently available, and some clinics utilize preoperative irradiation in patients with suspected or proven ovarian cancer.

THE M. D. ANDERSON HOSPITAL METHOD

At the M. D. Anderson Hospital, postoperative irradiation has been found to be most effective when directed to the entire abdomen. The moving strip technique is used, with supplemental pelvic irradiation with a 22-MeV betatron.[2]

The abdomen is divided into contiguous segments or strips 2½ cm wide. The field is increased by one strip every two days until four strips or 10 cm have been treated. The 10 cm segment is moved up 2.5 cm every two days until the last strip is reached. The field is then reduced progressively one strip at a time. On the last two days of treatment, a single 2.5 cm strip is irradiated. The kidneys are shielded from the posterior beam by two half-value layers of lead, and the upper portion of the liver is shielded front and back with one half-value layer of lead.

Each strip is treated for eight days by the main beam, and each strip receives what the equivalent of four additional treatments by the penumbra. An average tumor dose of 2600 rads is delivered to each strip.

RADIOISOTOPES

Radioisotopes have been widely used in ovarian cancer. They penetrate approximately 4 mm and are, therefore, only useful in patients with very early cancer who may have single cells or aggregates of cancer cells in the abdominal cavity. Two isotopes are frequently used. Radioactive gold emits 90% beta rays and 10% gamma rays and has a half-life of 2.7 days. Radioactive gold is a true colloid and is taken up by serosal macrophages, and about 90% of its ionizing irradiation is expended within the first few millimeters of the peritoneal surface. Müller[8] has estimated that 150 mC; of radioactive gold delivers approximately 6000 rads to the omentum and 7000 rads to the retroperitoneal and mesenteric structures; 750 rads are added for the gamma component. The poor penetration of gold and complications such as intestinal obstruction and dense peritoneal fibrosis have limited its usefulness. The control of ascites has been stated as one of the more favorable effects; however, Kettell and associates have[7] concluded from a study of 209 patients that the use of an alkylating agent has a much broader palliative effect and is almost as effective as gold in the control of ascites.

Hester and White[6] have accumulated experience with radioactive chromic phosphate in ovarian cancer. Radioactive chromic phosphate is a pure beta emitter, has a half-life of 14.5 days, and a maximum penetration of approximately 4 mm. In their experience, there was no evidence that the radioisotope prolonged survival. Furthermore, chemotherapeutic drugs appeared equally effective in controlling malignant effusion.

Decker and co-workers[1] have reported their experience from the Mayo Clinic. Intraperitoneal radioactive gold (Au 198) was given to 85 postoperative patients with epithelial ovarian cancers. Patients were chosen for treatment if the tumor showed definite evidence of peritoneal spread (implants did not exceed 2 mm in diameter), if rupture of the cyst had potentially contaminated the peritoneal cavity, or if the external surface of the malignant cyst was involved by the tumor. Unfortunately, the overall survival rate did not differ significantly from the overall survival figures for the entire series, and the authors claim that radioactive gold did not show a statistical advantage. They did, however, observe a marked improvement in survival in a selected group of patients (25 cases) whose cancer ruptured during surgical excision. The patients who received radioactive gold had an five-year survival rate of 80% as compared with 43% for a similar untreated group.

In summary, although the use of radioatcive isotopes is declining, a major indication for their use appears to be in those patients with Stage I lesions whose cancer ruptured at operation.

THERAPY GUIDE

Epithelial Cancers of the Ovary

PRINCIPLE

Survival is affected by the extent and histologic differentiation of the carcinoma: the more extensive and undifferentiated the cancer, the worse the prognosis.

STAGE I

1. Total abdominal hysterectomy and bilateral salpingo-oophorectomy is the standard treatment.

2. Since ovarian cancer is a disease of the entire abdominal cavity, additional therapy is recommended unless the patient has Stage IA, Grade I cancer. No additional treatment is indicated in the latter group.

3. Patients selected to receive external irradiation therapy have their entire abdomen treated plus a pelvic boost.

4. A unilateral oophorectomy may be performed in the young patient with a stage IA, well-differentiated (Grade I) encapsulated cancer. Although mucinous carcinomas would perhaps be the best choice, this conservative approach is not recommended with much enthusiasm.

STAGE II

1. Total abdominal hysterectomy and bilateral salpingo-oophorectomy are performed and pelvic implants are excised when possible.

2. These patients receive postoperative external irradiation to the entire abdomen plus a pelvic boost, if excision is complete or if no masses > 2 cm in diameter remain in the pelvis (recent treatment plans deemphasizing radiation therapy and favoring chemotherapy).

3. Patients with residual masses > 2 cm in diameter receive Alkeran 1 mg/kg orally in divided doses over a 5-day period and repeated every 30 days.[12]

STAGE III

1. The surgeon exercises clinical judgment, but is persistent and removes as much tumor as possible and, when feasible, performs a total abdominal hysterectomy and bilateral salpingo-oophorectomy.

2. Removal of an involved segment of bowel is recommended if complete removal of all recognizable cancer can be accomplished.

3. Multiple biopsies are taken in patients with unresectable carcinomas to insure adequate tissue for histological diagnosis.

4. Those patients with extensive cancers receive Alkeran 1 mg/kg orally in divided doses over a five-day period.

5. Careful selection guided by meticulous surgical exploration is essential if patients are chosen for external irradiation therapy (whole abdomen plus pelvic boost) (recent treatment plans deemphasizing radiation therapy and favoring chemotherapy).

STAGE IV

1. The same surgical approach as with Stage III cancers is performed.

2. All patients receive chemotherapy with Alkeran (same dose as in Stages II and III).

3. Patients with enlarged inguinal or supraclavicular nodes that do not regress with chemotherapy may receive supplemental irradiation since enlargement and ulceration of these nodes are painful and disfiguring.

REFERENCES

1. Decker, D. G., et al.: *Am. J. Obstet. Gynecol.* **115:** 751–758 (1973).

2. Delclos, L., and E. J. Quinlan: *Radiology* **93:** 659–663 (1969).

3. Delclos, Luis, and Julian P. Smith: *Textbook of Radiotherapy*, Gilbert H. Fletcher, Ed., 2nd edit. Lea & Febiger. Philadelphia, 1973.

4. Fletcher, Gilbert H.: *Textbook of Radiotherapy*, 2nd edit., Lea & Febiger, Philadelphia, 1973.

5. Hanks, C. E., and M. A. Bagshaw, *Radiology* **93:** 649–654 (1969).

6. Hester, L. L., Sr., and L. White: *Am. J. Obstet. Gynecol.* **103:** 911–918 (1969).

7. Keettel, W. C. et al.: *Am. J. Obstet. Gynecol.* **94:** 766–779 (1966).

8. Miller, J. H.: *Am. J. Roentgenol. Radium Ther. Nucl. Med.* **89:** 533 1963).

9. Munnell, E. W.: *Am. J. Obstet. Gynecol.* **100:** 790–805 (1968).

10. Rubin, et al.: *Am. J. Roentgenol.* **88:** 849–866 (1962).

11. Rutledge, Felix, and Beaury C. Burns, *Am. J. Obstet. Gynecol.* **96:** 761–772 (1966).

12. Rutledge, Felix, and Julian P. Smith, *Am. J. Obstet. Gynecol.* **5:** 691–703 (1970).

13. Wharton, J. T., et al.: *Am. J. Roentgenol.* **67:** 73 (1972).

CHAPTER 12 TREATMENT OF EPITHELIAL CANCER OF THE OVARY (Müllerian Origin)

FELIX RUTLEDGE, M.D.

Cancer of the ovary, the third most frequent cancer of the genital tract, is rapidly rising in the list of the most common causes of death from gynecologic cancer. Although advances in diagnosis and treatment for other gynecologic malignancies have improved results in recent decades, there is still very little improvement evident in the 5-year survival rates for patients with ovarian cancer (Figure 1). Too often generalized pelvic and abdominal spread of the cancer has been encountered at the time of exploratory laparotomy, making excision impossible. When operation is incomplete or when recurrences develop, irradiation or chemotherapy become necessary.

Current questions germane to total treatment of cancer of the ovary are:

1. Which patients should be treated with irradiation and which are best treated by chemotherapy?

2. Can postoperative irradiation be limited to the pelvis or must the whole abdomen be treated?

3. Which histological types of the epithelial cancers respond best to chemotherapy?

4. What clinical features are most favorable for irradiation treatment?

5. Which histological types of ovarian cancer are sensitive to radiotherapy?

6. What percent of patients will respond to chemotherapy? What is the duration of

remission expected from response obtained by chemotherapy?

7. Can sensitivity to irradiation therapy be improved by first reducing the bulk of the cancer using chemotherapy?

8. What is the value of a "second look" operation to guide management when there is no longer a palpable tumor because of complete chemotherapy response?

Although many studies and writings are devoted to the special tumors of the ovary, they do not pose such common management problems for the clinician as the epithelial tumors of müllerian origin (Figure 2). Thus, our discussion will only be concerned with epithelial tumors. Tumors of germ cell and ovarian mesenchyme (stem cell) origin will be discussed in Chapter 13.

EPITHELIAL TUMORS

This category includes serous adenocarcinoma, endometrioid, mesonephric, mucinous and undifferentiated adenocarcinoma.*

To provide a basis for assessing the accomplishments in management of this disease by the various modes of treatment, the clinical features of the disease in a series of

* In the Annual Report of Gynecological Cancers (Volume 15) FIGO lists endometrioid and mesonephric as two histological types of epithelial tumors of the ovary. We have considered them as histologic variants of serous carcinoma.

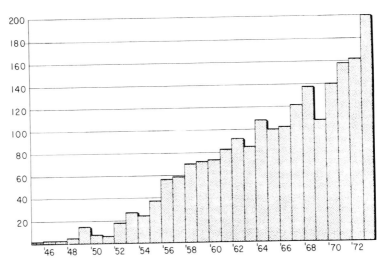

Figure 1 Ovarian cancer patients, M. D. Anderson Hospital, 1955–1793, 2079 patients. The number of patients admitted to the M. D. Anderson Hospital each year with ovarian cancer has increased because of our interest in treating these patients and because chemotherapy treatment often relieves pain and disability and provides extra years of comfortable life. Even when the cancer is extensive and not suitable for surgery or irradiation, patients can now be treated with chemotherapy.

Although most patients are treated by standard protocol, individualized planning is often necessary. The variety of treatment problems presented by many patients has taught our staff which patients of different histologic types respond best to irradiation and which to drug treatment. The gynecology staff uses this opportunity to perfect and devise new treatment methods through clinical investigation. New drugs and combinations of drugs are tested, the comparative benefits of chemotherapy against x-ray or the reverse order, and drug against drug are evaluated.

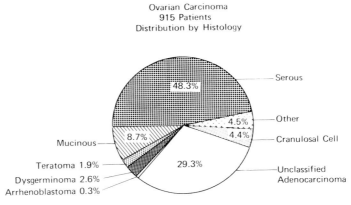

Figure 2 Epithelial tumors of müllerian origin—serous, mucinous and undifferentiated adenocarcinoma—account for 86% of the clinical problems at our institution. Endometrial and mesonephric carcinomas are infrequent varieties of müllerian tumors.

The germ cell tumors, dysgerminoma, embryonal and teratocarcinoma, are second to epithelial tumors in clinical importance. The primary ovarian choriocarcinoma of this group is extremely rare.

Interstitial or stem cell tumors are clinically important. The granulosa cell type is more common than the Sartoli-Leydig cell or arrhenoblastoma varieties.

Consistent with our teaching that all discussions of ovarian carcinoma should respect their differences and especially not consider them as a subject for statistical analysis, we have discussed the groups separately.

184

our patients are worthy of review.[1] The prevalence of epithelial tumors among the younger age group makes this disease especially distressing. Young women at the peak of their careers, often at the time when they are so important as mothers of young children and directors of households, are victims of this type of cancer. Regrettably, regular examinations for ovarian cancer do not fully protect many patients from developing untreatable disease. Rapid growth and spread had occurred in 63% of patients in our series, in 74% the disease had metastasized beyond the pelvis. Ascites, present in 50% of the patients, was frequently the first sign of the disease.

Among 201 patients (21%) exhibiting distant metastases, lymph node and pleural cavity spread was encountered most often (Table 1). Bone metastases were rare. A noteworthy clinical feature is the tendency for metastasis to nodes in the left rather than the right supraclavicular region (Table 2).

This observation has helped us to distinguish primary ovarian cancer from cancer of the breast, which commonly involves these nodes in both sides and often metastasizes to the ovaries. Metastasis to the ovaries from primary breast cancer in its advanced stage creates a pelvic tumor clinically similar to cancer of the ovary. The mechanism for ovarian cancer to metastasize to the inguinal nodes may be due to the vasculature of the round ligament connecting the two sites or may be caused by filling of the pelvic nodes and retrograde spread to the inguinal region. Pulmonary metastasis to the lung parenchyma was surprisingly low in view of the high incidence of pleural effusion. Only one-third of the patients with pleural effusion had pulmonary lung metastasis. Perhaps some direct communication between the peritoneal and pleural cavities affected the pleura without involving the parenchyma of the lungs.

Treatment

SURGERY

Operation is the single, most successful method for curing patients with cancer of the ovary. Additional patients with disease not completely excised may be cured with postoperative irradiation therapy. Chemotherapy, although less curative, offers a great opportunity to provide palliation and perhaps to potentiate the action of irradiation by making the disease masses smaller and more sensitive. The potential of these two treatments in combination is being investigated. Preirradiation chemotherapy may improve the action of irradiation therapy by shrinking the tumor masses, thereby improving the blood supply to the cancer cells situated near the center of the cancer masses. The efficiency of photons of external therapy to be cancerocidal requires adequate oxygenation of the entire cancer mass.

Table 1   Carcinoma of the Ovary

Distant Metastasis	No. of Patients	Percent
Node	106	11.6
Bone	22	2.4
Skin	4	0.4
Lung	69	7.5
Total	201	

Percent of total: 21.9

Table 2   Carcinoma of the Ovary: 915 Patients

	Nodal Metastasis (%)
Left inguinal	5.9
Right inguinal	2.1
Left supraclavicular	3.8
Right supraclavicular	0.9
Other	0.4

FACTORS THAT DETERMINE THE BENEFITS
OF RADIATION THERAPY

Spread. Cancer of the ovary causes special problems for the radiotherapist that are not usually present in other genital cancers. The large area that requires treatment and uncertainty about its boundaries are major obstacles to dosimetry. The surgeon often fails to gather the necessary data about metastasis during laparotomy. Often, the finding of disseminated ovarian cancer is so emotionally disconcerting that the experienced surgeon may close the abdomen before gaining all of the available information about the spread of the disease. This lack of information hinders the radiotherapists who must design postoperative therapy of maximum efficiency.

Sensitivity. To be cancerocidal the common müllerian tumors such as the serous, adenocarcinomatous, and mucinous epithelial types require irradiation dosage equal to that given to other epithelial tumors of the body. The amount may vary among patients influenced by cellular sensitivity and factors of tumor immunity. Large masses of tumor may be less radiosensitive because the blood supply is reduced within the tumor mass. The anoxic state of these cells increases their radioresistivity. Histologic types appear to respond equally.

DOSAGE RESTRICTION IMPOSED BY
SOME ABDOMINAL ORGANS

Absolute dosage tolerance levels for irradiation of the kidney must be respected to avoid producing renal insufficiency. Adequate portions of the liver must be shielded or this organ will be destroyed. Tolerance of the intestine and bone marrow restricts dosage less, and there is individual variation in the sensitivity of these organs. Still, all these tissues have a poor tolerance which limits the dosage and the area that can be safely irradiated. Adverse actions of irradia-

tion will be discussed later when the complications are listed.

Area of abdomen irradiated. The two general systems for postoperative irradiation for ovarian cancer employ treatment of the pelvic region alone or whole abdomen therapy (Figure 3). Some radiotherapists will readily admit defeat when the disease has spread diffusely through the abdomen and will want to treat only localized regions of the upper abdomen. They would prefer to restrict irradiation coverage to the general pelvic region, as this permits more conservative field (portals) sizes and reduces the side effects in the intestinal tract, lowers the rate of late complications, and permits concentration of a greater dose to the region most likely to harbor residual cancer and to develop recurrences. Our series of patients have been variously treated by x-ray therapy to the pelvic portal alone or to both the pelvis and the upper abdomen.[2] At present we advocate the latter method.

The moving strip technique is our preference for irradiation of the entire abdomen: it provides a more uniform distribution of irradiation, the treatment is better tolerated, and there are fewer interruptions of treatment because of abdominal cramps and diarrhea[3] (Figure 4). The whole abdomen is irradiated by the moving strip technique, delivering 2600 to 3000 rads in approximately two weeks of treatment by megavoltage machines plus 2000 rads to the pelvic region after the strip technique. This additional external therapy to the pelvic region is delivered through portals measuring 15 × 15 cm. Thus the total dose to the pelvic region is equal to about 5000 rads whole pelvis therapy. The moving strip technique employs a 4-in. portal of therapy that extends across the width of the abdomen. It is advanced upward 1 in. after each day of therapy. Each 1-in. strip receives four treatments directed from the patient's front and four directed from the back plus the equiv-

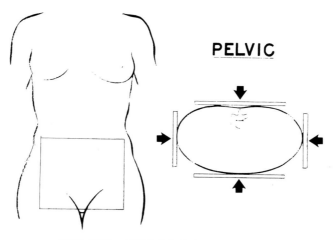

PELVIC

DOSE: 5000 – 6000 RADS IN 5 – 6 WEEKS

Figure 3 Radiotherapists are allowed considerable individual preference about the size and shape of the fields through which treatment is directed. Generally, the x-ray is carefully restrained to cover no more that the peritoneal cavity because unnecessary irradiation along the abdominal side walls or below the pelvic floor contributes additional irradiation side effects without purpose. Since ovarian cancer is free to migrate and theoretically can be in any part of the space around the abdominal cavity, shielding of the intestine and bone marrow is not practical if all the spaces potentially harboring cancer are to be covered. Although these organs are injured by irradiation, and dysuria, diarrhea, and depressed blood counts occur regularly, these effects heal within a few weeks posttreatment. The kidneys and liver do require protection. Beyond the 2000 rad level, irradiation nephritis and renal failure occurs, therefore about half the dosage planned for the abdomen is shielded from the kidneys. The liver is sensitive to irradiation and will not repair, thus an adequate portion must be protected.

In directing the x-ray the pelvic region is emphasized because the most often unresectable cancer remains here. Most often recurrences occur in the pelvic region postoperatively, and the organs in the pelvic region can tolerate a more nearly cancerocidal irradiation dose.

The difficulties with large-field portal irradiation of the abdomen are: marked systemic reactions of malaise, nausea, vomiting, diarrhea, and depressed blood values. These symptoms often force interruption and sometimes discontinuance of treatment, a "protraction" is usually necessary. Dosage levels beyond 3000 rads in 5 or 6 weeks becomes intolerable to large-field irradiation portals.

The moving strip technique may use any megavoltage x-ray machine (e.g., cobalt-60, linear accelerator), that treats from the pelvic floor to the diaphragm in 30–40 days and delivers 2400 to 2800 rads to each volume of tissue in 12 days. The dose to the tumor is within a shorter than usual treatment time and has a greater biologic effect than would be expected with this number of rads.

The strip technique accomplishes an equivalent cancerocidal effect with less toxicity and better possibility of completion.

alent of two additional treatments by "scatter" to the margins, as the field advances and departs in its progress up the abdomen. Approximately half of the delivery dose must be shielded from the kidney, and a significant segment of the liver must be protected from irradiation. This limited shielding of the abdominal cavity does provide some refuge for cancer cells in this region, making it impossible to completely irradiate

the whole abdominal cavity with the dosage needed to destroy epithelial carcinoma.

Isotopes. Although treatment with radioisotopes of gold or chromic phosphate is no longer popular, several centers report good results for early stage disease. Our results have been favorable when patients were carefully selected for suitability. The treatment has a significant record of bowel in-

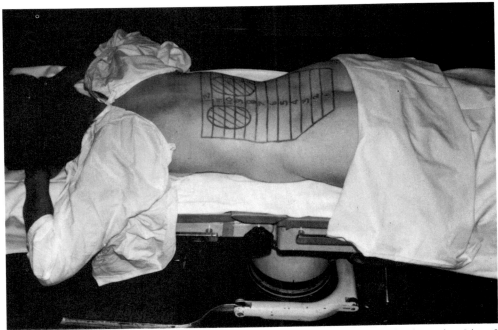

Figure 4 The region of the abdomen to be irradiated is divided into a series of adjoining strips. Lines 2.5 cm apart are marked upon the patient's front and back. Four of these lines (10 cm portal) are treated daily, each alternating front and back, advancing one strip after each treatment or each day.

A portion of the x-ray beam dose (penumbra) extends to adjoining tissues beyond the margins of the field being treated, and this must be counted as a contribution to the total dosage calculations. The penumbra adds about 50% of the daily dose to the abdomen along the upper and lower boundaries of the portal, although this tissue is not directly under the treatment portal.

jury; therefore unless good distribution seems assured, the material must not be placed into the abdomen. External therapy must not be used before or after, for the hazards of bowel injury are excessive.

Analysis. Multiple methods of irradiation therapy, including radioactive gold, have been used in this study group of 448 patients. There are enough patients treated with pelvic irradiation alone, whole abdomen irradiation alone, and whole abdomen plus an additional dosage boost to the pelvic region to evaluate each method for treating all three stages of ovarian cancer. This analysis allows us to answer the questions

posed earlier about selection of the optimum treatment for each stage.

The results of irradiation by stage after five years of observation show superior results for treating the whole abdomen (moving strip technique) followed by an additional boost to the pelvic region (Table 3). This superiority of the high-dose extended field irradiation therapy plan has been observed in all stages of the disease, especially in the Stage I and II lesions.

The late complications of large-field high-dose irradiation therapy have occasionally been serious (Table 4). Experience with similar high-dose irradiation to the whole pelvis for cervical cancer prepared us to anticipate some complications. Irradiation injury to bowel, progressing to obstruction, has required bowel resection or procedures to bypass these regions and can be attributed to irradiation therapy. This risk is unavoidable with such intensive treatment. In 7 patients technical errors that led to over-irradiating the liver probably contributed to their death from liver insufficiency. Leukopenia and thrombocytopenia occurred during irradiation, but bone marrow suppression severe enough to necessitate discontinuation of therapy was rare. We observed, however, that some reversible reduction of bone marrow reserve resulted. Although without additional stress the blood counts return to normal levels, in the patient who

has received irradiation to the whole abdomen, the ability to maintain adequate blood levels with chemotherapy diminishes. When the treatment plan uses both irradiation and chemotherapy the amount of bone marrow irradiation becomes a factor for decision. We must weigh the outcome by the improved survival rates when irradiation was given to both the abdomen and pelvis with less extensive, more localized pelvic region x-ray which conserves bone marrow and permits more effective chemotherapy.

The safety of the higher dose pelvic and abdominal irradiation must also be considered when planning individual treatment. For those with earlier stage disease a safer course may be justified, more limited irradi-

Table 3   Results of Irradiation Treatment by Stage: No Evidence of Disease, after 5 Years

| Treatment | Stage | | | | |
	I	II	III	IV	Total
Strip plus pelvic therapy	72.2%	34.4%	21.4%	0/1	35.5%
Strip	58.3%	21.4%	5.9%	0	25.6%
Gold	77.8%	18.8%	8.5	0/4	24.6%
Pelvis	4/5	17.6%	5.0%	0/1	18.6%
Abdomen	0/2	1/3	0/7	0/2	7.1%
Abdomen plus pelvis	3/3	2/6	2/7	0	43.6%

Table 4   Complications of Treatment

Treatment	Bowel Injury	Liver Injury	Bone Marrow Depression	Total Patients Treated
Strip plus total pelvis	7	13	8	148
Strip	2	4	3	60
Gold	5	0	0	87
Pelvis	2	0	0	47
Abdomen	0	0	1	14
Abdomen + pelvis	0	0	0	18
Other	0	0	0	9
Total	16	17	12	383

ation or chemotherapy. For those additional survivors the quality of life attributable to the more radical irradiation method must be acceptable. Serious bowel injury requires operations that may take long portions of the intestinal tract out of service. When this happens, life becomes difficult and unhappy. In weighing these adverse effects, we have concluded that whole abdomen and pelvic irradiation therapy eradicates the cancer better and is not unduly hazardous, considering the poor survival rate of patients with all stages of ovarian cancer.

We were especially anxious to find proof that irradiation therapy could destroy metastasis in the upper abdominal cavity, since some gynecologists have questioned the available supporting evidence. Table 5 records the sites of recurrences according to the stage of the disease at the time of treatment, but the data fail to answer this perplexing question. Often recurrent ovarian cancer was distributed too diffusely around the abdomen when recurrence was discovered to give a clue to its site of origin. When recurrences were clinically evident, both the pelvis and the upper abdomen were often jointly involved with tumor masses, so that

the source of treatment failure which caused regrowth was concealed.

Insensitivity of large masses of tumor. In advanced disease, large ascites was an obstacle to successful whole abdomen irradiation. The distended abdomen posed mechanical problems for the radiotherapy. Although paracentesis evacuated the ascites, it was difficult to maintain a flattened abdomen for the duration of treatment. For additional, baffling reasons patients with ascites did not respond to x-ray therapy as well as to chemotherapy. Patients with large upper abdominal masses responded poorly, and it was soon evident that irradiation of large masses rarely produced regression. This observation plus the availability of chemotherapy as a substitute for irradiation influenced our decision against the selection of such patients for irradiation therapy.

Preoperative irradiation. Initially most patients need a laparotomy to establish the diagnosis, amount, and location of the cancer; thus we have found little use for preoperative irradiation to make a carcinoma more resectable. If a patient has so much cancer at examination that it seems inoper-

Table 5   Site of Recurrence of Ovarian Cancer by Stage (260 Patients with Treatment Failure)

Site of Recurrence	Stage				Unknown	Total
	I	II	III	IV		
Abdomen	4	6	13	0	1	24
Abdomen + pelvis	8	29	91	6	1	135
Abdomen + distant metastases	0	2	1	0	0	3
Abdomen, pelvis + distant metastases	1	10	8	2	0	21
Pelvis	4	30	16	2	0	52
Pelvis + distant metastases	0	1	0	1	0	2
Distant metastases	0	3	1	1	0	5
Site unknown	3	6	9	0	0	18
Total	20	87	139	12	2	260

able, preoperative x-ray therapy is not the best choice.

Summary of postoperative irradiation management policies. Better survival statistics show the advantage of irradiating the upper abdomen for a maximum dose with an additional boost to the pelvic region. When the disease was thought to be limited to the pelvis, irradiation of the pelvis alone was less successful than irradiation of the whole abdomen and pelvis. Currently at M. D. Anderson Hospital, postoperative management of the common ovarian epithelial tumor is as follows: Stages I, II, and III disease with masses < 2 cm in diameter are treated by whole abdomen irradiation, using the moving strip technique, to a dose of 2600 to 2800 rads in two weeks followed by two weeks of x-ray therapy (an additional 2000 rads) to the pelvis. Patients with ascites and tumor masses larger than 2 cm in diameter are first treated with chemotherapy. If the disease is responsive to chemotherapy, the drug is continued as long as a response is maintained. For those patients with complete disappearance of all tumor, we have arbitrarily decided that after 12 to 18 courses of drug therapy reexploration of the abdominal cavity helps to plan future treatment. At "second look" laparotomy, masses of residual disease < 2 cm in diameter can be considered suitable for irradiation therapy by the conventional method of moving strip and pelvic boost if x-ray therapy or radioisotopes have not been used previously. Patients unsuitable for irradiation therapy are given more vigorous chemotherapy, often employing a different agent or combination of different drugs.

Chemotherapy

We have a special interest in chemotherapy for ovarian cancer since our institution is a referral center for patients with cancer and the majority of the patients we see have advanced stage disease. Our experience is sufficient to show clearly that chemotherapy is effective in the treatment for ovarian cancer.[6,7,8,9] After 10 years' experience melphalan remains the preferred standard drug for initial treatment, mainly because observations have shown that this agent causes tumor regression most regularly and with minimal toxicity.

Although almost 1000 patients have been treated to date, the last review of the series was in 1969 when there were 575 patients treated with melphalan.

We now regard epithelial ovarian cancers, for purposes of treatment, as being similar in behavior since these tumors seem to spread by the same mechanism and to have a similar response to both irradiation and chemotherapy. The prognosis differs however; therefore, in reporting results of treatment by chemotherapy the patients will be divided into three groups according to the histology of their tumor; that is, serous, mucinous, or undifferentiated adenocarcinoma. The response rate for each type will be noted.

DOSAGE OF MELPHALAN

The dose of melphalan for the entire series has been consistent for many years: 1 mg/kg body weight divided over five to six days. In earlier years the medication was given intravenously (Table 6). The 1 mg/kg body weight dose was administered as a slow intravenous drip of chilled dextrose solution over an 8-hr period. The oral preparation is now used routinely. By either route by administration, melphalan is repeated every four weeks if the WBC at that time is 3000/cu. mm. and the platelets are above 150,000/cu. mm. Almost every patient seen with an ovarian tumor that was unsuitable for irradiation or additional surgery was treated with chemotherapy. Although their physical condition may seem poor, these patients de-

Table 6 Chemotherapy Carcinoma Ovary of Müllerian Origin (Single Alkylating Agent Clinical Information)

Agent	Melphalan (sarcolysin, alkeran, L-phenylalanine mustard)
Dose	1 mg/kg body weight total dose
Administration	Oral, divided over 5 consecutive days
Interval	Repeat every 4 weeks if number of platelets are > 150,000 and WBC > 3000 on day of planned course

serve a trial of drug therapy because some astonishing remissions have been observed. Although it is obvious that this disease may reach a point at which any type of treatment will be futile, nevertheless, an occasional patient who seemed to be terminal did show favorable response to chemotherapy.

The response of 494 patients who had received melphalan as the initial chemotherapy was evaluated by the criteria of the National Cancer Chemotherapy Group. A complete response consisted of complete disappearance of malignancy for three months or longer, and a partial response consisted of a 50% decrease in volume of the tumor as determined on three separate examinations over three months or control of a serous effusion for three months or longer.

Approximately 45% of the patients with müllerian ovarian tumors had a partial or complete response after chemotherapy with melphalan (Table 7). An additional 10 to

20% not counted in the 46% response rate had tumors that did not increase in size. The lack of growth was not counted in the response rate, although it may be considered additional antitumor action. The individual tumor response to melphalan was approximately the same for the serous, mucinous, and undifferentiated adenocarcinoma histologic types. The duration of response correlated well with the rapidity of tumor regression. A rapid and impressive repression usually was more sustained. Histology was also a factor in duration of drug action. Patients with mucinous carcinoma had the least virulent cancer and the longest average duration of response. Patients with undifferentiated adenocarcinoma had the most virulent and the shortest average duration. Whether response occurs, the amount of tumor regression, and how long this action is sustained, varies with the individual patient. (Table 8).

ALTERNATE TO MELPHALAN

The problem of how to treat a patient who has failed to respond to the first trial of chemotherapy or who has developed a growing tumor mass after initial response to a drug is a matter of some concern. Almost every patient received melphalan, an alkylating agent, as initial chemotherapy. When a response was lacking or loss of control was evident, a new chemotherapeutic agent was selected. Usually an agent with a different antitumor action was chosen in preference to another alkylating agent. Ear-

Table 7 Response to L-Phenylalanine Mustard

Type	Patients	Complete Response	Partial Response
Serious	329	74 (22%)	88 (27%)
Mucinous	45	10 (22%)	10 (22%)
Undifferentiated adenocarcinoma	120	16 (13%)	35 (29%)
Total	494	100 (20%)	133 (26%)
			46%

Table 8 Survival—Stages III and IV Treated with External Therapy after Chemotherapy

		Range (months)	Mean (months)	Median (months)
Serous	43	5–75	27.3	23.0
Mucinous	2	14–15	14.5	14.5
Undifferentiated Adenocarcinoma	10	10–42	18.6	15.0
Total	55	5–75	25.2	21.0
Living	15	12–60	26.8	22.0
Dead	40	5–75	24.7	21.0

lier information indicated that second remission would rarely be induced by changing from melphalan to either chlorambucil, cyclophosphamide, or ThioTEPA because tumors form cross-resistance among these alkylating agents. (Cyclophosphamide now seems to be an exception.) Early in the study 5-fluorouracil was chosen as the alternate agent for cytotoxic action. Few responses were induced and, after an experience with 46 patients, 5-fluorouracil was replaced by a combination of drugs.

DRUG COMBINATIONS (ActFuCy)

A combination of drugs that have proved effective in tumors that do not respond to melphalan consists of Actinomycin-D, 5-fluorouracil, and cyclophosphamide, which we conveniently refer to as ActFuCy (Table 9). This combination was used in 47 patients and has been beneficial in 38% (Table 10). Toxicity of the combination drug treatment is greater than wtih melphalan.

Table 9 Triple Therapy (ActFuCy)

	Daily Regimen for 5 Days[a]
Actinomycin-D	0.5 mg IV push
5-Fluorouracil	8 mg/kg as IV drip
Cytoxan	7 mg/kg IV push

[a] A 5-day course is repeated every 4 weeks.

TOXICITY OF MELPHALAN

Serious toxicity was seldom encountered following treatment with melphalan. Only 1 patient who had been treated for several years died of irreversible bone marrow depression. Of the 4 patients who had life-threatening toxicity, it was due to thrombocytic depression in 2 patients and was an immediate allergic reaction in the others. Two patients developed leukemia during or following melphalan therapy. Of the 47 patients who received ActFuCy, 6 had serious toxicity due to the combination of drugs. The reaction either proved fatal or contributed to the patient's death in 3 patients. Both the hemopoietic and the gastrointestinal system may be adversely affected by this potent combination. Some of the serious reaction to ActFuCy was undoubtedly due to the fact that all the patients who received this combination had received prior doses of melphalan, and several of the patients were seriously disabled because of advanced cancer. Although there is greater risk in employing such drug combinations, the chance of benefit (35%) justifies their use when the course of the disease has become grave.

Many patients do well on melphalan and can tolerate multiple courses up to 3 years; however, the physician must eventually decide when the drug is no longer needed. In the absence of physical evidence of remaining cancer, the status of the abdomen may only be ascertained by laparotomy.

Table 10   Carcinoma of the Ovary: Response to ActFuCy

Type	Patients	Complete Response	Partial Response
Serious	34	3 (9%)	11 (32%)
Mucinous	5	0	0
Undifferentiated adenocarcinoma	8	1	3
Total	47	4 (9%)	14 (30%)
		(39%)	

"SECOND LOOK" ABDOMINAL LAPAROTOMY

The diagnosis and spread of carcinoma of the ovary cannot usually be determined without exploratory laparotomy, and for some patients reexploration after an interval of treatment helps the physician to ascertain if treatment has been successful. The exploratory laparotomy or "second look" procedure has become common practice at our institution, for treatments are designed and modified from these findings. Only 1 in 8 (12%) of our patients receiving chemotherapy qualified for the second look operation. In other patients the tumors either did not regress, or regression was of short duration, or their abdominal condition was obvious without laparotomy. The response of the ovarian cancer determined if and when the second look operation should be done. A dramatic regression of the tumor stimulated the physician to learn whether total regression had occurred, whereas a tumor that remained static during chemotherapy was a matter of concern to the physician. Patients with rapidly progressing disease were excluded because they were not expected to benefit by the second look operation. Since previous irradiation makes laparotomy more difficult and more prone to postoperative complications, patients who were treated by high-dose x-ray therapy did not undergo the second look procedure.

From March 1962 to March 1971, 800 patients with carcinoma of the ovary were treated with chemotherapy at the M. D.

Anderson Hospital. Of those with epithelial tumors, 103 patients had second look operations as part of the treatment.[4]

The number in the study group with each histologic cancer type retained the same proportional distribution as our total patient population admitted to the Department of Gynecology with ovarian cancer. The majority of patients had advanced disease, since late stages and very ill patients with ovarian cancer are most often treatable by chemotherapy. Also, these are the patients who are most likely to need the second look operation because their treatment is protracted and complex.

Observations. For each patient, the extended duration of the chemotherapy as well as a favorable tumor response were dominant indications for exploration of the abdomen to learn the status of the pelvic and abdominal disease. When tumor masses could no longer be palpated or, if still palpable, had ceased to change, laparotomy supplied valuable information about the effectiveness of treatment. Underestimating the remaining cancer could lead to discontinuation of an effective treatment such as melphalan; overestimating could lead to change to unduly drastic treatment when there is actually little or no carcinoma present. Clinical examination is less accurate for some patients and, especially after prior abdominal surgery, adhesions may result in a mass composed of intestine and omentum that can be mistaken for a cancer mass. Such masses do not regress with chemotherapy and can cause a misleading assessmen of drug action. Since ovarian cancer either grows or regresses, when lengthy chemotherapy produces no change the composition of the tumor guiding the physician needs investigation. As we gain experience with melphalan, we evaluate the time factor within which to expect regression and length of time it would be sustained. Although many patients respond for 12 to 18 months, few continue longer.

In the earlier part of this work, the minimum treatment time for clearing the abdomen completely was not evaluated. We were overly impressed by some patients who showed a prompt and a rapid tumor regression with melphalan, and were impatient to learn if a cure was possible or if conditions were favorable for a second try at resecting the cancer. In the early part of this study, after brief experience, we were less confident that patients could tolerate prolonged bone marrow injury by chemotherapy; thus the second look operations were done as soon as the tumor seemed smaller or resectable. Some patients were explored after a minimum of four courses of drug and, upon finding a "clean abdomen," melphalan was stopped. When the prematurity of this action became evident by regrowth of the ovarian cancer; this practice was changed for some patients. Now we continue melphalan until the clinical patterns of drug against cancer are established. (Table 11).

Patients who respond well are continued on melphalan for a minimum of 12 courses. This delay of the second look operation eliminates those patients who have a good but transient response to the drug. Although some patients may show a good initial response by tumor regression, there is a rapid redevelopment of cancer while still on the antitumor agent. Such patients will have a short survival and would not benefit from a second look operation.

There are several reasons for reexploration: (1) the patient may have had a sufficient amount of the drug; (2) the tumor may become more localized and possibly resectable for the first time; or (3) the benefit from the drug may be exhausted and it is time to switch to another drug; (4) the mass is now suitable for irradiation. (5) The mass that has served as a guide to the drug action is suspected not to be cancer as presumed. If such a tumor is composed of benign agglutinated organs rather than a neoplastic mass, the second look laparotomy may avert a clinical error. For patients with carcinoma of the ovary this operation has proved beneficial in a variety of conditions.

RESULTS AND FINDINGS OF LAPAROTOMY

The carcinoma at the second look laparotomy recorded in Table 12 for 23 patients with extensive prechemotherapy metastases about the abdomen disappeared completely. In 11 other patients there was no tumor large enough or sufficiently exposed to the peritoneal surface to be clinically apparent. However, within the tissue removed as a biopsy, there were microscopic size cancers. In 35 patients extensive carcinoma macroscopic in size was clearly evident at the second look operation, and in 34 patients the chemotherapy response was either much less complete or the tumor had reversed its

Table 11   Number of Chemotherapy Courses and Absolute Survival after Second Look Operation

Courses	1 Year	3 Years	5 Years
1–4	17/24 (70%)	7/24 (29%)	2/23 (9%)
5–9	29/40 (72%)	9/24 (37%)	6/19 (32%)
10 or more	40/45 (89%)	15/22 (68%)	8/10 (80%)

Table 12   Initial Treatment and Findings at Second Look Operation after Chemotherapy

| Initial Therapy | NED[a] | Findings at Second Look | | Unchanged or Progressive Carcinoma |
| | | Partial Responders | | |
		Micro Ca.	Marco Ca.	
Partial Removal	57	57	8	16	18
Biopsy Only	27	3	1	16	7
Surgery + Chemotherapy or X-Ray Therapy	19	5	2	3	9
Total	103	23	11	35	34

[a] No evidence of disease.

regression course, for the tumor masses were surprisingly large. These findings indicate that second look operations are unnecessary for most patients with ovarian cancer treated by chemotherapy. Further selectivity was advisable in this series for some patients who did not benefit.

Although we have little information to indicate that chemotherapeutic response is affected by the total neoplastic cell population, these observations on patients who had the second look operation are of interest. Sixteen patients had apparent total removal of their cancer at the first discovery abdominal operation. These patients developed recurrence and did well with chemotherapy, and 7 of the 16 were negative at second look operation. Among 41 patients with partial removal but a significant reduction in the total tumor by the primary operation, 8 were negative. Only 3 of 21 patients had a negative abdomen at second look operation, when no resection had been possible at first operation. We may postulate that the effectiveness of chemotherapy, like irradiation, is best when the cancer population is smaller and that older tumors are more prone to consume the host immunodefense mechanisms. Although patients with late stage or larger cancer cell population responded to chemotherapy with destruction of the por-

tion of the cells present, it was never complete. We must assume that the greater effort and ability for resection during the first operation is important, for the more complete the resection the better will be the response to chemotherapy. Further study of the reexploration finding as related to the findings at the original operation may ultimately perfect the use of chemotherapy for carcinoma of the ovary.

COMMENTS

Long-term remissions that may prove to be cures have been induced by melphalan therapy in approximately 6% of our patients. Those patients who originally had Stage III and IV disease now have shown several years of unsustained posttreatment remission and offer encouraging prospects for the future control of this disease by chemotherapy. The following case histories portray the potential of chemotherapy for selective patients:

M. McE., a 43-year-old patient with Grade III inoperable, serous carcinoma of the ovary and diffuse abdominal metastasis, was first treated with x-ray therapy, without significant improvement. When chemotherapy was initiated, there was a large pelvic mass spreading through the posterior fornix into the vagina, a positive left supraclavicular node, and positive pleural fluid. After melphalan was administered monthly for approximately a year and a half, all signs of cancer disappeared. Exploratory laparotomy was negative as was the excised cervix and the upper vagina, which contained the fungating lesion of metastatic ovarian cancer. The last chemotherapy was given 10 years ago and the patient remains well, demonstrating the curative value of chemotherapy.

L. Y., age 57, had diffuse carcinomatosis due to papillary serous carcinoma of the ovary in 1963. When melphalan was started, there was bilateral pleural effusion and an abdominal mass. After four courses of the drug the palpable tumor disappeared completely. Exploratory laparotomy was negative. Melphalan was discontinued for seven months, and a third exploratory laparotomy was also negative. The patient remained well for an additional two years without chemotherapy. Then, with evidence of recurrence, the fourth exploratory laparotomy showed a poorly differentiated adenocarcinoma in the omentum. A second remission was obtained by resuming melphalan therapy and the cancer was controlled for one year. The remission was lost, and attempts to use other medications failed.

This patient's tumor seemed unusually responsive to drug therapy. In retrospect, we conclude that the medication was discontinued prematurely. From this and similar experiences, we advise delaying second look laparotomy until 12 to 18 months of drug response is observed.

M. W., age 60, with a Stage IV inoperable serous carcinoma of the ovary, showed an excellent melphalan response. At the time of second look operation only small foci of residual disease were found in the right ovary. Whole abdomen strip irradiation and pelvic boost postoperative x-ray therapy were given. The patient remains well eight years from the date of external therapy.

Some patients clearly benefit by combined drug and irradiation treatment. The minute amount of residual cancer may also have been totally eradicated by continued chemotherapy.

B. T., age 34, was diagnosed as having Stage III papillary serous carcinoma of the cervix in 1965. After four courses of melphalan, second look exploratory laparotomy showed a small foci of cervical cancer is still present. The patient was then given 13 additional courses of the drug. The third laparotomy was negative, and the patient has remained well without chemotherapy for over five years.

Prolonged chemotherapy has proven very safe. We resorted to exploratory laparotomy or second look operations for some patients with long-term remissions on drug therapy, to help decide whether medication could be discontinued. We found that clinical appraisal was often insufficient to determine the status of the disease, especially when the tumor mass was too diminished to palpate. A palpable mass in the abdomen or pelvis, such as an adherent mass of omentum and intestine or a neoplastic mass, and may be a benign tumor. Thus, laparotomy may be the ony way to determine the extent of the disease.

SUMMARY

Operation is responsible for most cures of patients with ovarian cancer. Aggressive surgery has gained some favor and appears to have achieved improved results. Resection of intestinal segment is proper if almost complete removal of the cancer will result. Tenacious dissection to remove large pelvic masses of the cancer may result in remarkable success; however, such an approach necessitates good judgment, since hemorrhage or other injury to pelvic organs may be catastrophic. Such an effort seems logical as long as resection appears complete and control is maintained during the procedure.

There is no purpose in preserving the uterus as a radium receptacle. Intracavitary radium therapy for ovarian cancer has been replaced by megavoltage x-ray therapy. Only on rare occasions should an ovary be saved. For a Stage I mucinous carcinoma, this may be considered for the young patient with a strong desire to preserve fertility.[5] Patients with serous and undifferentiated cancer require bilateral resection.

Irradiation ranks second to surgery as curative treatment, although its applicability, like that of surgery, is limited to early stage disease or cases in which operation has almost completely excised the tumor. No doubt postoperative x-ray therapy adds to the survival of patients in all disease stages, especially those in Stages I and II. External roentgen therapy should be radical and inclusive. Generally, ovarian cancer can be expected to be more advanced than is clinically apparent. The high incidence of recurrence after apparent resection in Stage I and II disease indicates frequent subclinical spread in earlier stages. Positive peritoneal lavage with no apparent rupture of the tumor capsule points to early escape of cancer cells as an example. Lymphography demonstrates that lymphatic spread is common in ovarian cancer and much more prevalent than has been recognized. To explain the treatment failure incidence after seemingly total excision, subclinical residual tumor must escape detection often; therefore, postoperative irradiation is advocated.

This factor of unknown residual tumor must be considered when designating the area that will receive x-ray therapy. It is suspected that the entire peritoneal cavity harbors a potential for recurrence, and a maximum dose of tolerable irradiation must be administered early postoperatively. Ascites and large tumor masses, either pelvic or abdominal, are conditions which thwart radiotherapy. Integration of chemotherapy into the program provides an alternative method for sustaining treatment or is a preliminary to irradiation therapy.

Chemotherapy is an established treatment for cancer of the ovary. More patients should be offered this effective method for palliation (Figure 5). Although half of the patients with advanced disease will not benefit, the almost miraculous tumor regression achieved by some demands that the agent be tried when operation and x-ray therapy have failed. In the early years of our experience with chemotherapy, drug treatment was undertaken expecting only palliative effects. Today chemotherapy is proving as successful in curing cancer as x-ray therapy, and its position in the management scheme of ovarian cancer has advanced to replace x-ray therapy for some patients, and is now the first choice for treatment after surgery. In the beginning only patients with large tumor masses, widespread metastases, and long-term disease were given chemotherapy because drug toxicity was feared; thus its use was delayed for patients who had a favorable prognosis. As a result there is less information about the usefulness of melphalan for earlier stages. Comparison studies of melphalan and x-ray therapy for residual cancer of the ovary may prove the two equally effective.

The physician who treats patients for carcinoma of the ovary must be knowledgeable and skilled in all three treatment methods This knowledge must be current, since the management changes as new agents to chemotherapy are introduced. The cancerocidal drugs may reverse a disease with an apparent terminal course and restore a disabled patient to functional health. Each patient deserves a trial of treatment, since at present this is the only test of the individual's response. Preferably the oncologist who manages treatment should be capable

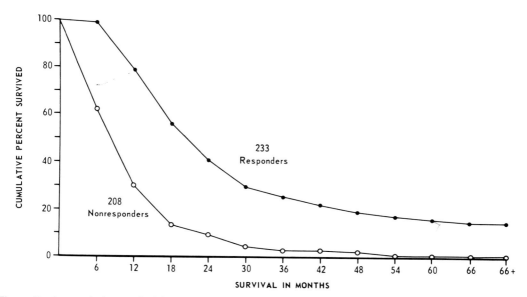

Figure 5 Accumulative survival in serous mucinous and undifferentiated carcinoma of the ovary treated with L-PAM by Berkson and Gage method, 441 patients.

Evidence that patients with advanced cancer of the ovary treated vigorously with chemotherapy survive longer is meager. Physicians readily accept chemotherapy for its success in palliative treatment, but most do not expect a cure.

The 5-year survival rates in recent years when the benefits of chemotherapy were available have improved little, yet some added life has been noted for those patients whose tumors are sensitive to chemotherapy.

The survival curve for patients who responded well to drug with regression of the tumor showed 22% increased in 5-year survival. At 2 years 35% more survived. This evidence indicates that chemotherapy is not merely palliative treatment, but actually prolongs survival.

in pelvic and abdominal surgery. Intestinal operations are frequently necessary to return the patient to adequate health so that she is eligible to receive chemotherapy or x-ray therapy. Often opportunities for palliative restoration are missed because of reluctance by physicians to perform operations.

This type of cancer illustrates a philosophy about oncology: a physician should accept a patient for the duration of her disease. If he does not wish to have this responsibility or feels unqualified and there is the possibility of referral, a decision should be made as early as possible. Mistakes in management, lack of courage in resection, distrust based upon antiquated knowledge, and insufficient interest are disservices physicians must strive to eliminate if we hope to reduce the disaster of ovarian carcinoma.

REFERENCES

1. Burns, Jr., Beaury C., Felix Rutledge, and H. Stephen Gallagher: *Obstet. and Gynecol.* **22:** 30–37 (1963).

2. Burns, Jr., Beaury C., Felix Rutledge, Julian P. Smith, and Luis Delclos: *Am. J. Obstet. Gynecol.* **98:** 374–386 (1967).

3. Delclos, Luis, and Gilbert H. Fletcher, *Clin. Obstet. Gynecol.* **12:** 993–1002 (1969).

4. Delgado, Gregorio, *"Second Look" Operations in Ovarian Neoplasms,* M D. Anderson Hospital, Houston, 1972.

5. Munnell, Equinn W., *Am. J Obstet. Gynecol.* **103:** 641–653 (1969).

6. Rutledge, Felix, and Beaury C. Burns, *Am. J. Obstet. Gynecol.* **96:** 761–772 (1966).

7. Rutledge, Felix, and Julian P. Smith, *Am. J. Obstet. Gynecol.* **5:** 691–703 (1970).

8. Rutledge, Felix, Julian P. Smith, and J. Taylor Wharton: *Cancer* **30:** 1565 (1972).

9. Rutledge, Felix, *Med. World News; Obstet. Gynecol.* 87–88 (1970).

CHAPTER 13 TREATMENT OF OVARIAN CANCERS

(Germ Cell and Mesenchymal Origin)

J. TAYLOR WHARTON, M.D.

There are two major groups of special ovarian tumors: tumors of germ cell origin and gonadal stromal tumors. Although these tumors are rare individually, they are common as a group. Gynecologists should be familiar with the pathological and clinical manifestations of each tumor because therapy is specific. Some tumors are minimally aggressive and can be treated while preserving fertility; others are very sensitive to irradiation, and others resist irradiation and are rapidly fatal. The origin of these cancers is vague, but a theoretical concept serves as a basis for clinical classification.

Although gonad embryology is complex, a simplified review of its development will provide some insight into the origin of the different elements contained. In the embryo the thickened coelomic epithelium along the ventromedial aspect of the mesonephros forms the genital ridge. During this process the underlying mesenchyme is incorporated and germ cells migrate to this area from the hindgut. All of these elements, or cells capable of producing them (pleuripotential cells), are retained by the adult ovary and cancers may arise from them. Thus, the normal ovary contains all of the components thought necessary for the genesis of a bewildering, diverse group of cancers. The abnormal gonad may also undergo malignant degeneration, since the same precursors are present.

The following scheme shown in Figure 1 is useful in demonstrating the histogenesis of germ cell tumors. Their highly malignant potential makes them extremely important.

GERM CELL TUMORS

The four basic types of germ cell tumors are: dysgerminoma, embryonal carcinoma, malignant teratoma, and choriocarcinoma. Any of these may present in pure form or as part of a mixed germ cell tumor. The mixed forms, such as dysgerminoma that contain elements of embryonal carcinoma or malignant teratoma, are troublesome because one of the components may be overlooked if histologic sampling is not extensive. Initial recognition of the different elements present is essential since the clinical course is determined by the most malignant components. To diagnose a mixed tumor or to be certain a tumor is pure, the pathologist must examine multiple sections and the surgeon must obtain multiple biopsies if the tumor is unresectable. Prompt and proper fixation of the surgical specimen is critical. When a large tumor is removed it should be sectioned immediately and promptly placed into a large volume of fixative. Inadequate fixation greatly hinders histologic interpretation which in turn can compromise therapy.

201

Germn Cell Tumor

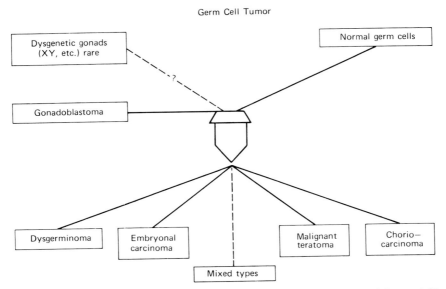

Figure 1 Germ cell tumors. From Gallagher, H. S., and R. P. Lewis: Sequential gonadoblastoma and choriocarcinoma. *Obstet. Gynecol.,* **41,** 123 (1973). Reprinted with permission.

Dysgerminoma

HISTOLOGY

This tumor has a distinct monocellular pattern, with nodules of uniform polyhedral cells with clear cytoplasm and regular round nuclei separated by fibrous septa variably infiltrated by lymphocytes. The degree of malignancy cannot be predicted from microscopic findings. Areas of eosinophilic necrobiosis, granuloma formation, or clusters of bizarre giant cells may be present. Such changes do not indicate a poorer prognosis.

CLINICAL FEATURES

The majority of dysgerminomas are tumors of youth and occur before the age of 30. Patients usually experience abdominal enlargement and pain or notice a palpable abdominal mass. An occasional patient will present as an acute abdominal crisis, secondary to torsion or an accident related to the tumors blood supply. Sometimes the first manifestation is metastasis. Bilateral

tumors are found in approximately 10% of cases.

Dysgerminoma may be found in patients with primary amenorrhea and are occasionally associated with an underlying gonadoblastoma. Such patients, especially those with abnormal sexual development, require chromosome analysis. The majority of patients with dysgerminoma, however, are normal females. The tumor may complicate a normal pregnancy.

There is some basic knowledge about the behavior of dysgerminoma that is helpful in planning therapy:

1. The pure form of the dysgerminoma is radiosensitive.

2. The lymphatic system is an important pathway of spread.

3. The tumor has a predilection for the young.

4. The tumor is usually unilateral and often large.

5. It may be associated with congenital defects.

6. The presence of an elevated gonadotropin titer is usually associated with an admixed choriocarcinoma within the tumor which significantly alters prognosis and treatment selection.

SPREAD PATTERN

These tumors spread by lymphatic extension. Regional and aortic node involvement is frequent. Dysgerminoma may involve nodes beyond the abdominal cavity (inguinal and left supraclavicular groups), and lung, liver, and upper abdominal metastases also occur.

In our experience the following features are poor prognostic signs: lack of encapsulation, infiltration of adjacent pelvic organs, metastasis to regional or aortic lymph nodes, bilaterality and ascites.

PREOPERATIVE OR POSTOPERATIVE EVALUATION

A chest x-ray, IVP, and lymphangiogram are the most helpful diagnostic tests. The lymphangiogram may detect lymph node metastasis in patients thought to have disease confined to only one ovary. Evaluation of the paraaortic nodes is particularly important since they are frequently the first group to be involved. The lymphatic channels accompany the ovarian veins, which drain directly into the left renal vein and the vena cava.

An elevated human chorionic gonadotrophin (HCG) titer is diagnostic of the presence of trophoblastic tissue (choriocarcinoma). A buccal smear or karyotyping or both are indicated.

TREATMENT

Dysgerminoma exhibits varied clinical behavior. Clinicians have different experiences, which accounts for the dissimilar reports from the various oncology centers.

Pedowitz and associates[8] noted only a 35% five-year survival rate for conservatively treated patients compared with 50% for those treated with complete excision. Malkasian and Symmonds[4] reported that conservative therapy may be justified in certain cases. However, the patients who were treated conservatively did not do as well in five-year survival rates as those in the complete excision group. Brody[1] recommends a conservative operation in patients with a favorable prognosis, followed by external irradiation administered to protect the remaining ovary. Most authors agree that patients with advanced disease should receive excision plus irradiation therapy.

We believe that unilateral oophorectomy is adequate therapy for the young patient with a unilateral, well-encapsulated tumor 10 cm or less in diameter. Patients with metastases or older patients who do not wish to have children are treated by total abdominal hysterectomy and bilateral salpingo-oophorectomy.

At the initial exploratory celiotomy the surgeon must search for metastases. Enlarged pelvic or paraaortic nodes should be biopsied and marked with radiopaque clips. Aggressive surgery that interrupts the bowel or the urinary tract is not indicated in patients with pure dysgerminoma because the cancer is responsive to radiation. It is wise to remove as much tumor as possible while sparing the adjacent structures since volume reduction has some advantages, and bulky lesions undoubtedly account for some radiation failures. Patients with mixed germ cell tumors containing elements of embryonal carcinoma or immature teratoma (teratocarcinoma) are also not subjected to bowel resection. A complication that delays inception of therapy in these patients is particularly detrimental because the growth rate can be extremely rapid.

Phenotypic female patients with negative smears and Y chromosomes may have a dysgenetic gonad or gonadoblastoma, and the contralateral gonad should be excised when the tumor is removed.[3]

THE M. D. ANDERSON EXPERIENCE

Our experience with 23 patients with dysgerminoma of the ovary also supports the belief that this disease is especially sensitive to irradiation, for postoperative treatment, prophylaxis, and treatment for recurrent disease. Table 1 gives the two-year survival figures for 23 patients treated with radiation postoperatively. It is noteworthy that patients with advanced dysgerminoma were also candidates for radiation, since 13 of the 23 patients treated had Stage III or IV cancers.

The protection provided by postoperative x-ray therapy can be observed in the results obtained in the 10 patients who had disease confined to the pelvis; there were only two recurrences.

Dysgerminoma often offers a second chance for cure. Of 5 patients with dysgerminoma that metastasized or recurred in the supraclavicular lymph nodes, 3 were treated successfully with radiation therapy.

The extent of the disease at recurrence is important for the overall prognosis, but advanced spread does not imply a hopeless situation. Since low-dose irradiation is possible, patients can tolerate large areas of treatment. Often the entire abdomen and also the mediastinal and supraclavicular node chains are irradiated.

Table 1 Dysgerminoma: Results of Postoperative Radiation, The M. D. Anderson Hospital

Stage	Number of Patients	2-Year Survival (%)
I	5	100
II	5	60
III	6	50
IV	7	43
Total	23	52.3

TECHNIQUE OF RADIATION THERAPY

Patients with pure dysgerminoma are given 2000 rads to the entire abdomen by the moving strip technique with the Cobalt-60 unit. An additional dose of 2000 rads is administered to the pelvis, the paraaortic nodes, or both, as indicated by the findings at surgery and/or by lymphangiography. If metastatic tumor is found in the paraaortic lymph nodes, prophylactic irradiation (2500 rads for three weeks) is given to the mediastinum and the left supraclavicular area after three to six weeks of rest.

Patients with unilateral dysgerminomas, especially young patients who want to maintain their fertility, are not given postoperative irradiation unless (1) the tumor is >10 cm in diameter, (2) there is lymph node involvement, (3) the capsule of the tumor was ruptured prior to surgery, or (4) there is malignant ascites.

Metastatic dysgerminoma in the liver, lung, or brain should be treated with irradiation. Usually the dose required to destroy the tumor does not exceed 2500 rads. Lesions that do not respond to irradiation are often mixed, and are an indication for exploration and tissue diagnosis. Mixed germ cell tumors require aggressive chemotherapy.

Gonadoblastoma

Gonadoblastoma is an extremely rare and well-defined histologically characteristic neoplasm that occurs almost exclusively in the gonads of intersexual patients.[12] Usually the patients are phenotypic females and have hypoplastic uteri and tubes. When gonads are recognizable, they are either fibrous streaks or immature testes.

PATHOLOGY

The tumor consist of clusters of germ cells mixed with immature Sertoli's cells which surround eosinophilic hyaline bodies. Calcification is common. Overgrowth by other germ cell elements such as dysgerminoma, teratocarcinoma, embryonal carcinoma, choriocarcinoma, or mixtures of these lesions may obscure much evidence of the existence of a gonadoblastoma. The presence of calcification in what appears to be dysgerminoma should raise a strong etiologic presumption of gonadoblastoma.

CLINICAL ASPECTS AND TREATMENT

Gonadoblastomas are only seen in individuals with gonadal disorders. Usually the individuals are sex-chromatin negative, phenotypic females with primary amenorrhea. The abnormal gonad may secrete significant amounts of androgen, thus further emphasizing abnormal development.

Although gonadoblastoma is a neoplasm of limited malignant potential, it frequently gives rise to or is associated with germinal neoplasia of grave prognostic significance.[3]

The opposite gonad should be removed in all cases of unilateral gonadoblastoma. This gonad is usually a streak or immature testis, and the principle of preserving ovarian function is not applicable.

Embryonal Carcinoma

The term embryonal carcinoma includes germ cell tumors of the endodermal sinus pattern and polyvesicular vitelline tumor pattern and also less well-defined epitheloid tumors of germ cell origin. It is probably the most common type of highly malignant ovarian neoplasm in young women under 25. A painful abdominal mass is the usual presenting complaint.[5] Mixtures with other types of germ cell tumors, such as dysgerminoma or immature teratoma, have been encountered. As with other germ cell cancers, it is imperative that the pathologist examine multiple areas of the tumor.

This tumor was mistakenly called ovarian mesonephroma by Schiller. Embryonal carcinoma and mesonephroma have nothing in common in their histogenesis, general architecture, incidence, or clinical behavior.

ENDODERMAL SINUS PATTERN

This histological pattern is the most common type and is composed of embryonal cells lining a network of microcysts which produces a honeycomblike appearance. The cells lining the spaces are usually flat, but in more differentiated areas they form characteristic papillary projections that have a mesodermal core with a capillary in its center. An additional feature of this tumor is the presence of intracellular and extracellular hyaline bodies.[14]

POLYVESICULAR VITELLINE PATTERN

This histologic variant is extremely rare and consists of vesicles that vary in form and size. The pure cancers of this pattern may go unrecognized as being of germ cell origin, and may thus delay therapy. This yolk-saclike pattern frequently overlaps the endodermal sinus pattern and has the same clinical features.

TREATMENT

Embryonal cancers grow rapidly. They are not as sensitive as the dysgerminomas to irradiation. Chemotherapy has caused dramatic reduction in tumor size, and aggressive and persistent use seems to have protected both pediatric and young adult patients who are presently under treatment at our institution. The chemotherapeutic regimen currently in use is shown in Table 2. The addition of a Bleomycin-Velban combination recommended by Samuels[10] for testicular germ cell cancers has also produced meaningful tumor regression in some patients who fail to respond to other chemotherpay combinations.

Although the tumor grows rapidly and reaches a large size, the contralateral ovary is rarely involved. Thus it is not important

Table 2   Combination Chemotherapy (VAC)

Drug	Dosage	
	Pediatric	*Adult*
Vincristine	2 mg M² B.S.A.[a] IV weekly for 8–12 wk, not to exceed 2 mg/wk	1.5 mg M² B.S.A. IV weekly for 10 wk, not to exceed 2.5 mg/wk
Actinomycin D	0.075 mg/kg/day (total dose) IV over 5–7 days, repeated every 6 wk for 1–2 yr	0.5 mg/day IV for 5 days, repeated every 4 wk for 2 yr
Cytoxan	40–60 mg/kg/day (total dose) IV over 5–7 days, repeated every 6 wk (given with Actinomycin D) for 1–2 yr.	5–7 mg/kg/day IV for 5 days, repeated every 4 wk for 2 yr

[a] Body surface area.

for the surgeon to remove the contralateral ovary that appears normal, since its presence is not decisive in the postoperative recurrence rate. The surgeon should excise the tumor as completely as possible, but do nothing that would prolong postoperative recovery and delay the initiation of chemotherapy.

The recurrence rate of embryonal cancer is so high that patients with unilateral tumor masses which have apparently been completely excised rarely remain free of disease. Therefore all patients, regardless of the stage, should receive chemotherapy.[13]

Teratomas

The usual classification of teratomas into two categories, solid and cystic, has been confusing to many gynecologists, partly because this nomenclature assumes that all solid teratomas are malignant and that cystic teratomas are usually benign. Although this is generally correct, the gross appearance can be misleading. Because of a rapid growth rate, immature solid teratomas may undergo necrosis and contain cystic areas. Cystic teratomas may also have mature elements that undergo malignant degeneration. Also, some solid teratomas that contain mature elements only have an excellent prognosis.[15] Therefore, a better understanding of their malignant potential and clinical behavior can be gained by examining the morphologic maturity (differentiation) of the various components contained within the teratomas.

IMMATURE TERATOMAS

Patients with an immature teratoma (also called embryonal teratoma or teratocarcinoma) usually notice an enlarging abdomen or palpate a mass. Occasionally, symptoms of small bowel obstruction or distention due to ascites may be present. The growth rate may be very rapid and tumor volume can double in a matter of four to five weeks.

Pathology. Immature teratomas may contain multiple malignant elements: embryonic mesechyme, anaplastic carcinoma, sarcoma of any type (rare), and neural elements (common). Frequently they are fatal, since most components are undifferentiated and very malignant. A possible exception is a teratoma with mature elements. The prognosis in such cases is reported to be better than for teratomas with immature components.[9, 15] The grading method proposed by

Thurlbeck and Scully aids in categorizing the tumors according to the degree and amount of immature elements within.[16]

Treatment. Initial treatment for immature teratoma is total abdominal hysterectomy and bilateral salpingo-oophorectomy. Since these tumors are rarely bilateral, reoperation is perhaps unnecessary if one ovary remains. In our opinion, all patients (with the possible exception of cancers having only mature elements) should receive VAC chemotherapy. We believe that these patients, like those with embryonal carcinoma, are less likely to be protected by radiation therapy alone.

Trophoblastic tissue may be present either alone or as part of a teratoma. HCG will detect the presence of choriocarcinoma, and combination chemotherapy is the recommended treatment. Recurrences of non-gestational choriocarcinoma after the HCG titer has returned to normal levels has been encountered at our institution and by others, and caution plus more persistent therapy is indicated.

MATURE TERATOMAS (DERMOID)

These tumors are usually cystic and contain adult tissues derived from all three germ layers. Approximately 2% are complicated by the development of a malignant tumor; 80% will be squamous carcinomas. Adenocarcinomas, thyroid lesions, sarcomas, carcinoid tumors, and melanomas also occur.

The carcinoid tumor may secrete serotonin (5-hydroxytryptamine) and produce the classic carcinoid syndrome even though it is confined to the ovary. The ovarian veins empty into the vena cava, which bypasses the liver amine oxidase system that would otherwise metabolize the serotonin.[2]

Tumors that contain predominantly thyroid acini are known as strum ovarii. These tumors may undergo malignant changes (5%) and may also cause clinical hyperthyroidism.

OVARIAN STROMAL TUMORS

These tumors are interrelated and arise from embryonic gonadal mesenchyme and/or sex cords. They may contain granulosa cells, theca cells, Sertoli cells, Leydig cells, or any of their precursors either alone or in combination. The stromal components or perhaps the cells themselves may produce androgens or estrogens that cause clinical manifestations of diagnostic significance. The majority of these tumors, however, are inactive hormonally and produce symptoms related primarily to their size and location. The overall malignant potential for the group is low and, although metastases and death occur, many of the reported highly malignant variants probably represent histologic misinterpretation.[11]

Granulosa Cell Tumor

On gross examination the tumor is usually a partly solid yellow mass with multiple cysts filled with clotted blood. The microscopic features show great variation. Numerous descriptive terms such as microfollicular, macrofollicular, cylindromatous, gyriform and sarcomatoid are given to the various patterns. The better differentiated forms show Call-Exner bodies, whereas the undifferentiated forms resemble sarcomas. Although the sarcomatoid pattern is believed to represent a more malignant lesion, the microscopic pattern is not a reliable indicator of malignant potential. In an analysis of tumors, Norris and Taylor[6] found it difficult to relate the microscopic appearance of stromal tumors to the clinical outcome.

CLINICAL FEATURES

Although stromal tumors may occur at any age they are more common in the 45 to 55-year-old group. Estrogen production can cause the early development of secondary sex characteristics in the very young, but this is rare. A hyperplastic endometrium with irregular bleeding is usual, and occasionally a concurrent adenocarcinoma of the endometrium is seen in the older age groups. Most tumors, however, are found on routine examination, for pelvic pain due to a mass, or as an emergency because a thin-walled cyst has ruptured producing a hemoperitoneum, or because of tumor infarction due to torsion. Since the malignant forms of these tumors have a peculiar habit of recurring within the abdomen or pelvis after the five-year postoperative interval, the physician responsible for postoperative care should be constantly alert.

TREATMENT

The unilateral, encapsulated granulosa cell tumor in the young is treated by conservative unilateral oophorectomy. This is justified because bilaterality is encountered in only 10% of patients and the tumor is relatively low in malignancy potential. The opposite ovary should be biopsied. A total abdominal hysterectomy and bilateral salpingo-oophorectomy are indicated when it is not felt necessary to preserve fertility.

Patients with metastatic granulosa cell cancers are treated in a similar manner to those with epithelial cancers. These tumors are radiosensitive, and radiation is indicated for pelvic or abdominal metastases when the residual masses are 2 cm or less in diameter and the liver and kidney areas are free of disease. We recommend treatment to the entire abdomen using the moving strip technique supplemented by a pelvic boost.

Combination chemotherapy (Table 2) is recommended at some point in treatment if the tumor has spread beyond the abdomen or when the patient has received previous radiation therapy. In our experience granulosa cell cancers are less likely to respond to single alkylating agents. However, a response can occur, and melphalan (Alkeran) may be tried before attempting

more toxic combinations when the clinical situation justifies less aggressive treatment.

Sertoli-Leydig Cell Tumors

These tumors contain Sertoli and Leydig cells and may produce hormones. The term arrhenoblastoma is frequently used to describe them, especially when masculinization is present. These tumors are so rarely seen that it is difficult for one medical center to accumulate enough experience to formulate scientifically valid treatment recommendations.

PATHOLOGY

Sertoli-Leydig cell tumors are grossly very similar to granulosa cell tumors. Histologically various developmental phrases of embryologic testicular elements are observed, and range from well-differentiated tubules to undifferentiated cords. The three principal patterns—tubular, intermediate, and undifferentiated forms—may be present as admixtures or pure. As with granulosa cell tumors it is not possible to correlate the histologic picture with prognosis.[7] It is thought that the Sertoli-Leydig cell tumor is more often malignant than the granulosa cell tumor.

TREATMENT

Young patients with a unilateral encapsulated tumor are treated with unilateral oophorectomy. This is justified since bilaterality is noted in 5% of patients. Other patients who do not desire more children are treated with a total abdominal hysterectomy and bilateral salpingo-oophorectomy.

Patients with pelvic or abdominal metastases receive radiation therapy as previously discussed for granulosa cell cancers. Although our experience with chemotherapy for patients with large masses or with spread beyond the abdomen is limited, combination chemotherapy (Table 2) plus radiation has been used in a few patients with some success.

REFERENCES

1. Brody, S.: Clinical aspects of dysgerminomas of the ovary. *Acta Radiol.* (Stockholm) **56:** 209 (1961).

2. Campbell, A. C. P., The pathological relationship of S-hydroxytryptamine. In *Modern Trends in Pathology,* New York, pp. 231–247, 1959.

3. Gallagher, H. S., and R. P. Lewis: Sequential gonadoblastoma and choriocarcinoma. *Obstet. Gynecol.* **41:** 123 (1973).

4. Malkasian, G. D., and R. E. Symmonds: Treatment of the unilateral encapsulated ovarian dysgerminoma, *Am. J. Obstet. Gynecol.* **90:** 379 (1964).

5. Neubecker, R. D., and J. L. Breen: Embryonal carcinoma of the ovary. *Cancer* **15:** 546 (1962).

6. Norris, H. J., and H. B. Taylor: Prognosis of granulosa cell cancer of the ovary, *Cancer* **21:** 255 (1968).

7. Novak, E. R., and J. H. Lang: Arrhenoblastoma of the ovary. *Am. J. Obstet. Gynecol.* **92:** 1082 (1965).

8. Pedowitz, P., et al.: Dysgerminoma of the ovary. *Am. J. Obstet. Gynecol.* **70:** 1284 (1955).

9. Robboy, S. J., and R. E. Scully: Ovarian teratoma with glial implants on the peritoneum. *Hum. Pathol.* **1:** 702 (1970).

10. Samuels, M. L., D. E. Johnson, and P. Y. Holoye: The treatment of stage III metastatic germinal cell neoplasia of the testis with Bleomycin combination chemotherapy. *Proc. Am. Assoc. Cancer Res.* **14:** 89 (1973).

11. Scully, Robert E.: Recent progress in ovarian cancer. *Hum. Pathol.* **1** (No. 1): 85–91 (March 1970).

12. Scully, Robert E.: Gonadoblastoma, a review of 74 cases. *Cancer* **25** (No. 6): 1340 (June 1970).

13. Smith, J. F., P. Rutledge, and W. W. Sutow: Malignant gynecologic tumors in children, current approaches to treatment, *Am. J. Obstet. Gynecol.* 261.

14. Telium, Gunnar: Special tumors of ovary and testis, J. B. Lippincott Company, Philadelphia & Toronto, 1971, p. 56.

15. Woodruff, D. J., P. Protos, and W. F. Peterson: Ovarian teratomas, relationship of histologic and ontogenic factors to prognosis, *Am. J. Obstet.* **102:** 702 (1968).

16. Thurlbeck, W. M., and R. E. Scully: Solid teratoma of the ovary, a clinicopathological analysis of 9 cases, *Cancer* **13:** 804 (1960).

CARCINOMA OF THE VULVA

CHAPTER 14 CARCINOMA OF THE VULVA

RICHARD C. BORONOW, M.D.

CONTROVERSIES

1. What is standard therapy and what is its basis?

2. Is there prognostic and therapeutic value in the FIGO staging?

3. Are there situations for departures from standard therapy?

Cancer of the vulva usually implies squamous cell carcinoma (at least 85% of cases). Vulvar melanoma accounts for approximately 5% of cases and will be discussed elsewhere. Bartholin's gland cancers, sarcomas, and unclassified malignancies of the vulva comprise most of the remaining neoplasms of these tissues. One to two percent are basal cell cancers. Carcinoma in situ or intraepithelial carcinoma of the vulva is recognized. Invasive squamous cell carcinoma occurs most commonly in older women.

While some vulvar cancers arise in chronic granulomatous disease, and others in a field of hypertrophic vulvar epithelium (leukoplakia), most appear to arise de novo from essentially unremarkable vulvar skin. Some observers have collected a small number of cases of vulvar and vaginal cancers with known antecedent condyloma acuminata, raising the question of viral etiology.

The disastrous results achieved by local excision of invasive squamous cell carcinoma are historically significant. The application of extensive surgery with vigorous management of the primary lesion as well as appropriate and planned resection of the regional spread pattern of this disease have improved results in terms of both total salvage and local control.

THE PATIENT

Age

Vulvar cancer is a disease of older women. Epidermoid or squamous cancer develops at a mean age of about 60 years. Although approximately 75% of cases occur in women 50 years or older, the disease may occur in young women. Reflecting the experience of a referral cancer institution, Rutledge and associates[1] reported 15 percent of cases in women under 40. Similar age patterns are noted in women with Bartholin's gland cancer and melanoma. The rare vulvar sarcomas appear to develop in a younger population.[2]

Venereal Disease

Syphilis in the patient's past history is reported in from 13 to 50% of cases[3,4] and exceeds that expected in the general population. Although it is probably not of etiologic significance, this is a venereal exposure marker.

Chronic vulvar granulomatous disease has been associated with squamous cancer of

213

the vulva. Although the incidence was quite low in the M. D. Anderson Hospital experience,[3] this association was observed in 60% of cases in the experience of Hay and Cole.[4]

Lymphopathia venerum (lymphogranuloma inguinale), thought to be caused by a virus, is one of the most common of the so-called granulomatous diseases. Further epidemiologic data suggesting not just one but several viral cofactors in possible carcinogenesis come from two sources. The interrelation of neoplasia of the cervix, vagina, and vulva is recognized. A recent series[3] reports that 15% of patients with vulvar cancer had (either a history or subsequently developed) carcinoma in situ or invasive cancer of the cervix. Merrill[5] noted a 34% association. Currently, herpes virus type 2 is under scrutiny as either a cofactor or the possible etiologic agent in cervical cancer. In addition, some authors report a history of condyloma acuminatum, and some have collected small prospective series of patients with vulvar and vaginal condylomata who have subsequently developed cancer.[6] We have observed 1 patient with an early cancer at age 25 and a history of extensive condylomata 10 years earlier.

Chronic Vulvar Dystrophies

Vulvar dystrophies, especially epithelial hyperplasia (formerly called leukoplakia), have been considered as possibly premalignant. In a recent survey[3] it was noted that although in retrospective studies up to 50% of women with untreated leukoplakia were believed destined to develop cancer, a more realistic figure is probably closer to one-tenth of that projection (5%). A far more meaningful interpretation of the prognosis of any vulvar dystrophy is afforded by an assessment of its typical or atypical nuclear features.[7] Clearly, a spectrum of malignant potential exists with these vulvar lesions as it does with cervical intraepithelial neoplasia.

Other factors associated with patients with vulvar cancer include obesity, diabetes, hypertension, and nulliparity.

Suspicion Demands Biopsy

From this brief review some semblance of the at risk patient has been developed. But it is equally apparent that medically healthy women with no history of venereal disease or chronic vulvar dystrophy represent the majority of those who develop vulvar cancer. Thus, any vulvar lesion must be biopsied. Unexplained and persistent pruritus demands further study as well.

Although reports of two and three decades ago underscored the significant role of both patient and physician delay, this is not just a phenomenon of past medical history. It is disturbing to note that in a recent report of 249 cases 60% of patients with untreated vulvar cancer gave a history of a vulvar mass or "sore" for an average of 10 months prior to diagnosis; 25% of patients were under medical treatment without biopsy; 30% of patients experienced a physician delay of three or more months.[1]

THE DISEASE

Histologic Types

The vast majority of vulvar cancers are epidermoid (squamous). In the collected data recorded in Table 1, 86.2% of cases were of the squamous variety, melanoma accounted for 4.8%, and Bartholin's cancers for 1.0%. Basal cell cancers were 1.4% of cases, and sarcomas were 2.2% of this series.[8]

SQUAMOUS CELL CANCER

The initial lesion may appear after an interval of persistent pruritus. The superficially ulcerative lesion or occasionally papillary growth may at first seem innocent

Table 1 Incidence of Vulvar Neoplasms by Histologic Type[8]

Histologic Type	Total	
	Number[a]	Percent
Epidermoid	1188	86.2
Melanoma	66	4.8
Basal cell	19	1.4
Bartholin's gland		
Squamous	5	0.4
Adenocarcinoma	8	0.6
Sarcoma	30	2.2
Adenocarcinoma	8	0.6
Unidentified or undifferentiated	54	3.9

[a] 1378 cases collected from 12 series from 1934–1964.

enough. Continued growth, exophytic or ulcerative, is gradually associated with some bleeding, secondary infection, and pain. A consensus has suggested that with invasive squamous cell vulvar cancer, the grade of undifferentiation has little prognostic significance.[8] Some current experience[9,10,15] supports the contention of Cherry and Glücksman[11] 20 years ago that poorly differentiated and anaplastic lesions (Figure 1) metastasize to regional nodes more quickly than well-differentiated lesions (Figure 2), and behave in a more virulent fashion.

BASAL CELL CANCER

These lesions usually occur on the labia major. They begin as a small nodule and tend to develop central ulceration (the so-called rodent ulcer). The epithelial infiltration into the underlying connective tissue is orderly and circumscribed. Like basal cell cancer elsewhere on the body, they do not invade lymphatics and local excision is adequate. The pathologist should not overlook

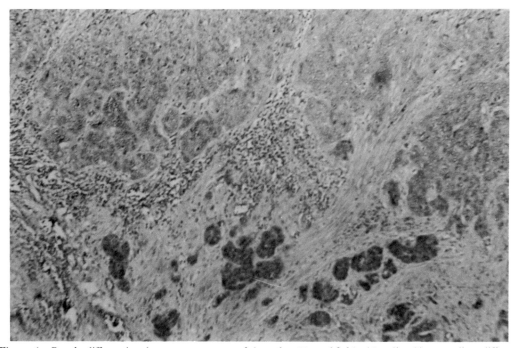

Figure 1 Poorly differentiated squamous cancer of the vulva. Top of field with cells of intermediate differentiation, lower field contains nests of more anaplastic cells.

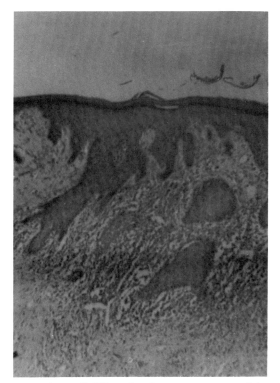

Figure 2 Well-differentiated squamous cancer of the vulva. Very superficial invasion.

a mixed component of the basosquamous cell variety, since this lesion behaves like a squamous cell cancer and local excision is inadequate.

MELANOMA

Melanoma arise from nevi containing a junctional component (either pure junctional nevi or compound nevi). Vulvar pigmented nevi appear to contain a higher than expected incidence of nevi with junctional components than most other areas of the body.[12] Accordingly prophylactic excision of vulvar pigmented nevi is appropriate. The anatomic site of origin of melanoma differs somewhat from squamous vulvar cancers because the labia major are somewhat less involved. The histologic picture is identical

to melanomas of other sites. Vulvar melanoma is discussed in detail elsewhere.

SARCOMA

From a recent review it appears that fewer than several hundred cases of this rare group of malignancies have been reported. The 12 cases recently reported included leiomyosarcoma (3), rhabdomyosarcoma (3), neurofibrosarcoma (3) and fibrosarcoma (1). Others reported in the past include myxosarcoma, mixed mesodermal sarcoma, hemangioendothelioma and hemangiosarcoma. Occasionally, apparently localized lymphoma has been reported.[8] The mean age of patients with soft tissue sarcomas is younger than for the epithelial malignancies, and most occur between 30 and 50. The mean age reported by DiSaia et al. was 38 years.[2] Extensive local surgery is indicated and distant recurrence is common. Although the role of lymph node spread and lymph node dissection is not clear at this time, it deserves further study.

PAGET'S DISEASE

Extramammary Paget's disease has been reported arising in the vulva in approximately 100 cases. The slightly raised, red, eczematoid area with patches of white epithelium is usually associated with long-standing pruritus. The epithelium is infiltrated with characteristic large Paget cells apparently arising from the underlying apocrine glands, but the precise site of origin is unknown.[13] Adjacent, normal appearing epithelium is often involved microscopically. Wide vulvectomy is indicated because of the frequency of local recurrence after simple excision. The specimen must be studied for underlying invasive adenocarcinoma, found in about 25% of reported cases. Appropriate regional node surgery is indicated if cancer is found. However, in the limited experience accumulated, node dissection may be more prognostic than therapeutic.[14]

BARTHOLIN'S GLAND CANCER

This is a rare lesion, comprising approximately 1% of vulvar cancers. Among 176 collected cases,[8] 40.9% were of the epidermoid variety (Bartholin's duct epithelium and possibly from squamous metaplasia), 42.6% were adenocarcinoma, 5.1% sarcoma, 0.6% melanoma, and 10.8% were unknown. Because of the deep site of origin, diagnosis may be delayed until ulceration of vulva or vagina occurs. A hard lump in the Bartholin's area must be viewed with suspicion. Lymphatic spread is to both the inguinal and pelvic nodes. Surgery must be more locally extensive than for most vulvar cancers, and inguinal and pelvic lymphadenectomies are indicated. While this author's only experience with Bartholin's cancer was one case treated radically eight years ago (currently alive without evidence of disease), the literature contains only 14 reported five-year cures according to a recent survey.[8]

Local Growth and Spread Pattern

The majority of vulvar squamous cancers appear to arise primarily on the labium majus (Table 2). Other primary sites, in order, are labia minor, clitoris, and perineum or posterior forchette. Occasionally the lesion is so extensive that the precise site of origin cannot be determined. Urethral cancer is excluded from this discussion. The lymphatic drainage of the vulva is depicted in Figure 3. The primary route of spread is to the inguinal nodes (the superficial and deep femoral, or groin, nodes). From there, an orderly embolic spread to the external iliac and obturator nodes, and the common iliac and aortic nodes is customary.

Metastasis to pelvic nodes, while bypassing the groin nodes, is anatomically possible (Figure 3) and was observed in 3% of Way's first 143 cases.[15] In his next 263 cases, however, he observed no case of vulvar cancer with pelvic nodes metastases in the absence of inguinal metastases.[16] The latter condition has also been reported recently by others. [1,17]

The lymphatic system of the vulva is regarded as an extensively anastomosing network. While small, unilateral lesions usually have ipsilateral groin metastases, contralateral involvement may occur. Larger lesions, particularly lesions located more anteriorly and those involving midline structures, are especially liable to bilateral groin node metastases.

Among 1122 cases of vulvar cancer treated by radical vulvectomy with groin and pelvic node dissection (16 series reported from 1941 to 1963) there were 517 cases (46.1%) with positive nodes.[8] As patient and physician awareness increases, the diagnosis of vulvar cancer will be made earlier and the incidence of nodal metastases should decrease. Two relatively recent series report 37 percent of cases with nodal metastases.[1,18]

Progressive local growth may involve the urethra, vagina, anus, and occasionally the bladder or rectum. Although in some instances these structures may be involved early in the course of disease, this state

Table 2 Location of Primary Vulvar Malignancy[8]

Location	Total Number[a]	Percent
Labia	1094	71.2
Majora	457	
Minora	156	
Both	94	
Clitoris	210	13.7
Vestibule	10	0.7
Perineum, fourchette	69	4.5
Prepuce	13	0.8
Bartholin's gland	14	0.9
Urethra	48	3.1
Unclassified or extensive	79	5.1

[a] 1537 cases collected from 15 series from 1929–1964.

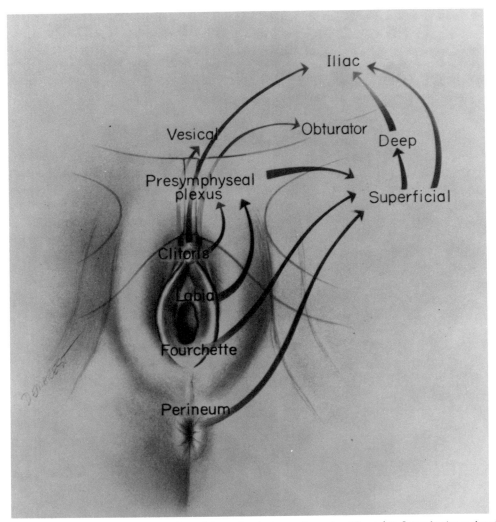

Figure 3 General schematic representation of the major drainage channels of the vulva. Lymphatics and regional nodes of perineum, forchette, and labia are located within the subcutaneous fatty tissue of the vulva, mons veneris, and femoral triangle. The clitoris, on the other hand, drains to primary lymph node sites within the pelvis. From Plentl, A. A., and E. A. Friedman: *Lymphatic System of the Female Genitalia*, W. B. Saunders Company, Philadelphia, Pennsylvania, 1971. Reprinted with permission.

usually reflects significant delay. With such locally advanced disease, additional lymphatic pathways may be involved (communication with vaginal lymphatics draining to the pelvic nodes, and also communication to the hemorrhoidal system draining to the aortic nodes). This is described further in Chapter 17.

THERAPY AND STAGING

Contemporary Therapy

The anatomic data reviewed provide the basis for contemporary therapy. Extensive local resection is required for local control. The status of the regional nodes appears pivotal in terms of curability, as demonstrated in the collected experience recorded in Table 3. The impact of age and associated infirmities takes a significant toll. Negative groin nodes carry an even better prognosis after definitive surgery than the data of Table 3 indicate: Way[15] noted no cancer deaths among 44 patients with negative lymphadenectomy; Franklin and Rutledge[9] reported no deaths of cancer among 53 patients with negative lymphadenectomy.

Radical surgery for vulvar cancer is established (Figure 4). Local measures appear to save fewer patients than radical surgery, even in the presence of nodal metastasis (Tables 3 and 4).

That some patients have pelvic node metastasis and that some of these patients can be cured is established (Table 5), but

whether pelvic lymphadenectomy should be routinely employed remains a matter of controversy. [1,17]

Further discussion on therapy of these invasive lesions is found in Chapter 16.

The Utility of Clinical Staging

There have been a variety of efforts to evolve a clinical staging system for vulvar cancer. Taussig[19] proposed five groups based on size and anatomic extent of the primary lesion coupled with clinical assessment of the groin nodes. McKelvey[20] proposed four groups based on the surface area of the lesion and the anatomic extent. He excluded clinical assessment of the groin nodes because he considered this method completely unreliable. Even up to recent years, most believed: ". . . consider the operating findings in lieu of and in preference to clinical features. That this is appropriate for carcinoma of the vulva is based on the recognized unreliability of clinical observation in this disease."[8]

FIGO STAGING

For these reasons, vulvar cancer is the last of the major gynecologic cancers to be assigned an international staging system. The recently adopted FIGO staging is noted

Table 3   Comparative Survival Rates in Vulvar Cancer According to Regional Node Involvement[8]

Status of Node	Number of Patients	5-Year Survival Number[a]	5-Year Survival Percent
Negative	314	237	75.5
Positive	236	98	41.5

[a] 550 cases collected from 12 series from 1941–1963.

Table 4   Vulvar Cancer Survival by Treatment Plan[8]

Modality	Patient Treated	5-Year Survival Number[a]	5-Year Survival Percent
Radiotherapy	836	109	13.0
Simple vulvectomy	334	103	30.8
Vulvectomy plus radiotherapy	659	214	32.5
Radical vulvectomy and femoral lymphadenectomy	449	250	55.7
Radical vulvectomy and femoral and pelvic lymphadenectomy	440	278	63.2

[a] Cases collected from 36 series from 1934–1965.

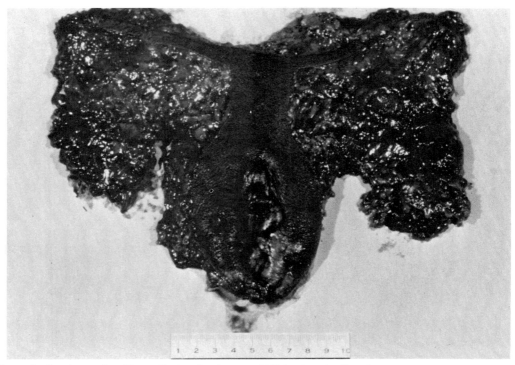

Figure 4 Specimen of en bloc radical vulvectomy and bilateral groin dissection.

Table 5   Incidence and Survival for Pelvic Node Metastases in Vulvar Cancer[3]

Incidence of Nodes

	Total Positive Nodes		Positive Pelvic Nodes	
Number of Patients[a]	Number	Percent	Number	Percent
477	176	36.9	56	11.7

Survival with Complete Lymphadenectomy

	5-Year Survival	
Number of Patients[b]	Number	Percent
42	9	21.4

Operative Mortality with Complete Lymphadenectomy

	Operative Deaths	
Number of Patients[c]	Number	Percent
974	74	7.6

[a] Collected from 8 series from 1938–1963.
[b] Collected from 5 series from 1957–1963.
[c] Collected from 17 series from 1937–1963.

Table 6   TNM Classification and Clinical Staging of Carcinoma of the Vulva Adopted in 1970 (to Be Used from January 1, 1971)[21]

A. TNM Classification

   Primary tumor (T)

   T1   Tumor confined to the vulva, 2 cm or less in larger diameter.
   T2   Tumor confined to the vulva, > 2 cm in diameter.
   T3   Tumor of any size with adjacent spread to the urethra and/or vagina, and/or anus.
   T4   Tumor of any size infiltrating the bladder mucosa, and/or the rectum mucosa, or both, including the upper part of the urethra mucosa and/or fixed to the bone.

   Regional lymph nodes (N)

   N0   No nodes palpable.
   N1   Nodes palpable in either groin, not enlarged, mobile (not clinically suspicious of neoplasm).
   N2   Nodes palpable in either one or both groins, enlarged, firm and mobile (clinically suspicious of neoplasm).
   N3   Fixed or ulcerated nodes.

   Distant metastases (M)

   M0   No clinical metastases.
   M1a Palpable deep pelvic lymph nodes.
   M1b Other distant metastases.

B. Clinical Stage Groups

Clinical Stage	TNM Classification	Descriptive Characteristics
I	T1 N0 M0 T1 N1 M0	All lesions confined to the vulva with a maximum diameter of 2 cm or less and no suspicious groin nodes.
II	T2 N0 M0 T2 N1 M0	All lesions confined to the vulva with a diameter > 2 cm and no suspicious groin nodes.
III	T3 N0 M0 T3 N1 M0 T3 N2 M0	Lesions extending beyond the vulva but without grossly positive groin nodes.
	T1 N2 M0 T2 N2 M0	Lesions of any size confined to the vulva and having suspicious groin nodes.
IV	T1 N3 M0 T2 N3 M0 T3 N3 M0 T4 N3 M0	Lesions with grossly positive groin nodes regardless of extent of primary.
	T4 N0 M0 T4 N1 M0 T4 N2 M0	Lesions involving mucosa of rectum, bladder, urethra, or involving bone.
	M1a M1b	All cases with distant or palable deep pelvic metastases.

in Table 6, and is the only FIGO staging using the TNM system.

The primary purpose of any clinical staging system is for the uniform accumulation of clinical experience and the comparison of results. The secondary purpose is to identify, if possible, areas of refinement of current therapy within certain subsets of the disease. To reject all pretreatment clinical evaluation as totally unreliable is to deny the opportunity to refine our clinical acumen and understanding of the disease. One recent series of vulvar cancer was critically retrospectively restaged by the FIGO criteria to test the utility and applicability of pretreatment staging.[1,9,22]

Tumor (T). The size of the lesion is a crucial factor in predicting nodal metastasis. Lesions 2 cm or less in diameter (T1) had 15% groin node metastasis as contrasted to 38 percent in lesions > 2 cm (T2).[1,9,22] This appears to be somewhat more accurate than the previously reported 3 cm diameter differential in predicting nodal metastasis.[10,23] Extension beyond the vulva (T3) increased the nodal metastases (22% of lesions 2 cm or less and 50% for lesions larger than 2 cm).[1,9,22]

Although Green[17] cautions that even 1 cm lesions had 32% positive nodes and histologic Grade 1 lesions had 48 percent positive nodes, recent reports suggest that small, superficial and well-differentiated lesions are at extremely low risk for node metastases.[9] More data are needed.

Tumor extension beyond the vulva (T3 and T4) has a significantly poorer prognosis, as reported in the past[19,20,24] and this was reflected both in local failure and overall salvage in recent reports from the M. D. Anderson Hospital.[1,9,22]

The one area of controversial results was within the T3 category and involved perineal extension. Perineal extension from the vulva did not worsen the prognosis. But perineal extension with vaginal or anal involvement did indicate a poor prognosis.[1]

Nodes (N). Clinical assessment of nodes remains controversial. Of 605 patients collected from 12 series[8] (1929 to 1963), 38% of patients with clinically suspicious, palpable nodes (N2, N3) were actually free of tumor. Among cases with clinically nonsuspicious groins (N0, N1), 35% revealed metastatic cancer. Recent critical studies suggest that we can be somewhat more accurate in clinical assessment.[9,10,18] Although suspicious (N2 and positive (N3)

nodes may be negative in 22 to 30% of cases[9,10,18] it is noteworthy that occult disease was found in only 11, 12 and 14% of nonsuspicious groins (N0, N1).[9,10,18]

COMMENT

Careful critical TNM pretreatment staging for vulvar cancer deserves our support. The FIGO system seems valid. Inherent in the system is the recognition of decreasing salvage based on local and regional spread. Radical vulvectomy and groin dissection should be performed in all operable cases. Pelvic lymphadenectomy should be included for N2 and N3 cases and added later, if not done, when N0 and N1 cases are found to have metastatic disease. Although histologic differentiation and depth of invasion are not included in the FIGO systems, these features should be collected. We need further data for guidance, especially for the high-risk patient with a small lesion. Inherent in this staging is the opportunity to define subsets for further therapeutic trials: as preoperative groin radiation (N3), or as extended vulvectomy, pelvic exeneration, or preoperative radiation in locally advanced cases (T3, T4).

REFERENCES

1. Rutledge, F., J. P. Smith, and E. W. Franklin: Carcinoma of the vulva. *Am. J. Obstet. Gynecol.* **106:** 1117 (1970).

2. DiSaia, P. J., F. Rutledge, and J. P. Smith: Sarcoma of the vulva. Report of 12 patients. *Obstet. Gynecol.* **38:** 180 (1971).

3. Franklin, E. W., III, and F. Rutledge: Epidemiology of epidermoid carcinoma of the vulva. *Obstet. Gynecol.* **39:** 165 (1972).

4. Hay, D. M., and F. M. Cole: Primary invasive carcinoma of the vulva in Jamaica. *J. Obstet Gynecol. Br. Commonw.* **76:** 821 (1969).

5. Merrill, J. A.: Discussion in Rutledge F., J. P. Smith, and E. W. Franklin: Carcinoma of the vulva, *Am. J. Obstet. Gynecol.* **106:** 1117 (1970).

6. Woodruff, J. D.: Personal communication.

7. Woodruff, J. D., J. S. Baens: Interpretation of atrophic and hypertrophic alterations in the vulvar epithelium. *Am. J. Obstet. Gynecol.* **68:** 713 (1963.)

8. Plentl, A. A., and E. A. Friedman: *Lymphatic System of the Female Genitalia,* W. B. Saunders Company, Philadelphia, 1971.

9. Franklin, E. W., III, and F. Rutledge: Prognostic factors in epidermoid carcinoma of the vulva. *Obstet. Gynecol.* **37:** 892 (1971).

10. Garcia, C. C., Jr., and R. C. Boronow: Carcinoma of the vulva: anatomic and histologic prognostic factors. *South Med. J.* **65:** 237 (1972).

11. Cherry, C. P., and A. Glücksman: Lymphatic embolism and lymph node metastasis in cancers of the vulva and of uterine cervix. *Cancer* **8:** 564 (1955).

12. Allen, A. C.: The skin. In *Pathology,* 3rd edit., W. A. D. Anderson, Ed., C. V. Mosby Company, St. Louis.,

13. Fenn, M. E., G. W. Morley, and M. R. Abell: Paget's disease of the vulva. *Obstet. Gynecol.* **38:** 660 (1971).

14. Boehm, F., and J. McL. Morris: Paget's disease and apocrine gland carcinoma of the vulva. *Obstet. Gynecol.* **38:** 185 (1971).

15. Way, S.: Carcinoma of the vulva. *Am. J. Obstet. Gynecol.* **79:** 692 (1960).

16. Way, S.: Personal communication.

17. Green, T. H., Jr.: Discussion in Rutledge, F., J. P. Smith, and E. W. Franklin: Carcinoma of the vulva. *Am. J. Obstet. Gynecol.* **106:** 1117 (1970).

18. Merrill, J. A., and N. L. Ross: Cancer of the vulva. *Cancer* **14:** 13 (1961).

19. Taussig, F. J.: Carcinoma of the vulva. *Am. J. Obstet. Gynecol.* **40:** 764 (1946).

20. McKelvey, J. L.: Malignant tumors of the vulva. In *Treatment of Cancer and Allied Diseases, Tumors of the Female Genitalia,* 2nd edit., Vol. 6, Pack, G. T., and I. M. Ariel, Eds. Harper and Brothers, Hoeber Medical Division, New York, 1962.

21. Kottmeier, H. L., Ed.: *Annual Report on the Results of Treatment in Carcinoma of the Uterus, Vagina and Ovary,* Vol. 15, Stockholm, Sweden, 1973.

22. Franklin, E. W., III: Clinical staging of carcinoma of the vulva. *Obstet. Gynecol.* **40:** 277 (1972).

23. Collins, C. G., J. H. Collins, D. L. Barclay et al.: Cancer involving the vulva. A report of 109 consecutive cases. *Am. J. Obstet. Gynecol.* **87:** 762 (1973).

24. Green, T. H., H. Ulfelder, and J. V. Meigs: Epidermoid carcinoma of the vulva. An analysis of 235 cases. *Am. J. Obstet. Gynecol.* **75:** 834 (1958).

CHAPTER 15 INTRAEPITHELIAL CARCINOMA OF THE VULVA

FELIX RUTLEDGE, M.D.

INTRODUCTION

Untreated intraepithelial carcinoma of the vulva progresses to invasive cancer? Topics of current interest include: the incidence of progression to invasion, the rate of progression, the frequency of spontaneous regression, the etiologic agents, and the cause of an apparently increased incidence of intraepithelial cancer of the vulva. A consequence of better understanding of the pathogenesis of intraepithelial cervical cancer has been increased interest in intraepithelial cancer of the vulva. Increased attention has stimulated more careful research for these lesions. Since more patients with intraepithelial carcinoma of the vulva are being diagnosed at an earlier age, the responsibility for proper treatment is of immediate concern.

Clinical experience suggests that a reappraisal of our management of intraepithelial cancer is needed because this disease, like other gynecologic cancers, permits individualized treatment. The demonstration in recent years that some lesions can be made to regress by topical therapy suggests that this type of cancer may not be firmly established in all patients. Only localized areas of the vulva may be affected. A slow rate of growth is characteristic of the lesion, and the adverse effect of complete vulvectomy

upon a young woman's sexual functions is given important consideration in deciding the type of treatment to be used.

In recent years we have been less dogmatic in our belief that treatment should provide adequate excision of the lesion plus prophylactic removal of the vulva, which may be prone to develop similar lesions subsequently. In earlier years there was a prevalent opinion among our staff that once a neoplasia became evident in the vulva, the whole region should be committed to treatment. Thus vulvectomy was necessary, and to do less was to risk losing the opportunity for definitive treatment of an early detected cancer of the vulva. Today this view seems too rigid. Although it is still applicable to some patients, it is not required for all. A more conservative excision has demonstrated that the affliction can be singular and local, and although a new lesion may emerge after conservative, limited excision, some patients are cured.

Conservatism in management is only safe if a careful posttreatment surveillance can be maintained to observe the remaining vulva for new lesions that may develop. Local resection of intraepithelial carcinoma may be acknowledged as a decision with calculated risk by both the physician and the patient. The patient should be aware that repeat local resection or vulvectomy may become necessary if other lesions appear, and that even though the treatment has been fairly simple she should not underestimate the seriousness of the condition. The patient treated by local excision remains at a higher risk, therefore any neglect or delay in the treatment of a new lesion could well lead to the development of an invasive carcinoma. Thus, conservatism is safe only when the patient joins with the physician in a program of examinations at regular intervals for the possible detection of additional lesions.

Conservative management can only be employed when the remaining vulva appears healthy. Often intraepithelial carcinoma develops in the vulva, where its appearance is already abnormal because of a preexisting pathosis. Leukoplakia of either the hypertrophic or atrophic variety may extend outward around the intraepithelial lesion to obscure its borders. Unless the boundaries of the neoplasms are fairly distinct, complete excision is not assured. Similar confusion is created by condyloma acuminata, granulomatous lesions, and even hypertrophic changes due to chronic vulvitis. Where these conditions conceal early detection of new lesions, definitive treatment by vulvectomy should be considered.

The patient's age should be a factor in the individualization of treatment, although a single small, distinct and demarcated lesion may be treated by local excision in patients of all ages. Complete vulvectomy may be more disturbing emotionally to the younger woman. Each treatment has its advantages. The fact that a vulvectomy can be performed safely and heal well, and ample assurance that it will permanently rid the patient of the problem is often worth the additional resection.

In recent years we have modified our treatment of intraepithelial cancer of the vulva from a routine complete vulvectomy for all lesions that show the characteristic cellular changes to a more individualized

conservative operation for the patient whose lesion is smaller and well circumscribed. Factors to be considered when planning treatment are:

1. The amount and location of the involvement of the vulva. (Small lesions or large? Local or diffuse? Accessibility for removal?)
2. The health of the remaining vulva. (Are associated vulvar dystrophy, leukoplakia, kraurosis, or chronic vulvitis present?)
3. Patient's personal factors. (Age, crippling effects of a complete vulvectomy should be considered more seriously for the young; sexual activity, emotional values of the genitalia, and maturity of the patient for understanding her disease.)
4. The practical factors for follow-up care. (Is the patient dependable for follow-up examination? If topical application is selected, will she apply the medication conscientiously?)
5. Is the lesion intraepithelial carcinoma? (Although the histologic changes appear to be neoplastic, could they actually be a reactive change to some agent? Will this lesion regress with observation?)

CLINICAL FEATURES

Intraepithelial carcinoma of the vulva presents a variegated change in the skin. The lesion may become evident by a different color, either brown, red, or white. When not distinguished by color, the physical difference is the clue: the texture of the lesion is often firmer than the adjacent skin. Microscopic patterns among patients are often dissimilar. These differences are expressd by terms such as Bowen's disease, erythroplasia, Paget's disease and atypical leukoplakia. The names and the variable appearance are not, however, important in clinical management. (Figure 1).

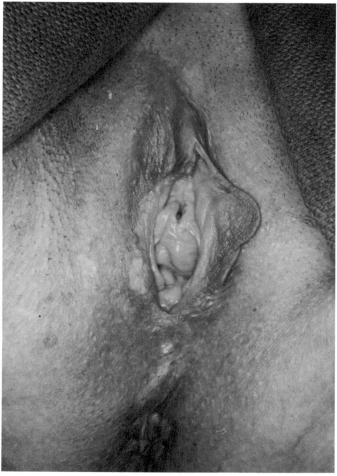

Figure 1 Intraepithelial carcinoma of the valvu confined to the right. This is the second appearance of the disease. Previous treatment excised the right labia minora. A patient like this who demonstrates a trait should be treated next with vulvectomy.

TREATMENT

Vulvectomy

The majority of our patients have been treated by vulvectomy with excision of the labia, the clitoris, and part of the mons with the underlying fibrofatty tissues that give form to the vulva. The skin is removed from the labiocrural folds laterally to the hymenal ring mesially. The tissues underlying the skin are not essential in treatment of intra-epithelial carcinoma because there is no concern about lymphatic spread. However, the operation is easier when the tissue plane behind these structures is followed, also the skin margin and the vaginal mucosa are less separated for closure. These excision lines, shown in Figure 2, are ample because hemorrhage is minimal and good healing is usual.

Complete Skin Excision

Excision of an equal area of vulvar skin excised without the underlying glands and

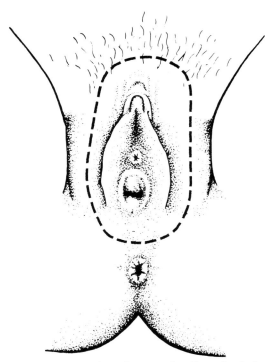

Figure 2 Operations for removing the vulva lesion have names such as simple vulvectomy, complete vulvectomy, total vulvectomy, and radical vulvectomy. These are variously defined among authors and imply different limits of resection among surgeons.

The dashed line on this sketch of the vulva shows the directions usually followed for the outer limits of the simple or complete vulvectomy. To include more peripheral disease these boundaries could be extended to resect wider, and still this type of vulvectomy would not be counted as radical.

fibrofatty tissue serves as well as vulvectomy.[1] The skin is loosely attached where there is no hair, thus following the plane provided by the dartos fascia, from which it can be stripped off. Except when fixed by scar tissue of disease or injury, the skin of the vulva slides freely over the dartos fascia. Sometimes there is sufficient redundancy of the boundary skin when undercut mobility allows coverage of the defect (Figure 3). If the intraepithelial lesions are diffuse a wider skin excision is necessary. Therefore mobili-

zation of skin about the inner thighs is inadequate for the size of the defect, and a graft is necessary. Because skin graft will serve well to cover larger denuded area; provisions for grafting may encourage the surgeon to be more certain that the specimen margins are ample.

SKIN EXCISION AND GRAFTING

Skin grafting to preserve the contour and form of the vulva produces superior results. (Figures 4, 5, and 6). Generally patients are pleased with both their appearance and sexual sensitivity after this operation. Yet the operation is more complex, the hospitalization period is longer, and postoperative recovery is more uncomfortable than in simple vulvectomy.

LIMITED EXCISION

There is less opportunity for local excision than for the above methods for reasons already discussed. In addition, the surgeon should consider the size of the defect and whether primary closure is feasible. Will a scar in this area produce dyspareunia? Will the excision margins be clear of intraepithelial carcinoma? These simple reminders are suggested in an effort to place this less orthodox treatment in perspective with more established treatments by complete vulvectomy.

Topical Chemotherapy

Most experience with topical therapy uses 5-fluorouracil, now available commercially. Pharmacists may dissolve the 5-fluorouracil in a base of propylene glycol; a 5 to 20% preparation is preferred. Although our experience is small, regressions have been observed if the patient applies the medication regularly, until the 5-fluorouracil causes an uncomfortable inflammatory reaction.

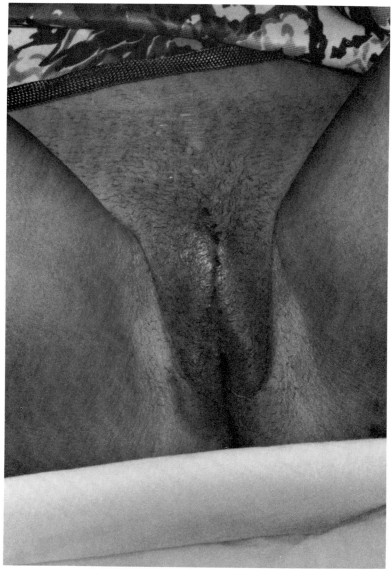

Figure 3 The vulva skin has been excised and the denuded area covered with skin beyond the excision line. By undercutting, this skin is mobilized and moved medially. A sulcas is reestablished over the symphysis by suturing the skin margins to the periosteum. The remaining skin margins are sutured to the edge of the vaginal mucosa.

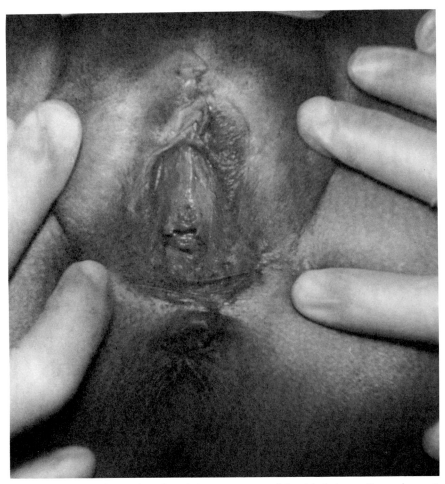

Figure 4 Intraepithelial carcinoma has altered the appearance of the skin between the vagina and anus rather subtly. Since the area was too large for local excision and primary closure, treatment was by skin excision and graft. Multiple sites of intraepithelial cancer were proven by biopsy of the labia, therefore the entire vulva was stripped and the skin replaced by graft.

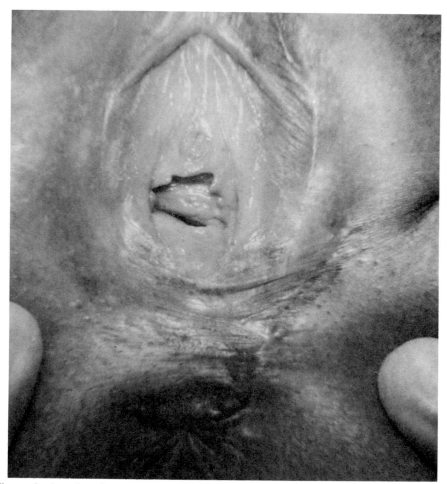

Figure 4 (*continued*)

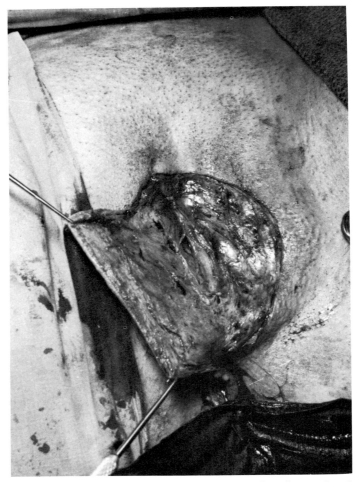

Figure 5 For the skin excision and graft operation, the depth of the dissection reaches the dartos fascia. The skin is loosely attached to this fascia, thus when the correct plane is followed, blunt dissection progresses easily. Vulvar shape is preserved by not excising the fibrofatty tissue which is covered by a skin donated from the inner thigh or buttocks.

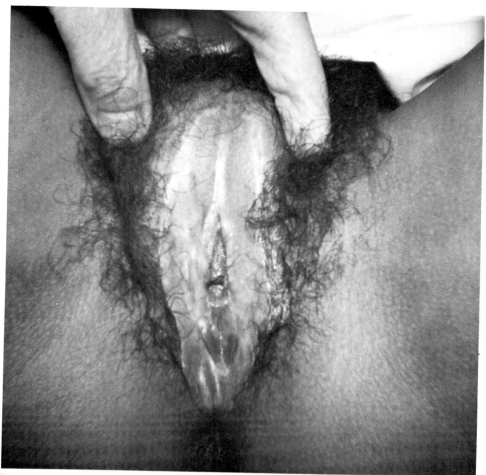

Figure 6 Postoperative appearance of skin excision and graft. After excision the lesions around the perineum (Figure 4) required a graft back to the anus. When the (retracted) labia returns to usual position, the vulva appearance is scarcely altered.

SUMMARY

Acceptance of vulvectomy as proper treatment for intraepithelial carcinoma is based on the well-known tendency of this kind of cancer to be multicentric and the frequent association of other pathologic vulvar conditions that may obscure the presence of additional cancerous foci. Since the operation is disfiguring, and the resulting deformity could be a detriment to normal sexual expression, less than total vulvectomy may be permissable for those patients in whom the lesion is confined. Some flexibility in management to permit individualization of treatment seems a warranted change in current practice.

REFERENCE

1. Sinclair, Marga H., *Am. J. Obstet. Gynecol.* **6:** 806–818 (1968).

CHAPTER 16 THERAPY OF INVASIVE CARCINOMA OF THE VULVA

J. TAYLOR WHARTON, M.D.

Squamous carcinoma is the most frequent type of primary cancer of the vulva. Although malignant melanomas are also seen, they are rare. Squamous lesions represent a broad spectrum of epithelial changes and may present clinically at any phase in the spectrum. The early changes may be characteristized by discrete or diffuse hypertrophic areas on the vulva that show dysplastic changes at biopsy, or as areas of carcinoma in situ. Chronicity is a common denominator, since a high percentage of patients have long-term symptoms such as pruritus or chronic irritation. These changes may progress, and recognition of the initial invasive phase is particularly important since early diagnosis favors cure. Minimal difficulty is experienced in diagnosing the large invasive carcinoma that has destroyed the vulva. However, therapy results are remarkably good for these advanced lesions, and a negative viewpoint on the part of the physician is frequently unjustified.

The standard treatment for invasive carcinoma is radical vulvectomy and lymphadenectomy.[1,2,3,4,6] There is a place for less than radical operation, and therapy is individualized based on the size and histologic features of the cancer.[7,9] The diagnostic and therapeutic aspects of cancer of the vulva will be discussed herein. A lesion of the older population group, cancer of the vulva will perhaps occur more frequently since women in our society are living longer.

DIAGNOSIS

Delay in diagnosis is a major problem in carcinoma of the vulva. Often the cancer is quite advanced when the initial diagnosis is made. There are many reasons for delay. Some patients are shy and simply neglect themselves and refuse examination. Occasionally a physician will prescribe topical medications without performing an examination. Many patients have had symptoms such as pruritus or repeated inflammatory processes for years preceding actual invasion, and this chronocity accounts in large measure for loss of awareness and for neglect. Persistence is wise on the part of the physician and any mass, pigmented lesion, ulcer, or hypertrophic process should be biopsied and rebiopsied at yearly intervals if not resolved. A punch type instrument or simple knife excision is well suited for the purpose and requires only a local anesthetic. The correct biopsy method will include adjacent subcutaneous tissue, thus permitting the depth of invasion to be determined.

PATHOLOGY

Squamous carcinoma has a wide variety of clinical appearances. The cancer may resemble a simple ulcer, an innocuous white plaque, a subcutaneous mass, or a polypoid lesion with or without necrosis. The appearance may be masked by a chronic granulomatous process or condylomata. Microscopically, squamous carcinomas of the vulva are indistinguishable from squamous cancers in other locations. The degree of histologic differentiation is variable, and histologic grading does not influence therapy plans.

It is generally believed that squamous carcinoma of the vulva, like carcinoma of the cervix, originates as an intraepithelial process then extends laterally and invades deeply over an indeterminate period. The microinvasive phase of cervical cancer is well documented. Data are available that suggest there is a similar category for cancer of the vulva that can be diagnosed when the carcinoma has invaded the stroma to a depth of 5 mm or less. This definable stage has clinical significance because the incidence of spread beyond the vulva is quite low. In the authors' series none of the patients with microinvasive carcinoma of the vulva had metastatic cancer in lymph nodes.[9]

MALIGNANT MELANOMA

Melanomas of the vulva are usually quite aggressive and resemble melanomas arising in other areas of the body. Early diagnosis is possible if any pigmented lesion is biopsied, and biopsy is particularly important when junctional nevi or pigmented areas that are changing are encountered. Patients with multiple pigmented lesions may represent a high-risk group. Unfortunately, melanomas are usually not associated with preexisting clinically detectable abnormalities. Melanomas are treated by radical vulvectomy and bilateral inguinal and pelvic lymphadenectomy.[5]

SPREAD PATTERN

Vulvar cancer spreads by direct invasion of adjacent structures and by invasion of the lymphatics. The spread pattern is complex when the vagina, urethra, or anus are involved. The lymphatic drainage pattern is precise and has been studied in detail.

The lymphatics from the labium majus and minus drain anteriorly toward the mons veneris and follow within the lateral aspect of the labiocrural fold. Contralateral lymphatic spread occurs and both groins are at risk. The channels converge and empty into the superficial inguinal nodes, which usually consist of 8 to 12 nodes lying in the superficial fascia. From the superficial nodes, vessels terminate in the deep inguinal nodes or the lower external iliac nodes. The deep inguinal nodes are located in the femoral canal medial to the femoral vein and average one to three in number. The uppermost node is the most constant (nodes of Cloquet or Rosemüller), and has clinical significance in serving as an indicator of the status of the pelvic nodes. The efferent channels of the deep inguinal nodes are confluent with the external iliac nodes. Involvement of the pelvic lymph nodes is usually an extension of cancer in the inguinal nodes, and pelvic node metastasis without involvement of the inguinal nodes is rare.

It should be understood that lymphatic metastasis in cancer of the vulva progresses in an orderly manner.

PREOPERATIVE EVALUATION OF REGIONAL LYMPH NODES

Clinical evaluation (palpation) by an experienced examiner will detect metastasis in 60 percent of patients.[6] Those patients with associated inflammatory conditions of the vulva or infected carcinomas are particularly hard to evaluate since node enlargement may be caused by underlying infection.

Lymphangiography may be useful in evaluating the pelvic nodes. Preoperative knowledge of involvement would indicate extensive lymph node disease and might be an indication for preoperative radiation therapy. In our opinion the value of lymphangiography in evaluating the inguinal nodes needs additional study.

We do not hesitate to biopsy questionable inguinal lymph nodes in certain clinical situations. Assurance that a node is negative allows vulvectomy alone for patients in poor medical condition or of advanced age. Knowledge of the amount of cancer in nodes is of value when preoperative radiation therapy is planned, since a less intense dose is indicated for microscopic foci of cancer than would be necessary for the 2 to 3 cm mass.

PROGNOSTIC FACTORS

Size of the Lesion

The size of the lesion and involvement of adjacent structures are important factors in deciding if a cure is possible. Generally the larger lesion implies that the disease has been present for a longer period, allowing greater opportunity for lymphatic involvement and for direct extension to the vagina, perineum, or urethra. The possibility of local recurrence is high following removal of these massive cancers, since a surgical margin free of tumor is not easily obtained.

Positive Lymph Nodes

This is the most important factor in determining the possibility of cure. However, metastatic carcinoma to the inguinal and pelvic nodes does not necessarily mean that death will result from disease, since patients are cured by surgical dissection. There is, however, an indirect relationship between survival and degree of nodal involvement.

SURGICAL TREATMENT

Carcinoma of the vulva is ideally suited for en bloc surgical removal. The classical tenets of cancer surgery can be rigidly adhered to because the primary lesion and pathways of potential spread can be re-moved in a one-stage procedure. As discussed previously, anatomy and orderly lymphatic drainage guide the surgeon along proper planes. The standard treatment is radical vulvectomy and bilateral lymphadenectomy. The limits of the operation include the mons veneris and resection along the labiocrural folds crossing the perineum above the anus. The inner incision follows the hymenal ring, leaving a minimal margin of mucosa around the urethral meatus. The deep fascia limits the depth of the vulva excision, but excision of the urogenital diaphragm and dissection of the ischiorectal fossa and paravaginal spaces as well as partial amputation of the urethra are sometimes necessary. Inguinal lymphadenectomy is performed prior to the vulva portion of the operation, and the skin is closed as much as possible. This sequence protects the inguinal dissection site from possible bacterial and tumor contamination that may result from manipulation of the vulva lesion, the vagina, and the perineum. The stripped femoral artery and vein in the femoral triangle are vulnerable to injury if postoperative skin necrosis is extensive. These structures are always protected with the sartorius muscle, which is detached from its origin on the anterior superior iliac spine and sutured to the inguinal ligament.

Pelvic lymphadenectomy should not be considered as part of the standard operation. The most important group of patients to receive pelvic lymphadenectomy are those with positive inguinal nodes. Preoperative evaluation and microscopic study by frozen section of suspicious nodes (especially Cloquet's node) during surgery is helpful. Patients with extension of the primary cancer to the urethra, clitoris, vagina and/or anus are treated by pelvic lymphadenectomy.

POSTOPERATIVE CARE

Primary closure of the incision is usually performed since the skin flaps are mobile, having been undermined to allow complete removal of the subcutaneous fat overlying the nodes in the femoral triangle. Suture line tension at the closure junction is usually pronounced but will frequently lessen when the patient is taken out of the stirrups. A fluffed gauze dressing is applied, and pressure is added by securing with elastoplast tape. It is important to build multiple layers of fluffed gauze over the femoral triangle area because pressure in this location will secure apposition of the skin flaps to the underlying structures.

The patient should be placed on prophylactic antibiotics. The wound is at risk for both gram-positive and gram-negative organisms, and comprehensive coverage is advised. Tissue necrosis of the traumatized, partially devascularized, skin flaps is greatly augmented if infection intervenes. The dressing should remain in place for five days unless persistent temperature elevation indicating wound cellulitis is observed.

Although the skin incision may heal by primary intention, some degree of necrosis is usual. The devascularized area may demarcate and slough exposing the underlying structures, or it may form a hard eschar. The firm eschar is an ideal barrier for protection against infection, and should not be removed unless the adjacent skin becomes infected. The eschar will demarcate toward the end of the third week, as granulation tissue progresses at its periphery. When extensive necrosis is experienced the wound will be moist and infected. This type of wound should be opened and debrided daily. A perineum light source can contribute dry heat and aids in wound care. Fluffed gauze placed in the wound pulls adjacent necrotic tissue from the wound borders when the dressings are changed (several times a day). A clean, dry wound is mandatory.

Repeated episodes of lymphangitis of the lower extremities are common in the postvulvectomy patient because obstruction by the operative procedure impairs normal circulation. The fibrosis that results from repeated infections produces chronic lymphadema of the lower extremities. This sequence of events may be lessened by prophylactic Bicillin injections or equivalent antibiotic coverage for the first two years of the postoperative period. Support hose are also of value, and routine use is advised. Early institution of physical therapy is also helpful.

COMPLICATIONS

The major postoperative complication is wound necrosis which occurs to some degree in 75% of patients. Tissue loss may be extensive and healing requires time. Life-threatening infection is rare, and only 1 patient died of infection in the M. D. Anderson series.[6] Hemorrhage from the femoral vessels is unlikely because the sartorius muscle provides protection. The incidence of life-threatening pulmonary emboli is surprisingly low considering patients' age and length of time spent in bed. Although patients have not required prophylactic anticoagulation, elastic stockings are used regularly during the postoperative period.

RADIATION THERAPY

A reappraisal of modern irradiation methods for cancer of the vulva is overdue. Supervoltage therapy given by a direct perineal portal produces desirable dose distribution, and the tolerance is superior to that encountered with orthovoltage therapy. The role of preoperative irradiation may aid in controlling advanced cancer of the vulva by transforming unresectable lesions into operable ones. The primary lesion can be treated as well as the regional lymph nodes. Recurrent cancers are suitable candidates for radiation therapy.

RESULTS OF SURGICAL TREATMENT

Various authors have reported a survival rate of 40 to 60%.[1,2,3,4,6] The survival rate improves in those cases without nodal involvement. Way reports an 80% five-year survival rate in patients without positive nodes compared to a 50% rate with positive superficial inguinal nodes.[8] Rutledge and associates report a 39% five-year survival in patients with positive inguinal nodes.[6] Both Way and Rutledge and co-workers reported survivors when the deep pelvic nodes were involved.

THE M. D. ANDERSON HOSPITAL EXPERIENCE

At the M. D. Anderson Hospital from 1944 to 1970 204 patients with histologically proven invasive squamous carcinomas have been treated; 175 patients were treated for cure; 29 were treated for palliative purposes because the cancer was too advanced or because of age and infirmity. Radical vulvectomy and lymphadenectomy were performed in 137 patients; 49 (36%) had positive nodes (Table 1). The disease was confined to the superficial nodes in 36 patients, and to the superficial and deep nodes in 10 patients. All of the patients with positive deep pelvic nodes had positive inguinal nodes, and in these patients the inguinal nodes were clinically palpable.

Table 1 Incidence of Lymph Node Metastasis, The M. D. Anderson Hospital (204 Patients)

Number of patients receiving lymphadenectomy	137
Number of patients with positive nodes	49
(a) Positive inguinal nodes	36
(b) Positive inguinal and pelvic nodes	10

Survival rates for the 175 patients treated for cure was 80.9% at three years and 77.3% at five years (Table 2). The three-year posttreatment period affords accurate evaluation of treatment methods because 93% of deaths from vulvar cancer occur within this interval.[6] The cure rate for patients in the group with positive lymph nodes was 40% (Table 3).

From March 1944 through June 1974 210 selected patients with squamous carcinoma of the vulva were reviewed. Thirty-nine (19%) developed recurrent invasive carcinoma and 20 are dead from cancer. Information was precise for the recurrence site in 36 of these patients (Table 4). Regrowth in the vagina, urethra, or perineum accounted for 22 of the 30 recurrences within the boundaries of the initial operation (treatment area) and 14 of these patients were cured by a second excision or irradiation. No cures were obtained when groin or pelvic wall recurrences were diagnosed.

Of the 60 patients treated by vulvectomy alone, 84% survived three years or more.

Table 2 Survival Data, The M. D. Anderson Hospital (175 Patients)[a]

Year	Month	Total	Dead of Disease	Dead Other	W.A.[b]	Survival Percent
< 1	0–11	175	19	1	12	88.7
1	12–23	143	8	2	17	83.4
2	24–35	116	1	1	13	82.7
3	36–47	101	2	3	11	80.9
4	48–59	85	0	2	11	80.9
5	60–71	72	3	2	6	77.3

[a] Berkson Gage method.
[b] Withdrawn alive.

Table 3   Influence of Positive Lymph Nodes on Survival, The M. D. Anderson Hospital (175 Patients)

Positive Node Group	Number of Patients	Number of Survivors[a]
Unilateral inguinal	25	11 (44%)
Bilateral inguinal	8	2 (25%)
Inguinal and deep pelvic	7	3 (43%)

[a] 36-month survival.

Table 4   Site of Recurrence, The M. D. Anderson Hospital (210 Patients)

Location	Number of Patients
Treatment area	30
Distant metastases	4
Treatment area and distant metastases	2
Total	36

(Table 5). The majority of these patients had lesions 2 to 3 cm in diameter and no evidence by clinical evaduation of inguinal node metastasis; 13 patients had microinvasive cancers.

Table 5   Survival — Radical Vulvectomy Alone as Curative Therapy for Invasive Carcinoma, The M. D. Anderson Hospital[a]

Interval (yr)	Total	Dead of disease	Survival %
< 1	60	3	94.8
1	52	4	86.7
2	38	1	84.2

[a] No deaths due to disease after 36 months.

A special effort was made to study the biological potential of small invasive cancers and to look for factors that would permit less than radical therapy. Among 45 patients who had carcinomas 2 cm or less in diameter, histological examination showed that the stroma was penetrated to a depth of 5 mm or less in 25 patients. It is believed that these patients represent a special category because no evidence of lymph node metastasis was detected and none died of recurrent cancer, whereas 3 patients died in the group of 20 with stromal penetration greater than 5 mm (Table 6). Clearly, however, the decision to treat patients conservatively must be based upon the most meticulous surgical planning and histological examination.[9]

Table 6   Survival Rates Microinvasive and Invasive Carcinoma of the Vulva, The M. D. Anderson Hospital[9]

	Microinvasive	Invasive
Total number of patients	25	20
Dead of intercurrent disease	1	1
Survived less than 5 years postoperatively	4	1
Dead due to vulvar cancer	0	3
Absolute survival (%)		
3 years	96	80
5 years	95.2	73.7
Determinate survival (%)		
3 years	100	84.2
5 years	100	82.4

REFERENCES

1. Brunschwig, A., and A. Brockunier, *Obstet. Gynecol.* **29:** 362 (1969).

2. Collins, C. G., J. H. Collins, D. L. Bareay, and E. W. Nelson: *Am. J. Obstet. Gynecol.* **87:** 762 (1963).

3. Green, T. H., Jr., H. Ulfelder, and J. V. Meigs: *Am. J. Obstet. Gynecol.* **75:** 848 (1958).

4. McKelvey, J. L., and L. L. Adcock: *Am. J. Obstet. Gynecol.* **26:** 455 (1965).

5. Morrow, C. P., and F. Rutledge: *Obstet. Gynecol.* **39:** 745–752 (No. 5) (May 1972).

6. Rutledge, F., J. P. Smith, and E. W. Franklin: *Am. J. Obstet. Gynecol.* **106:** 1117 (1970).

7. Rutledge, F.: In *Cancer Medicine,* James F. Holland, and Emil Frel, Eds., Lea & Febiger, Philadelphia, 1973.

8. Way, S.: In *Modern Radiotherapy Gynecological Cancer,* J. T. Deeley. Ed., Butterworths, London, 1972, p. 203.

9. Wharton, J. T., S. Gallagher, and F. N. Rutledge, *Am. J. Obstet. Gynecol.* **118:** 159 (1974).

CHAPTER 17 THERAPY OF ADVANCED CARCINOMA OF THE VULVA

RICHARD C. BORONOW, M.D.

CONTROVERSIES

1. Should these patients be treated with exenterative surgery or extended radical vulvectomy?

2. Does radiation remain obsolete in the management of vulvar cancer?

Locally advanced vulvar cancer implies extension of the primary lesion beyond the confines of the vulva. As seen in Table 6, Chapter 14, T3 (FIGO) tumors are lesions of any size with adjacent spread to the urethra and/or vagina, and/or perineum, and/or anus. T4 lesions may be any size and infiltrate the bladder mucosa, and/or the rectal mucosa or both, including the upper part of the urethral mucosa and/or fixed to the bone. N3 nodal disease is fixed or ulcerated.

ANATOMIC CONSIDERATIONS

When locally advanced vulvar cancer presents, there are several anatomic aspects of the therapeutic problem: (1) With extensive permeation of tissue a vigorous therapeutic effort directed at the primary disease is necessary; (2) vulvovaginal cancer has not just one regional spread pattern but two well-defined regional spread patterns and access to a third.[1] Figure 1 illustrates the

intercommunications possible between the primary vulvar spread to the lymph nodes in the groin and the femoral system, and the vaginal and cervical lymphatic drainage to the hypogastric system, its tributaries, and associated lymph nodes. Clearly in the lower vagina and in the area of the introitus, this dual-spread pattern is particularly likely, although intercommunications can occur at any level of the vagina. In addition, lesions of the perineum, fourchette, and posterior wall of the vagina can gain access to the superior hemorrhoidal system of lymphatic drainage.

THERAPY

Locally advanced vulvar cancer represents a difficult management problem. Since it is not a common clinical problem, there are few reports of more than a limited experience in managing such cases. Current therapy in the United States consists primarily of two surgical methods:

1. Conventional: This constitutes an extension of the radical vulvectomy. It is not truly conservative surgery inasmuch as it involves radical vulvectomy with appropriate node dissection and with extension of the resection to include segments of vagina

243

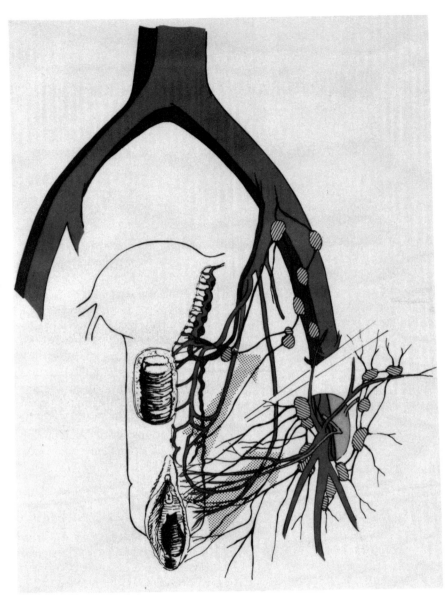

Figure 1 The dual lymphatic pathways of vulvar drainage to the groins and vaginal drainage to the deep pelvic nodes, with evident anatomic intercommunications of vulvovaginal cancer. From Boronow, R. C.: Therapeutic alternative to primary exenteration for advanced vulvovaginal cancer. *Gynecol. Oncol.* **1**: 233 (1973). Reprinted by permission.

and/or urethra, and/or anus but with preservation of the bladder and rectum.

2. Extended: The extended surgical approach primarily involves an exenterative (total, anterior, or posterior) procedure with en bloc radical vulvectomy, groin dissection and, usually, pelvic node dissection This therapeutic approach has gained prominence in a number of centers in recent years. Some lesions are so locally destructive that exenterative surgery is necessary (Figure 2).

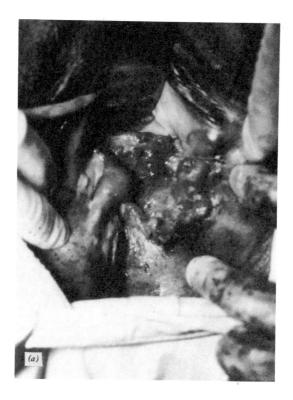

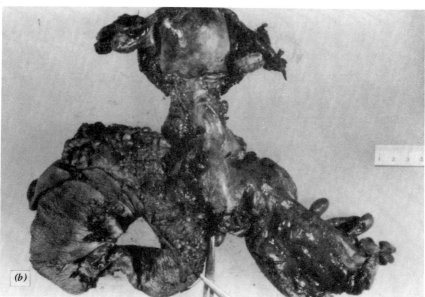

Figure 2 (*a*) Locally advanced vulvar lesion infiltrating anal sphincter (T4). (*b*) Posterior exenteration and radical vulvectomy specimen.

Table 1 records qualitatively some of the advantages and disadvantages of these two therapeutic approaches. The conventional approach has less operative morbidity and mortality, and preserves bladder and/or rectal function. However, the central resection margins may be compromised, and local failure might be greater, thus reducing the cure rate. The extended procedure, although less likely to compromise central resection margins (thus less likely to be coupled with local failure and, therefore, providing an increased possibility of cure) does nevertheless lose some of its effectiveness because of major operative morbidity, significant operative mortality, and sacrifice of bladder and/or rectum.

Conventional Surgery

Proper application of radical vulvectomy and groin dissection yields fairly comparable and quite satisfactory results when the disease is confined to the vulva. This, however, is not the subject of these considerations. Thus, while we have defined conventional surgery for locally advanced vulvar cancer as "radical vulvectomy and appropriate node dissection with extension of the resection to include segments of the vagina and/or urethra, and/or anus, but with preservation of the bladder and rectum," a survey of the available literature provides insufficient data to evaluate the efficacy of the procedure. As noted in Table 1, central

Table 1   Surgical Approaches for Locally Advanced Vulvar Cancer[2]

Parameter	Conventional	Extended
Operative mortality	Small	Significant
Operative morbidity	Small	Significant
Resection margins	May be compromised	En bloc
Local failure	Greater	Less
Bladder/rectum	Preserved	Sacrificed

resection margins may be compromised and central local recurrence may be greater. It has, however, been difficult to document this statistically from the literature. Although great emphasis has been placed upon the peripheral spread of the cancer (i.e., the regional lymph nodes), little comment is made regarding the central resection margins. Comments are often qualitative in nature. For example, Rutledge and coworkers[3] noted: ". . . several recurrences at the vaginal margins may have been due to inadequate excision of the vaginal mucosa."

Some reports suggest validity of this view with some degree of quantitation. Among 48 surgically treated patients reported by Shingleton and associates,[4] there were 15 recurrences, 11 of which were local, and 4 with distant metastasis. No description of the local extent of these lesions was given. Goplerud and Keetel[5] stated that 58% of their recurrences were in the vulvar area, but they too did not provide descriptive information.

In the critical review of the current M. D. Anderson experience[6] node metastases, local recurrence, and survival were significantly influenced by extension beyond the vulva. Pelvic or vulvar recurrence occurred in 6% of T1 or T2 tumors (confined to the labia). The incidence of pelvic or vulvar recurrence rose significantly for lesions in the T3 categories: with extension to vagina 18%, with extension to urethra 30%, with extension to anus 17%, with extension to perineum with anal or vaginal involvement 14%, but with perineal extension only from vulva, 4%. Thus their data confirmed all the features of poor prognosis of the FIGO T3 definition with the exception of involvement of the perineum (also without anal or vaginal involvement).

The largest report on the importance of this problem is the analysis by Green and associates[7] of 238 cases. Like others, they documented the trend toward reducing the cure rate with the increasing size of the primary lesion. But they noted: ". . . the local extension beyond the vulva itself, so frequently encountered with these larger lesions, is perhaps more important from the standpoint of curability than size per se." Further, ". . . approximately one-third of the failures were associated with local recurrence, in spite of so-called adequate surgery." Among 36 cases with urethral involvement, only 5 patients (14%) were five-year survivors; of 51 with vaginal involvement only 3 (6%) were five-year survivors, and of 26 with perineal, rectal, or ischiorectal fossal involvement, 3 (12%) were five-year survivors. Of these latter 6 cases, 2 patients were cured by posterior exenteration. This report, then, reviewed exenteration experience in advanced vulvar cancer to that date, lending credence to the therapeutic utility of the extended (exenterative) surgical approach. In a pure sense, these statistics provide ample evidence for the highly unfavorable prognosis of central extent beyond the vulva proper.

Extended (Exenterative) Surgery

In 1956 a therapeutic alternative was introducd with the initial report of Brunschwig and Daniel[8] (Table 2). This was the first

Table 2   Initial Report of Exenteration in Vulvar Cancer[8]

Operations	27
Deaths from operation (47%)	13
Total exenterations (7)	
Postoperative deaths (57%)	4
NED[a] at 56 mo	1
Anterior exenterations (16)	
Postoperative deaths	7
Hospital deaths (56.4%)	2
NED at 56 mo	1
Posterior exenterations (4)	
Postoperative deaths	0
NED at 19, 29 mo	2

[a] No evidence of disease.

published experience of exenterative surgery in advanced vulvar cancer. Morbidity was major, and the operative mortality was 47% in a series of 27 cases. Morbidity and mortality have been reduced as experience has accumulated.

The literature on vulvar cancer (excluding melanoma and sarcoma) and the exenteration experience has been reviewed from 1960 to the present time and is summarized in Table 3. In this effort to assess the combined experience with exenteration for primary vulvar cancer, several problems were encountered: (1) When the vulvar exenterations were reported in a larger series of exenterative procedures (usually for recurrent cervix cancer), the authors did not always indicate whether the exenteration was primary therapy or a secondary operation. When not specified they were excluded. (2) Some authors did not specify the type of exenterative procedures carried out. (3) Although all authors indicate their five-year survivors, or (often) the number of patients surviving at various time intervals, there is very incomplete information regarding postoperative deaths, major complications, and local recurrence. (4) Finally, the data from the citations recorded cannot be added because some represent an updating of previously reported experience. With these considerations in mind, some tentative conclusions can be drawn regarding the total number of exenterative procedures performed; a very minimal operative mortality figure can be calculated as well as a reasonably accurate five-year survival figure; but there remain totally incomplete data regarding major complications and local recurrence.

The primary exenterations reported from 1960 to the present time for locally advanced vulvar cancer are recorded in Table 3. Correcting for the duplications, 75 exenterations were performed (15 total, 12 anterior, 36 posterior, and 12 not specified). Eight postoperative deaths were recorded

Table 3 Primary Exenteration in Vulvar Cancer[2]

Author	Year	Type	No.	Postop Deaths	Other (major)	Local Recurrence	5-Year Survivors (and survivors beyond 3 yr)
Thornton, Flanagan[9]	(1973)	Total	7	1	1	1	2
		Anterior	1	0	0		1
		Posterior	2	0	1		1
Boutselis[10]	(1972)	Posterior	2	0	?a	?	0
		Anterior	1	0	?	?	0
Collins, Lee, Roman-Lopez[11]	(1971)	Total	1	?	?	?	?
		Anterior	3	?	?	?	?
		Posterior	3	?	?	?	?
Galante, Hill[12]	(1971)	Not specified	1	1	—	—	0
Daily, Kaplan, Kaufman[13]	(1970)	Total	2	0	5	5	0 (1 NED*b* 4 yr 11 mo)
		Posterior	7	1	—	—	1 (1 NED 4 yr 7 mo)
Rutledge, Smith Franklin[3]	(1970)	Total	1	?	?	?	0 (10 NED 3 yr)
		Anterior	3	?	?	?	
		Posterior	9	?	?	?	
Shingleton, Fowler, Palumbo, Koch[4]	(1970)	Total	1	?	?	?	?
		Posterior	5	?	?	?	?
Hay, Cole[14]	(1969)	Total	1	1	?	?	0
		Posterior	6	?	?	?	2
Barclay, Collins, Hansen[15]	(1967)	Not specified	11	?	?	?	1 (NED 4½ yr)
Brunschwig, Brockunier[16]	(1967)	Total	3		?	?	1
		Anterior	7	25%*c*	?	?	1
		Posterior	5		?	?	2
Collins, Collins, Barclay, Nelson[17]	(1963)	Not specified	10	4	?	?	0 (2 NED at 2+ yr)

a Not specific in manuscript.
b No evidence of disease.
c 6/24 in total series: fresh and recurrent.

for a 10.7% mortality rate. (Although the Brunschwig and Brockunier report indicated a 25% operative mortality, primary and secondary operations were grouped, so that no figure is available for a precise breakdown). Five major complications were re-

ported in one citation involving 9 exenterations. And in spite of the extensiveness of the resections, 5 local recurrences occurred in one report.[13] There were a total of 12 (16%) reported five-year survivors and an additional 13 patients were alive without evidence of disease beyond 3 years (a 33% total three-year survival rate.

Radiation Therapy

In the past, results with radiation therapy for primary vulvar cancer were poor. Painful injury, ulceration and fibrosis, failure to cure local and groin disease, suggested to the gynecologists of recent decades that radiation therapy had no place in the management of vulvar cancer.

A number of selected references on primary radiation therapy for vulvar cancer are recorded in Table 4. The much quoted report of Stoeckle[26] in 1930, with a five-year salvage rate of 12%, helped to hold this modality in disrepute. His material was collected from 126 cases treated by radiation therapy at different institutions employing different radiotherapy techniques and representing primarily cases considered unsuitable for definitive surgery. Yet it must be recalled that surgical therapy at that time yielded almost comparable results.

The additional experience of Berven[24] with a five-year salvage rate of 13%, and Tod,[25] with 25% did little to improve the image of radiotherapy in vulvar cancer.

Currently, with recent reports from Europe describing modern radiotherapy treatment modalities, there is a distinctly more favorable picture. Frischbier and Thomsen[20] reported a 70% five-year cure among 33 patients in Stage I and II disease; and a 33% five-year salvage rate among 85 patients in Stages III and IV. The recent report of Backstrom and associates[18] of 19 patients with local Stage IV lesions and 4 (25%) five-year survivors is also impressive.

It seems pertinent to reflect on the latter two series of five-year cure rates of 25% and 39% reported with radiation therapy only for primary, locally advanced vulvar cancer in contrast to the overall 16% five-year cure for primary exenteration in vulvar cancer (presumably for Stage III and IV lesions)

as collected from the data reviewed earlier and recorded in Table 3.

Combined Treatment

As a therapeutic alternative to primary exenterative surgery, we presented[2] a rationale for and results of a series of cases based on the established success of radiotherapy in vaginal cancer (and its spread pattern) utilizing vaginal radium (Figure 3) and external beam therapy, split parametrial portals, or whole pelvic portals (Figure 4), and based on the established success of surgery, radical vulvectomy, and groin dissection (Figure 5) for the vulvar primary and its spread pattern.

Considerable therapeutic individualization has been used. The vagina is treated with one or two suitable radium systems. Uterine tandems are used when the upper vagina (or cervix) is involved. Although external beam therapy was utilized in our first case, with both whole pelvis and parametrial portals because of cervical involvement, external beam treatment has not always been employed. More recently we have used the total pelvis technique if external beam therapy seemed indicated. Of 15 patients treated, 5 have had external beam therapy: 1 for cervical involvement, 2 for N3 groin disease (Figure 6), 1 for N2 groin disease, and 1 for extensive T3 disease.

Initially, radium dosage was usually calculated to deliver a maximum of 4500 to 5000 rads at 1 cm deep to the vaginal surface, fractioned in two applications 10 to 14 days apart. More recently, we have calculated vaginal surface maximum dose and aimed at approximately 9000 rads minus any contribution from external beam therapy. This is an effort to make a safe, yet therapeutic extrapolation from radiation therapy for vaginal cancer. This feature has been common to all cases treated. Additional individualization has been carried out with surgical procedure.

Table 4 Primary Radiation in Vulvar Cancer[2]

Author	Year	No.	Stage	Modality	Major Complication	5-Year Survivors (additional survivors)
Backstrom, Edsmyr, Wicklund[18]	(1972)	19	T4	Cobalt-60	Primary reactions very slight, late reactions few	25%
Nobler[19]	(1972)	2	IV	Cobalt-60	?[b]	0% (1 NED[a] 11 mo)
Frischbier, Thomsen[20]	(1971)	33	I + II	Electron beam (16 MeV betatron)	24% vulva, 8% groins	70%
		85	III + IV			39%
Gusberg, Frick[21]	(1970)	3	Advanced	22.5 MeV betatron	?	0% (all had good palliation for more than 1 yr)
Schubert, Hohne[22]	(1965)	27	All stages	Electron beam	?	44%
Renner[23]	(1965)	?	?	Electron beam	?	41%
Berven[24]	(1949)	30	?	Radium and roentgen rays	?	13%
Tod[25]	(1949)	116	Total	Interstitial radium implants	?	25%
		71	early			33%
		45	late			14%
Stoeckel[26]	(1930)	126	?	X-ray or radium	?	12%

[a] No evidence of disease.
[b] Not specific in manuscript

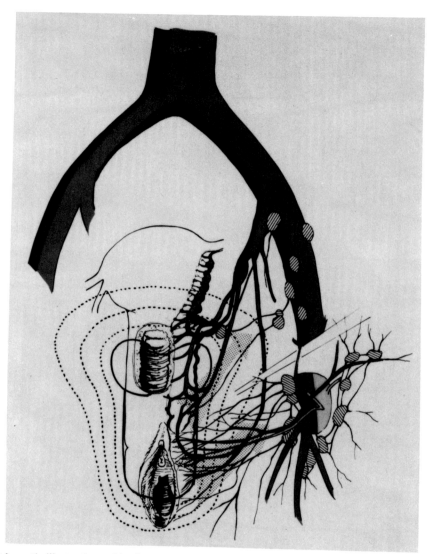

Figure 3 Schematic illustrations of isodose curve around vaginal Bloedorn radium applicator. From Boronow, R. C.: Therapeutic alternative to primary exenteration for advanced vulvovaginal cancer. *Gynecol. Oncol.* **1**: 233 (1973). Reprinted by permission.

The factors primarily considered in this individualization (both of surgery and radiation plan) were the initial clinical extent of disease and, secondly, occasional modification in treatment plan introduced because of the patient's age and general condition. Radical vulvectomy and groin dissection were performed in 10 patients, pelvic node dissection was added in 5 cases, and 5 patients had extensive vulvectomy without node dissection. All of these were patients with NO groins. Their ages were 81, 80, 76, 73, and 60, and all were in fragile states of health. The youngest (60) had a chronic brain syndrome and was bedfast. Today, 4 patients survive without evidence of disease

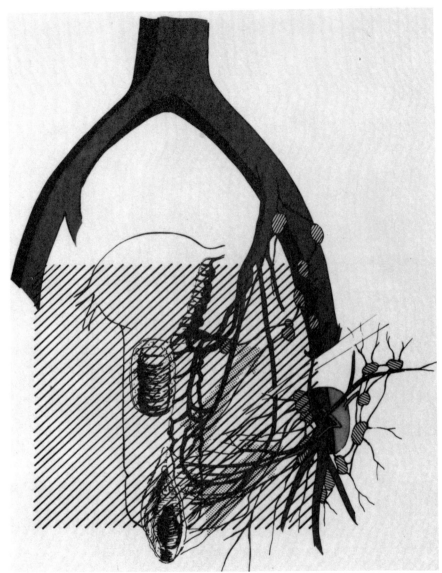

Figure 4 Schematic illustration of a total-pelvis external beam portal for preoperative therapy. From Boronow, R. C.: Therapeutic alternative to primary exenteration for advanced vulvovaginal cancer. *Gynecol. Oncol.* **1:** 233 (1973). Reprinted by permission.

at 4, 1½, 1, and 1 year. One patient became psychotic and died inexplicably without evidence of disease two months after therapy.

The results are given in Table 5. There was no treatment mortality, one instance of local recurrence, 3 cancer deaths (20%) and 2 (13.3%) five-year cures; 10 patients (66.7%) are without evidence of disease, 5 for more than 2½ years. The absence of treatment mortality, the preservation of bladder and rectal function, and the infrequency of both local failure and treatment morbidity validate our preliminary experience. We are encouraged to explore this

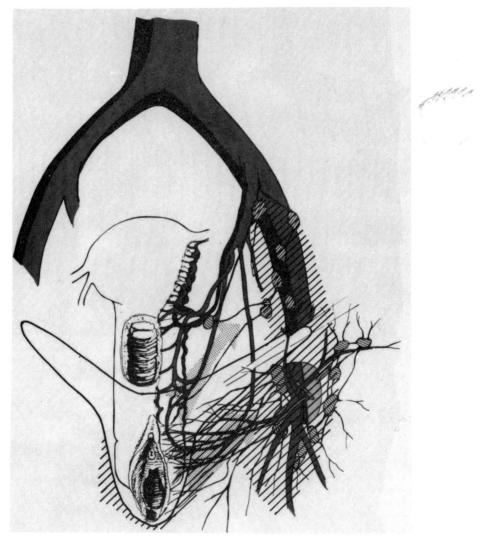

Figure 5 Schematic illustration of the addition of radical vulvectomy and groin and pelvic node dissection (dashed lines of deeper dissection) for completion of combined treatment. From Boronow, R. C.: Therapeutic alternative to primary exenteration for advanced vulvovaginal cancer. *Gynecol. Oncol.* **1**: 233 (1973). Reprinted by permission.

therapeutic approach with additional suitable cases.

COMMENT

Stage III and IV vulvar cancers have a poor prognosis but increasing numbers of patients appear salvageable by careful application of one of several treatment modalities. Despite the generally discouraging experience reviewed herein, some do achieve reasonably good results[27] with conventional, but locally more extensive, surgery. As experience increases, good results with exenterative surgery are found in the contemporary literature.[3,9,13] The combined radiation and

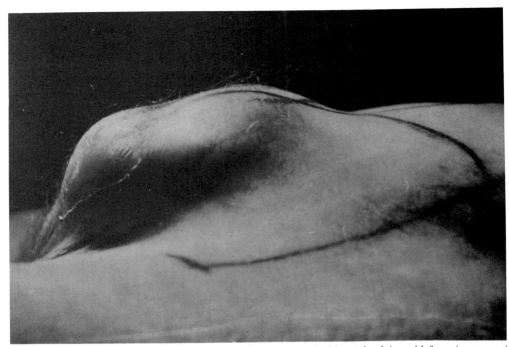

Figure 6 Lateral view of huge left groin node mass in case treated with total pelvis and left groin mass prior to radical resection. This patient is alive and well and without evidence of disease at 4 yrs. From Boronow, R. C.: Therapeutic alternative to primary exenteration for advanced vulvovaginal cancer. *Gynecol. Oncol.* **1:** 233 (1973). Reprinted by permission.

Table 5   Results of Combined Treatment

	Number
Case treated	15
Operative/treatment mortality	0
Local recurrence	1
Dead of disease (5, 10, 40 mo)	3
Dead of other cause, NED[a] (2, 8 mo)	2
5-year survivors, NED	2
Other survivors, NED (1, 1, 1, 1½, 1½, 2½, 3½, 4 yr)	8

[a] NED — no evidence of disease

radical surgery experience reported herein is viscera-preserving and holds promise for a reasonably good cure rate. Clearly, individual selection factors are operative in each institution and comparing one series with another is not completely valid. Further, the experience from Europe with good results with radiation therapy alone challenges us for clinical trials, as, for example, the use of preoperative radiation therapy for locally massive (T3 and T4) lesions and for significant nodal disease (N3).

REFERENCES

1. Plentl, A. A., and E. A. Friedman: *Lymphatic System of the Female Genitalia. The Morphologic Basis of Oncologic Diagnosis and Therapy.* W. B. Saunders Company, Philadelphia, 1971.

2. Boronow, R. C.: Therapeutic alternative to primary exenteration for advanced vulvovaginal cancer. *Gynecol. Oncol.* **1:** 233 (1973).

3. Rutledge, F., J. P. Smith, and E. W. Franklin: Carcinoma of the vulva, *Am. J. Obstet. Gynecol.* **106:** 1117 (1970).

4. Shingleton, H. M., W. C. Fowler, Jr., L. Palumbo, G. G. Koch: Carcinoma of the vulva: Influence of radical operations on cure rate. *Obstet. Gynecol.* **35:** 1 (1970).

5. Goplerud, D. R., and W. L. Keetel: Cancer of the vulva. Review of 156 cases. *Am. J. Obstet. Gynecol.* **100:** 550 (1968).

6. Franklin, E. W., and F. N. Rutledge: Prognostic factors in epidermoid carcinoma of the vulva. *Obstet Gynecol.* **37:** 892 (1971).

7. Green, T. H., H. Ulfelder, and J. V. Meigs: Epidermoid carcinoma of the vulva: An analysis of 238 cases. Part II. Therapy and end results. *Am. J. Obstet. Gynecol.* **75:** 848 (1958).

8. Brunschwig, A., and W. Daniel: Pelvic exenterations for advanced carcinoma of the vulva. *Am. J. Obstet. Gynecol.* **72:** 489 (1956).

9. Thornton, W. N., and W. C. Flanagan: Pelvic exenteration in the treatment of advanced malignancy of the vulva. *Am. J. Obstet. Gynecol.* **117:** 774 (1973).

10. Boutselis, J. G.: Radical vulvectomy for invasive squamous cell carcinoma of the vulva. *Obstet Gynecol.* **39:** 827 (1972).

11. Collins, C. G., F. Y. L. Lee, and J. J. Roman-Lopez: Invasive carcinoma of the vulva with lymph node metastasis. *Am. J. Obstet Gynecol.* **109:** 446 (1971).

12. Galante, M., and E. C. Hill: Pelvic exenteration: A critical analysis of a ten-year experience with the use of the team approach. *Am. J. Obstet. Gynecol.* **110:** 180 (1971).

13. Daily, L. J., A. L. Kaplan, R. H. Kaufman: Exenteration for advanced carcinoma of the vulva. *Obstet. Gynecol.* **36:** 845 (1970).

14. Hay, D. M., and F. M. Cole: Primary invasive carcinoma of the vulva in Jamaica. *J. Obstet. Gynaecol. Br. Commonw.* **76:** 821 (1969).

15. Barclay, D. L., C. G. Collins, and L. H. Hansen: Problem patients with vulvar malignancy. *Clin. Obstet. Gynecol.* **10:** 641 (1967).

16. Brunschwig, A., and Brockunier, A., Jr.: Surgical treatment of squamous cell carcinoma of the vulva. *Obstet Gynecol.* **29:** 362 (1967).

17. Collins, C. G., J. H. Collins, D. L. Barclay, and E. W. Nelson: Cancer involving the vulva: a report on 109 consecutive cases. *Am. J. Obstet. Gynecol.* **87:** 762 (1963).

18. Backstrom, A., F. Edsmyr, and H. Wicklund: Radiotherapy of carcinoma of the vulva. *Acta Obstet. Gynecol. Scand.* **51:** 109 (1972).

19. Nobler, M. P.: Efficacy of a perineal therapy portal in the management of vulvar and vaginal cancer. *Radiology* **103:** 393 (1972).

20. Frischbier, H. J., and K. Thomsen: Treatment of cancer of the vulva with high energy electrons. *Am. J. Obstet. Gynecol.* **111:** 431 (1971).

21. Gusberg, S. B., H. C. Frick, II: *Corscaden's Gynecologic Cancer,* 4th edit. Williams and Wilkins Company, Baltimore, 1970.

22. Schubert, G., and G. Hohne: Spatergebnisse, nach supervolt-therapie gynakologischer karzinome. *Sonderb. Strahlenther.* **67:** 143 (1965).

23. Renner, K.: Behandlungsergebnisse an der strahlenklinik janker unter besonderer berucksichtigung der ergebnisse mit energier-eichen strahlen. *Sonderb. Strahlenther.* **61:** 138 (1965).

24. Berven, E.: The treatment of cancer of the vulva. *Br. J. Radiol.* **22:** 498 (1949).

25. Tod, M. C.: Radium implantation treatment of carcinoma of the vulva. *Br. J. Radiol.* **22:** 508 (1949).

26. Stoekel, W.: Zur therapie des vulvakarzinoms. *Zentral. Gynecol.* **54:** 47 (1930).

27. Masterson, J. G.:

CARCINOMA OF THE VAGINA

CHAPTER 18   CARCINOMA OF THE VAGINA

J. TAYLOR WHARTON, M.D.

Primary carcinoma of the vagina comprises 1 to 2% of gynecologic malignancies. Squamous carcinoma predominates and usually occurs in the older age group.[5] Adenocarcinomas are rarer and are most often found in teenagers and patients in their early twenties. The adenocarcinomas are described histologically as clear cell cancers and frequently there is a history of maternal stilbestrol ingestion. Primary adenocarcinomas of the vagina also occur in older patients and can show the clear cell configuration.

A variety of treatment plans are available for these cancers, since it is difficult for one individual or center to collect sufficient treatment data to make specific recommendations. We have been fortunate in accumulating experience in the management of these cancers and have formulated a guide to therapy based on tumor location, volume, and potential for spread. The following discussion will present basic concepts and management ideas for primary carcinoma of the vagina.

SQUAMOUS CARCINOMA

Spread Pattern

Usually squamous carcinomas are moderately undifferentiated histologically. The most frequent site is the posterior vaginal wall. The size and extent of the cancer has a direct relationship to the incidence of lymph node metastasis. Carcinomas 2 to 3 cm in diameter and confined to the vagina (Stage I) have a low incidence of node involvement that has been verified by a high cure rate with conservative therapy.[1] Larger or infiltrating cancers have a much higher incidence of nodal metastasis and more radical therapy is indicated. Metastases occur primarily in the regional nodes that drain the area of the vagina where the tumor is located. Lesions in the lower third near the introitus spread to the inguinal nodes similar to cancer of the vulva. Cancers in this area will often involve both the vulva and vagina and their exact site of origin is unknown. Carcinomas of the upper vagina may utilize pathways available to the cervix and can be expected to behave in a similar manner. Staging should be according to the recommendations of the Cancer Committee of the International Federation of Obstetricians and Gynecologists (Table 1).

Diagnosis

Invasive lesions usually have an exophytic component and are accessible to direct biopsy, which is simple, safe, and can be done as an outpatient procedure. Although

259

Table 1   Staging of Carcinoma of the Vagina[a]

Preinvasive Carcinoma of the Vagina

Stage 0   Carcinoma in situ, intraepithelial carcinoma.

Invasive Carcinoma of the Vagina

Stage I   The carcinoma is limited to the vaginal wall.

Stage II   The carcinoma has involved the sub-vaginal tissues but has not extended to the pelvic wall.

Stage III The carcinoma has extended to the pelvic side wall or to the public symphysis.

Stage IV   The carcinoma has extended beyond the true pelvis, or has involved the mucosa of the bladder or rectum. A bullous edema as such does not permit allotment of a case to stage IV.

[a] Source: Kottmeier, H. L.: Problems relating to classification and stage grouping of malignant tumors in the female pelvis. In *Cancer of the Uterus and Ovary*, Chicago, Year Book Medical Publishers, 1966, p. 25.

Table 2   Carcinoma In Situ Vagina (Concomittant or Previous Conditions)

	Number of Patients
Post hysterectomy for carcinoma in situ cervix	14
Post hysterectomy for invasive carcinoma cervix	4
Post hysterectomy for benign disease	4
Multicentric carcinoma in situ vagina, vulva, or cervix	4
Concomittant invasive squamous carcinoma cervix	3
Concomittant invasive squamous carcinoma vulva	1
In situ carcinoma vagina with normal intact uterus	4
Total	34

vaginal cytology is frequently positive, it is not a substitute for biopsy.

Carcinoma in situ of the vagina is frequently multicentric and is often associated with other squamous cancers of the female genital tract. The lesions are usually detected by exfoliative cytology, since the in situ changes may not be clinically obvious. Lugol's solution is helpful in locating the abnormal area(s). Colposcopy is an additional diagnostic instrument and, in skilled hands, is quite accurate in locating abnormal areas. In patients with a previous history of in situ cancer of the cervix, the in situ changes are frequently found at the apex of the vagina (Table 2).

It is sometimes difficult to examine the entire vagina: the speculum blades can hide a lesion on the anterior or posterior wall; the young or nulliparous patient may experience pain and be uncooperative. The knee-chest position offers an advantage in most situations, and the large Kelly air cystoscope is particularly valuable for examining the vagina of the young patient.

Treatment

CARCINOMA IN SITU

Carcinoma in situ anywhere in the vagina may be treated locally by irradiation or may be excised. Prophylactic treatment of the entire vagina or total vaginectomy is extremely radical and should be applied only in select situations in which extensive or multifocal in situ carcinoma is noted. Patients with extensive disease and a need for maintaining function are treated by vaginectomy and skin graft. A flexible management plan should be followed according to the size of the lesions, their locations, and the patient's desire to maintain a functional vagina.

We prefer radiation therapy in most situations because a high cure rate has been obtained. Therapy has been individualized and vaginal function preserved whenever possible.

If the lesion is localized to the vault and the cervix is present, irradiation can be given with an intrauterine tandem and colpostats; the vault mucosal dose is 6000 to 7000 rads in 72 hr or 8000 to 9000 rads in two insertions of 48 hr each separated by one week.

If the cervix is absent, colpostats or a specially designed vaginal applicator (colpostat(s) plus vaginal cylinder(s), the so-called "Bloedorn" applicator) are utilized to deliver 6000 to 7000 rads vaginal surface dose in 72 hr.

Care must be taken to avoid overtreatment, which can lead to severe mucosal reaction and/or vaginal stenosis. Full-length vaginal irradiation may cause marked stenosis. Every effort should be made to avoid this in the sexually active patient. Multifocal areas demand comprehensive therapy, and the physician must be aware of the tendency for the surrounding structures such as the cervix, vagina, and vulva to develop separate primary cancers over a period of time.

Results with irradiation at the M. D. Anderson Hospital have been good. Only 4 of 34 patients treated have developed recurrent carcinoma in situ in the irradiated area. Excision biopsy was adequate treatment in 2 patients, vaginectomy in 1, and the remaining patient died of intercurrent disease.[1]

In summary, carcinoma in situ of the vagina may be surgically excised or irradiated. The therapy is designed to treat the involved area and spare the remaining vagina.

INVASIVE CARCINOMA OF THE VAGINA

The management of invasive carcinoma is determined by both the extent and location of the tumor. We usually prefer radiation therapy for all vaginal cancers; however, surgery is an acceptable alternate and is equally effective for early cancers. Large cancers, especially those of advanced stage, are best treated with radiation therapy.[2,5]

The preservation of a functional vagina is a decision that mainly involves the management of early (Stage I and II) cancers. Surgical management consists of a radical vaginectomy of all but lesions at the apex or introitus. Vaginal function is then restored, usually by skin graft. Radiation therapy with interstitial needles or tandem and ovoids spares a portion of the vagina and function is preserved. This is a distinct advantage. In advanced cancers function is destroyed by radical surgery or radical radiation.

Surgical management is straightforward but the proximity of the bladder and rectum allow minimal tissue for adequate margins. Irradiation therapy preserves adjacent structures but is quite individualized and may require the use of whole pelvis or transvaginal cone irradiation followed by colpostats and tandem, colpostats alone, vaginal cylinder, after-loading radium or 192 Iridium needles.[6]

The methods used for treatment based on location of the cancer are as follows:

CARCINOMA INVOLVING THE UPPER VAGINA

Irradiation therapy. Cancers of the upper vagina (Stage I or II) in patients with an intact uterus are treated with techniques similar to that for carcinoma of the cervix: 4000 rads external irradiation (12 × 12 cm parallel opposed fields) with a megavoltage unit is used initially and will reduce the tumor mass. This will render intracavitary radium more effective, since the radiation dose from cylindrical vaginal applicators (which falls off sharply) will be required to treat a smaller volume. If the vault is large enough, vaginal ovoids plus intrauterine tandem (ovoids alone if cervix is absent) can be utilized to deliver a total surface dose of 8000 rads in two applications of 48 hr each separated by two weeks. Carcinomas anterior or lateral to the cervix that show incomplete regression following external therapy may best be treated with interstitial radiation. A suprapublic incision and open-bladder technique will facilitate proper placement of the interstitial needles.[2]

Surgery. Radical hysterectomy or its equivalent, for patients who have had a previous simple hysterectomy, and lymphadenectomy with partial vaginectomy will allow en bloc removal of the upper one-third to one-half of the vagina. Total vaginectomy is unnecessarily radical for small lesions confined to the vaginal apex.

Large lesions that invade the bladder or the rectum require more extensive surgery, and anterior or posterior exenteration becomes necessary.

CARCINOMA INVOLVING LOWER
TWO-THIRDS OF THE VAGINA

Irradiation therapy. Small carcinomas (2 cm or less) may be treated entirely with interstitial irradiation. A single, double, or volume implant is used depending on the location of the cancer; 6000 to 7000 rads in five to seven days is the required dose.

Larger cancers require 4000 to 5000 rads external irradiation followed by 3000 to 4000 rads in three to four days from interstitial needles. Often the lesion is too long or not in the proper position for standard radium needles of 4.5 cm active length. Stainless steel hollow needles of greater length (4.5 to 8 cm) after-loaded with 192 Ir can be used.

Surgery. Small lesions confined to the anterior or posterior wall may be treated by a radical vaginectomy. Larger lesions may require anterior or posterior exenteration (in addition to vulvectomy), depending on their location.

Carcinomas at the introitus are treated in the same manner as vulvar carcinomas (radical vulvectomy and inguinal lymphadenectomy).

ADVANCED CARCINOMA

Stage III and IV lesions anywhere in the vagina are treated initially with 5000 rads external radiation in five weeks. The deep pelvic nodes are included in the treatment fields, since large tumors have a higher incidence of lymphatic metastasis than Stage I and II cancers. The patient is reevaluated after 5000 rads external therapy and may receive: (1) an additional 1000 to 2000 rads external therapy through reduced 10 × 10 cm fields, or (2) an interstitial implant to deliver 2500 to 3000 rads in three to four days.

Tumors involving the distal third of the vagina can metastasize to the inguinal nodes. These nodes are usually treated by radical inguinal dissection. A dosage of 4000 rads of external radiation is given preoperatively if the nodes are large or matted or have been biopsied recently. If excision is not contemplated, 5000 rads in five weeks appears to be a minimal cancerocidal dose. The control rate will be low with this dose if the nodes contain more than microscopic aggregates of cancer cells.

The results of treatment for invasive carcinoma of the vagina at the M. D. Anderson Hospital are shown in Table 3.

ADENOCARCINOMA

Primary adenocarcinoma of the vagina is rare and may occur in any age group. The cancer is most frequent in teen-agers and women in their early twenties. The recent association of adenocarcinoma of the vagina with maternal ingestion of stilbestrol during pregnancy has focused attention on this disease.[3] Bulletin Number 22 from the American College of Obstetricians and Gynecologists notes that all nonsteroidal synthetic estrogens have been implicated in the material histories and there does not seem to be a specific dose-time relationship. It is also known that not all incidences of

Table 3   5-Year Survival of Patients with Invasive Squamous Cell Carcinoma of Vagina[1]

Stage	Absolute	Intercurrent Disease or Lost to Follow-up	Determinate
I	11/16 (69%)	3 (1)[a]	11/13 (85%)
II	13/19 (68%)	2 (1)[a]	13/17 (76%)
III	4/15 (27%)	5	4/10 (40%)
IV	0/11	2	0/9

[a] Lost to follow-up in parentheses.

adenocarcinoma of the vagina are related to stilbestrol ingestion.

Pathology

The most frequently reported histologic type of primary adenocarcinoma is mesonephroma or clear cell carcinoma. Microscopically it resembles renal cell carcinoma and shows characteristic large cells with abundant, clear cytoplasm. The cancer is identical morphologically with clear cell carcinoma which occurs in the ovary, broad ligament, and cervix. The origin of the lesion has been considered to come from mesonephric remnants. However, some authors provide evidence in support of müllerian origin.[4] There is a frequent association with adenosis vaginae. Adenosis is observed in patients whose mothers ingested stilbestrol, but may also be seen in those patients with a negative hormone history. Its hyperplastic glandular pattern may be confused with cancer.

Spread Pattern and Factors Influencing Spread

Small lesions (< 3 cm in diameter) confined to the vagina (Stage I) probably have a low incidence of lymph node metastasis. Our clinical experience, which consists of local therapy, suggests this is true because a local or regional lymph node recurrence has not been encountered.[7] We know that early squamous carcinomas of the vagina behave

in this manner. Although the depth of invasion is also a factor in determining the potential for spread, data are insufficient for a definite correlation.

Involvement of the cervix offers additional pathways for spread, and documentation of cervical involvement requires more intense therapy.

Clinical Considerations

Abnormal vaginal bleeding or discharge is the most common clinical symptom. One patient in our series was asymptomatic, and the diagnosis was made by examination after the mother had read about the association with stilbestrol. Another patient whose mother had not taken hormones was noted to have a visible lesion while having a routine examination to obtain oral contraceptives. Routine vaginal cytology is not reliable and is not a substitute for a careful pelvic examination. Schiller-staining and biopsy of abnormal areas that fail to stain can be done as an office procedure. Patients in their early teens can be placed in the knee-chest position, and the cervix and vagina can be examined with a Kelly air cystoscope.

Current Concepts in Therapy

The treatment of choice is radical hysterectomy, vaginectomy, and pelvic lymphadenectomy. More radical excision has been employed for advanced lesions that have spread beyond the vagina. A major decision in planning therapy is whether or not the entire vagina is at risk. If this is the case or if multifocal lesions are frequent, a total vaginectomy is indicated.

Radiation therapy is an effective treatment for this cancer and offers certain advantages. In our own series, we have used radiation as primary therapy in both early and advanced cancers.[7]

Clinical Material:
The M. D. Anderson Hospital

Of 23 patients with primary adenocarcinoma of the vagina who have been treated at the M. D. Anderson Hospital (Table 4), 10 (Group I) were 15 to 23 years of age. The histologic pattern was the classic clear cell configuration and 8 of the 10 carcinomas originated in the upper third of the vagina (Table 5). The older patients (Group II) showed a variable histologic pattern, and 9 of 13 cancers were in the mid and lower vagina (Table 5).

Techniques of Radiation Therapy:
Table 7

Early cancers (3 cm or less in diameter) confined to the vaginal apex are treated with a transvaginal cone; 6000 rads in 20 treatments (140 kV unit) of 300 rads each or its equivalent was effective in 3 patients. When 4 patients with early cancers limited to the vaginal walls were treated with interstitial needles, 6000 to 7000 rads given in 6 or 7 days proved successful. The use of vaginal cylinders or other types of surface applicators is undesirable because full-length vaginal irradiation produces stricture.

Bulky or infiltrating cancers require combination radiation therapy. External therapy precedes local radiation, since it is essential to reduce the size of the cancer prior to applying interstitial or intracavitary applicators. The rapid fall off in intensity from radium or cesium sources due to the inverse square law makes these sources unsuitable for the initial treatment of large cancers. Thirteen patients were treated with com-

Table 4   Primary Adenocarcinoma of the Vagina: Clinical Material, The M. D. Anderson Hospital

	No. Patients	Histology	Age Range (Yr)	Average Age (Yr)
Group I	10	Clear cell	15–23	19.6
Group II	3	Clear cell	30–67	48
	10	Papillary	40–63	

Table 5   Primary Adenocarcinoma of the Vagina: Location of Carcinoma, The M. D. Anderson Hospital

Position	Group I Location			Total
	Upper 1/3	Mid 1/3	Lower 1/3	
Anterior	6	—	—	6
Posterior	1	2	—	3
Lateral	1	—	—	1
	—	—	—	—
Total	8	2	—	

Table 6   Primary Adenocarcinoma of the Vagina: Location of Carcinoma, The M. D. Anderson Hospital

	Group II Location			
Position	Upper 1/3	Mid 1/3	Lower 1/3	Total
Anterior	—	3	2	5
Posterior	—	1	—	1
Lateral	1	2	1	4
Apex	3	—	—	3
Total	4	6	3	

Table 7   Primary Adenocarcinoma of the Vagina: Treatment Techniques, The M. D. Anderson Hospital

Technique	Group I	Group II	Total
Transvaginal radium	3	0	3
Interstitial radium	2	2	4
Intracavitary	—	1	1
Combination	5	8	13
Surgery	—	2	2

bination therapy and 11 received external radiation prior to interstitial or intracavitary radiation or wide excision (1 patient). Field size varied because of the location of the cancer and the desirability of treating the regional node groups. Stage III or bulky carcinomas received whole pelvis radiation (superior border of field at L-5 vertebrae). The risk of lymph node metastasis is thought to increase in direct proportion to the volume and extent of the tumor.

Results

At the M. D. Anderson Hospital, 17 patients are 24 months or more posttherapy, and 16 have been free of disease from 24 to 115 months. Two deaths have occurred: 1 patient died following the removal of interstitial needles from a pulmonary embolus, and 1 died 30 months posttherapy from recurrent cancer. Eleven of the patients have survived three years or longer (Table 8).

No recurrences have been encountered in the Group I patients. The death from recurrent cancer occurred in a 40-year-old patient in Group II with a mucin-producing adenocarcinoma.

Table 8   Primary Adenocarcinoma of the Vagina: Treatment Results, The M. D. Anderson Hospital

	Evaluable 24 mo.	Alive[a]	Dead of Disease	Dead of Other Causes
Group I	8	7	—	1
Group II	9	8	1	—
Total	17	15	1	1

[a] Free of disease 24–115 months.

Summary

Primary adenocarcinoma of the vagina may be treated successfully with radiation therapy. Therapy can be individualized, and patients with small cancers can be treated with local therapy which preserves the vagina and adjacent organs and leaves ovarian function intact. This is particularly desirable in younger patients.

METASTATIC CARCINOMA OF THE VAGINA

Vaginal extension from a lesion of the endometrium or cervix is frequent. Since whole pelvis irradiation is usually employed initially, the lower extent of the disease is marked with a lead-tipped lucite probe and included in the therapy fields. Following external radiation, a vaginal cylinder or interstitial implant is used to supplement the treatment to the lower vagina.[2]

REFERENCES

1. Brown, G. R., G. H. Fletcher, and F. N. Rutledge, Cancer, 28, 1278 (1971).
2. Fletcher, Gilbert H., Textbook of Radiotherapy, Lea & Febiger, Philadelphia, Pennsylvania, 1973.
3. Herbst, A. L., and R. E Scully, Cancer, 25, 745 (1970).
4. Herbst, A. L., H. Ulfelder, and D. C. Poskanger, New Engl. J. Med. 284, 878 (1971).
5. Rutledge, F. N., Am. J. Obstet. Gynecol., 97, 635 (1967).
6. Wharton, J. T., et al. Davis Obstetrics and Gynecology, Harper & Rowe, Hagerstown, Maryland (1972).
7. Wharton, J. T., et al. The Treatment of Clear Cell Adenocarcinoma in Young Females, Obstet. and Gynecol. 45, 365 (1975).

INDEX